KU-262-377

PALLIATIVE MEDICINE SECRETS

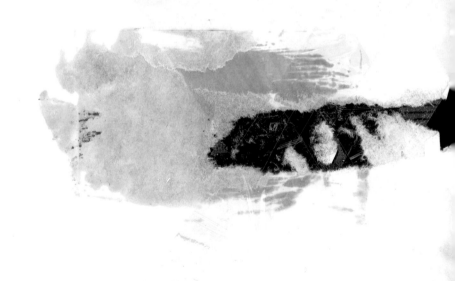

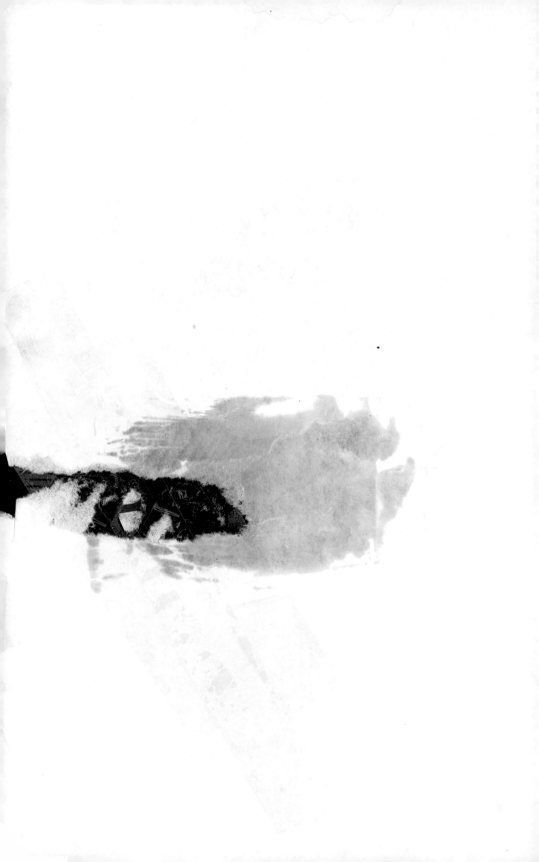

PALLIATIVE MEDICINE SECRETS

SURESH K. JOISHY, MD, FACP
Palliative Medicine Specialist
Former Staff, Palliative Care Unit
Department of Hematology and Oncology
The Cleveland Clinic Foundation
Cleveland, Ohio

HANLEY & BELFUS, INC./ Philadelphia

Publisher: HANLEY & BELFUS, INC.
                  Medical Publishers
                  210 South 13th Street
                  Philadelphia, PA 19107
                  (215) 546-7293; 800-962-1892
                  FAX (215) 790-9330
                  Web site: http://www.hanleyandbelfus.com

Note to the reader: Although the information in this book has been carefully reviewed for correctness of dosage and indications, neither the authors nor the editor nor the publisher can accept any legal responsibility for any errors or omissions that may be made. Neither the publisher nor the editor makes any warranty, expressed or implied, with respect to the material contained herein. Before prescribing any drug, the reader must review the manufacturer's current product information (package inserts) for accepted indications, absolute dosage recommendations, and other information pertinent to the safe and effective use of the product described.

Library of Congress Cataloging-in-Publication Data

Palliative medicine secrets / edited by Suresh K. Joishy.
        p.   cm. — (The Secrets Series®)
    Includes bibliographical references and index.
    ISBN 1-56053-304-8 (alk. paper)
      1. Cancer—Palliative treatment—Miscellanea.   I. Joishy, S. K.,
    II. Series.
      [DNLM: 1. Palliative Care examination questions.   WB 18.2 P167
    1999]
    RC271.P33P355   1999
    616.99'406—dc21
    DNLM/DLC
    for Library of Congress   98-43418
                                                         CIP

PALLIATIVE MEDICINE SECRETS   ISBN 1-56053-304-8

Last digit is the print number: 9   8   7   6   5   4   3   2   1

CONTENTS

CONTRIBUTORS

Bharati D. Bhate, MD
Medical Director, Illinois Regional Cancer Center, DeKalb, Illinois

Harvey Max Chochinov, MD, PhD, FRCPC
Professor, Department of Psychiatry and Family Medicine, Division of Palliative Care, University of Manitoba, Winnipeg, Manitoba, Canada

Christine Duelge, CRNH
Albany Community Hospice, Albany, Georgia

Geoffrey Parker Dunn, MD, FACS
Medical Director, Great Lakes Hospice; Active Staff, Department of Surgery, Hamot Medical Center, Erie, Pennsylvania

Kathleen S. Ellis, PT
Women's Health Team Leader, Phoebe Memorial Hospital, Albany, Georgia

Gerri Frager, RN, MD, FRCPC
Assistant Professor of Pediatrics; Faculty Scholar, Open Society Institute's "Death in America" Project, Dalhousie University, Halifax, Nova Scotia, Canada

Jane M. Griffiths, MD, CCFP
Assistant Professor, Departments of Palliative Care Medicine and Family Medicine, Queen's University, Kingston, Ontario, Canada

Geoffrey Arthur Thomas Hawson, MBBS, FRACP, FRCPA
Clinical Associate Professor, Department of Pathology, University of Queensland, Brisbane; Director of Oncology/Palliative Care, Redcliffe Hospital, Redcliffe, Queensland, Australia

Sharon Bean Heidecker, BSN, CRNH
Hospice Patient Care Coordinator, Great Lakes Hospice, Erie, Pennsylvania

Kym Annette Irving, PhD
Developmental Psychologist, Faculty of Education, Queensland University of Technology, Brisbane, Queensland, Australia

Suresh K. Joishy, MD, FACP
Palliative Medicine Specialist; Former Staff, Palliative Care Unit, Department of Hematology and Oncology, The Cleveland Clinic Foundation, Cleveland, Ohio

Mark Lander, MD, FRCPC
Associate Professor, Department of Psychiatry, University of Manitoba, Winnipeg; Staff Psychiatrist, Health Sciences Center, Winnipeg, Manitoba, Canada

James B. Ray, PharmD
Clinical Pharmacist, Department of Oncology/Pain Management, Pharmacy and Drug Information Services, Hamot Medical Center, Erie, Pennsylvania

Mary Raymer, MSW, ACSW
President, Raymer Psychotherapy and Consultation Services; Chair, Social Work Section, National Hospice Organization, Acme, Michigan

Reverend Stephen Rosendahl
Chaplain, Great Lakes Hospice, Erie, Pennsylvania

Tadaaki Sakai, MD
Medical Director, Life Care System, Tokyo, Japan

Charles G. Sasser, MD
American Board of Hospice and Palliative Medicine; Medical Director, Mercy Hospice, Conway, South Carolina

Martha L. Twaddle, MD
Assistant Professor of Clinical Medicine, Northwestern University Medical School, Evanston, Illinois

PREFACE

This book has been written to educate the medical community about the philosophy and practice of palliative care and hospice. The goals of palliative care are symptom control and patient comfort. With the support of an interdisciplinary team, palliative care strives to improve quality of life for patients with advanced cancer and other incurable diseases. In addition to the patient's physical state, his or her psychological, emotional, and spiritual conditions are addressed. The family is included in the team taking care of the patient. Bereavement follow-up is offered.

Over the past decade, increasing attention has been given to the needs of dying cancer patients and their families. The growing hospice movement in the United States rivals the proliferation of high technology that typified medicine in the 1970s and 1980s. Textbooks on palliative care have appeared since 1993, mainly from across the Atlantic Ocean. An appreciation for "high-touch" palliative care is now evident. Since November 1996, hospice and palliative medicine has been recognized as a subspecialty in the United States with the establishment of a board by the American Academy of Hospice and Palliative Medicine.

In *Palliative Medicine Secrets,* my co-authors and I reveal the "secrets" of palliative care. We were very selective in choosing the subjects to be presented, in part because we did not want to duplicate other textbooks on palliative medicine. However, we have not compromised our goal to benefit a broad-based audience of physicians, medical students, hospice and palliative care nurses, and other supportive healthcare professionals.

This book is a handy resource that can be used with ease to tackle any symptoms facing an advanced cancer patient. All of the chapters focus on what *must* be known and *should* be known. It is hoped that this book will teach healthcare professionals how to assess the patient quickly, apply a commonsense approach, and develop gold standards for palliative care treatments. The role of each team member is clarified for better patient care. The question-and-answer format addresses problems arising on the wards, in home hospice situations, and in the board examinations.

We hope *Palliative Medicine Secrets* helps caregivers solve the day-to-day problems they encounter and encourages interdisciplinary team members to display a cooperative spirit toward patients and their families. We also hope that the principles outlined in this text will kindle further interest in the field of palliative medicine.

Suresh K. Joishy, M.D., F.A.C.P.

Dedication

To my mother, Susheela Joishy, for giving me physical and spiritual health, and to my late father, Keshav Joishy, whose profession inspired me to become a physician.

Acknowledgements

I am grateful to my wife, Muktha, for sharing the hardships in making a book.

To my daughter Mahima and son Mahanth for relentless drafting of the manuscripts.

Thanks to Marie Miller, transcriptionist, for express typing of many manuscripts.

OVERVIEW: THE EVOLUTION OF PALLIATIVE MEDICINE IN THE UNITED STATES

Suresh K. Joishy, M.D., F.A.C.P.

This author has been taking care of patients with advanced cancer in the United States since the early 1970s. Medical schools in the 1970s focused on curing patients at any cost regardless of how advanced the cancer was. It meant giving patients toxic chemotherapy irrespective of side effects, and no one mentioned the words "quality of life" to the patients. Meanwhile, as high-technology diagnostic tools were developed, extensive cancer was more precisely diagnosed, resulting in more toxic therapies. Oncologists were able to tell the patients that a decrease in the size of the tumors in millimeters was sufficient to justify more of the same treatment and more side effects. Still there was no consideration of quality of life. Further, clinical trials became fashionable. It seemed that any oncologist could join any cooperative oncology group and even conduct clinical trials sponsored by the National Cancer Institute (NCI). The NCI had to show the government how it was spending its money by the number of patients who were "accrued" in clinical trials, but the government never asked how many patients were cured.

Traditionally, hospitals in the U.S. established cancer care programs with the intent of curing malignant disease. With the rapid development of diagnostic tools and advances in surgery, radiotherapy, and chemotherapy, comprehensive cancer centers were established in almost every major city. In a zeal to cure cancer, the control of symptoms that were due to morbidity of advanced cancer assumed secondary importance. Despite having cured a handful of cancers in early stages and relatively rare cancers, we still have a long way to go to cure most common cancers in adults. Pioneering efforts by physicians in England, Australia, and Canada have helped to formulate policies and procedures to control symptoms in advanced cancer, the foremost of which is pain. The synthesis of these efforts has resulted in the emergence of a new discipline in medicine called palliative care. In essence, palliative care is an all-encompassing discipline of medicine geared toward the control of symptoms in advanced cancer and other endstage incurable diseases.

The U.S. was the first country to declare medical oncology a specialty. Cancer patients previously had been treated by internists, surgeons, and radiotherapists. With the establishment of hematology as a specialty and success with hemopoetic neoplasms, hematologists took over the treatment of more and more solid tumors. This in turn led to the establishment of a board of medical oncology. Still, palliative care of cancer patients was nowhere in sight.

Dramatic cure rates did occur in children with leukemia and young adults with Hodgkin's disease and testicular cancers. However, the biology of these tumors is markedly different than that found in the most common adult cancers, such as lung, breast, and colon cancers. Many oncologists seemed blind to this reality, and they intensified successful chemotherapies that were used for hemopoetic tissues and germ cells and applied them to other solid tumors, achieving no meaningful survival benefits or cure. Rather than trying to find other types of innovative cures, research was intensified to treat side effects of chemotherapy such as nausea, vomiting, and cytopenia so that more and more futile chemotherapy could be given. Almost every patient on chemotherapy today receives prophylactic antiemetics and hemopoetic growth factors, which add enormous cost to the treatments but little improvement in survival. Even when lives are prolonged, suffering also is prolonged, and there is no improvement in quality of life.

Pain is one of the major symptoms in patients with advanced cancer. Oncologists taking a curative approach with chemotherapy or surgeons contemplating major surgery traditionally had little knowledge concerning how to relieve intense pain in cancer patients. Morphine in large doses was avoided for fear of addiction or side effects; morphine was saved for the patient's death bed. Almost all patients died with pain, anorexia, nausea/vomiting, fatigue, and dyspnea. Finally,

Dr. Cicely Saunders in England came to the rescue of advanced cancer patients. Her empathy toward terminally ill patients was unmatched. She defied all notions of high-tech medicine to focus on relieving patients' symptoms and suffering irrespective of the underlying diagnosis. Dr. Saunders also realized the importance of treating the patient as a person rather than just treating the disease. She understood that when a patient suffers, the family suffers too. Her tireless efforts led to the notion of "hospice" care for terminally ill patients. This author had the privilege of meeting Dr. Saunders, a great physician of this century, and hearing directly from her the best approach to patients with life-limiting illness.

Economy dictates health care in the U.S. Money for cancer care became limited in the 1980s with the advent of diagnosis-related grouping for reimbursement and more scrutiny of costs by insurance companies. Many cancer patients sought alternative therapies and spiritual care. With limited reimbursements for hospital stays in the 1990s, homecare became popular. These events produced the perfect time and setting for hospice to take over the care of these patients from homecare. Hospice care in the U.S. is mainly homecare rather than institutional care. Once Medicare came forward to bear the expense of home hospice patients on a per diem basis with a 6-month limit, home hospice care in the U.S. grew phenomenally. Specialized inpatient hospice units are being established gradually.

The type of care given to patients in hospices, focusing on symptom control rather than the disease process, came to be known as palliative care. Palliative care eventually became a specialty in Europe known as palliative medicine. Palliative medicine was readily accepted in Canada and grew rapidly in both clinical and research fields. In the U.S., many oncologists remain skeptical about enrolling patients in palliative care programs or hospices.

Many patients with advanced cancer still need hospitalization for the treatment of acute symptoms mainly related to complications of cancer, including hypercalcemia, malignant effusions, pathologic fractures, and cord compression. A new model, in addition to hospice, has emerged for inpatient palliative care. One can aptly call it "tertiary" palliative care because the care is generally given for acute symptoms in a tertiary-care hospital setting. The goal is to improve the patient's quality of life for a reasonable time. Palliative surgeries for obstructive bowel, tubes, stents, and prostheses are examples of high technology applied in tertiary palliative care to control symptoms.

It is the conviction of this author that all cancer care programs must include palliative care as part of their multidisciplinary and team approaches. It is hoped that the information in this book clarifies the principles of palliative care and motivates hospitals to establish palliative care programs.

Historical Perspective

DECADE	PROFESSIONALS TAKING CARE OF LIFE-LIMITING ADVANCED CANCERS	APPROACH
1960s	Internists Surgeons	Hospital-based Curative
1970s	Hematologists Surgeons Radiotherapists	Hospital-based Moderately aggressive Multimodality
1980s	Hematologists/oncologists Surgical oncologists Radiation oncologists	Hospital-based Aggressive Radical
1990s	Oncologists Surgical oncologists Radiation oncologists Palliative care physicians (?)	Effective antiemetics Hemopoetic growth factors Intensive chemotherapy Bone marrow transplants Limited surgeries Palliative care (?)

(Table continued on following page.)

Historical Perspective (Continued)

DECADE	PROFESSIONALS TAKING CARE OF LIFE-LIMITING ADVANCED CANCERS	APPROACH
The future (author's version)	Palliative care physicians Palliative care surgeons Palliative care radiotherapists Hospice medical directors	Home-based hospice Hospital-based hospice Acute tertiary palliative care units Medical, spiritual and psychosocial care

BIBLIOGRAPHY

1. Cassell CK, Vladeck BC: ICD-9 code for palliative or terminal care. N Engl J Med 335:1232–1233, 1996.
2. Doyle E, Hanks GWC, McDonald N (eds): Textbook of Palliative Medicine. New York, Oxford University Press, 1993.
3. Meier DE, Morrison RS, Cassell CK: Improving palliative care. Ann Intern Med 127:225–230, 1997.
4. Roy DJ: Palliative care: A fragment towards its philosophy. J Palliat Care 13:3–4, 1997.
5. Saunders C (ed): Hospice and Palliative Care. An Interdisciplinary Approach. London, Edward Arnold, 1990.
6. Twycross RG: Palliative care. The joy of death. Lancet 350(suppl III):20, 1997.
7. Waller A, Caroline NI: Handbook of Palliative Care in Cancer. Boston, Butterworth-Heineman, 1996.

1. PALLIATIVE CARE: DEFINITIONS AND DOMAINS

Suresh K. Joishy, M.D., F.A.C.P.

1. What is the definition of palliative care?

The World Health Organization has defined palliative care as "the active total care of patients, controlling pain and minimizing emotional, social, and spiritual problems at a time when disease is not responsive to active treatment." However, considerable confusion exists as to the meaning of palliative care. The word *palliative* is derived from the Latin word *pallium*, which means cloak, as worn by a priest at church. A cloak hides or covers something. Perhaps the word was chosen to indicate the protection of patients who suffer from the complex symptoms of incurable diseases. Terms such as *supportive care, hospice care,* and *terminal care* are sometimes used interchangeably to explain palliative care. Palliative care is associated with treatment given to advanced cancer patients and also applies to other advanced diseases, such as AIDS and end-stage pulmonary, cardiac, renal, and central nervous system disorders. Palliative care is a global approach to controlling suffering and seeks to give patients their highest possible quality of life.

2. What is supportive care?

Supportive care is frequently confused with palliative care. Supportive care is given to any patient with any disease and not exclusively to patients with advanced incurable diseases. Intravenous fluids, blood component therapies, and enteral or parenteral nutrition are examples. Supportive care measures are justified in palliative care when absolutely necessary for symptom control, but generally for limited times. Several modalities of palliative treatments are also given to support the patient. The term *supportive care* falls short of the all-inclusive meaning of palliative care.

3. Do palliative care and terminal care mean the same thing?

There is a misconception that palliative care is suitable for patients in the terminal, actively dying state. Dying patients require palliative care only when symptom control becomes an issue. Terminal care is just one component of palliative care.

4. How do you distinguish terminal status from actively dying status?

It is unfortunate that the word *terminal* is used loosely by health care professionals. The moment patients are told they have a terminal cancer, they are instilled with profound fear. They feel death is imminent. Terminal status may last for weeks to months depending upon the type of the disease and stage. It is the performance status of the patient that distinguishes terminal status from actively dying status. A simple and helpful performance scale is used by the Eastern Cooperative Oncology Group (ECOG). The scale is graded 0 to 4. Zero means that the patient is asymptomatic, eating well, and fully ambulatory. At 4, the patient is completely bedridden and incapable of self care. The prognosis is grave, and the patient will probably enter the actively dying state.

Characteristics of Patients at Grade 4 on the ECOG Performance Scale

- In bed all of the time
- Incapable of self care; need total nursing care
- Eating less than 800 calories in 24 hours, the least amount of energy needed for heartbeat, respiratory movements, and other involuntary functions
- Drinking less than 800 ml of fluids in 24 hours, the minimum amount of fluid needed to replenish daily loss of body fluids.
- Has an incurable disease. Patients with newly diagnosed lymphomas and acute leukemias, even if in ECOG 4, may be salvageable because they have a curable disease. On the other hand, pancreatic cancer with ECOG 4 is terminal, and the patient may be actively dying.

5. What are the goals of palliative care?

1. To provide relief from pain and other distressing symptoms in advanced cancer and other incurable endstage diseases.

2. To maintain the quality of life while neither hastening nor postponing death.

3. To integrate psychosocial and spiritual aspects of patient care with medical and surgical care.

4. To offer supportive systems to help the family during the patient's illness and bereavement.

6. What is hospice care? Is it the same as palliative care?

The term *palliative care* encompasses a broad range of services directed at controlling and preventing symptoms in cancer patients. The care given in the hospice setting is also palliative. However, hospice care involves extremely ill patients mainly in the terminal stage. The goals of hospice care and palliative care are the same.

What is now a worldwide hospice movement was pioneered in England in 1967 by Dr. Cicely Saunders, whose idea of palliative care was to take care of dying patients with incurable diseases and intractable symptoms. The word *hospice* is derived from the Latin word *hospitum*, meaning hospitality. The care given to hospice patients whether in the hospital or at home is palliative. Hospice care is the component of palliative care in which the patient's total comfort takes precedence over all other goals. Treatments are simplified, and invasive diagnostic or treatment procedures are rarely indicated. The patient becomes a team member along with the family in the decision-making process. The plan of support, not only to the patient but to the family, is emphasized.

7. What are the justifications for referring to palliative care as a subspecialty?

1. A great deal of cancer care is actually palliative—aimed at reducing tumor burden and eliminating symptoms rather than cure. In fact, 70% of the oncologist's time is probably spent in palliative care. Only 30% of cancer therapy with curative intent involves surgery, radiotherapy, and chemotherapy in adult patients.

2. Palliative care is not an extended care or a rehabilitation service, nor is it a referral service for dying patients only.

3. It involves medical and nursing staff in taking care of extremely ill patients. In the fullest sense, palliative care can be called an intensive care.

4. While good medicine is a major component of palliative care, patients are treated in such a way that the symptomatic benefits clearly outweigh any disadvantages of the treatment.

5. Palliative care can affirm life, yet regards dying as a normal process.

6. Palliative care becomes a major responsibility of physicians when the curative treatment ceases to have a rational basis. Palliative care is able to identify specific measures to keep the patient comfortable. Cessation of palliative care is never an option.

Since the foundation of the hospice movement in 1967, palliative care has become a subspecialty in the United Kingdom, Europe, Australia, and Canada. Although the hospice movement has been growing in the U.S., palliative care is just being recognized as a specialty. A specialty board has been established by the American Association for Hospice and Palliative Medicine, and the first examination was given in November 1996.

8. How is palliative medicine different from medical oncology?

Many cancer treatments, such as chemotherapy, given with curative intent by medical oncologists, are in reality palliative; they are aimed at reducing the tumor burden and consequently eliminating symptoms rather than achieving a cure. When cancer progresses, the continuation of such treatments ceases to have a rational basis. Many oncologists hesitate to stop treatments that have a curative intent. Treatments may continue to the point of futility, whereas the benefits of palliative care always outweigh any disadvantages of treatment. Palliative care is able to identify specific measures to keep the patient comfortable. Cessation of palliative care is never an option. In this regard, palliative care is distinct from oncology. The table compares the principles of modern oncology and those of modern palliative care.

Principles of Oncology and Palliative Care

PRACTICE ITEMS	TRADITIONAL ONCOLOGY CONCEPTS	PALLIATIVE CARE CONCEPTS
Goal	To cure	To care
History-taking	Not focused	Focused on symptoms
Symptoms	Separated from body and mind	May not be separable; holistic
Timeframes	Acute or chronic	Never stop caring
Basis of decisions	Physical	Physical, emotional, spiritual, social, ethical
Orders not to resuscitate	Rarely	Almost always
Diagnosis	Instrumental	Minimize
Members of medical care team	Professionals	Professionals, patient, and family
Futility	Ignored	Honored
Side effects of treatment	Ignored	Never ignored
Spirituality	Ignored	Honored

9. What is palliative treatment?

Specific measures or interventions aimed at symptom control and improved quality of life of a patient with incurable disease. Modern palliative care treatments fall into distinct domains, which are discussed in subsequent chapters and summarized below.

- Palliative medical treatments
    - Control of pain with opioids and nonopioid drugs
    - Control of nausea, vomiting, constipation, and other gastrointestinal (GI) symptoms
    - Control of symptoms related to fluid, electrolyte imbalance
    - Treatment of anxiety, depression, and delirium
- Palliative radiotherapy
    - Control of pain due to bone metastasis, cord compression, and plexopathy
    - Relief of airway, GI, or gastrourinary obstruction
    - Control of hemorrhage from tumors
- Palliative surgery
    - Bypass surgeries and ostomies for GI obstruction
    - Insertion of feeding tubes
    - Insertion of drainage tubes for malignant effusions
    - Stents for biliary or ureteric obstruction
- Psychosocial support
    - Feeling of isolation in advanced cancer can be a major source of psychosocial problems for the patient. Social services can offer psychosocial support and recognize the emotional and financial needs of the patients and family members in dealing with the cancer.
- Spiritual support
    - Patients with advanced cancer may be experiencing a sense of failure, guilt, or fear. The palliative care team, including clergy members, can offer indispensable spiritual support.

10. Is palliative care given exclusively to cancer patients?

Generally, palliative care is the care of advanced cancer patients. Most patients enrolled in hospice have terminal cancer. However, suffering related to any advanced disease is equally important. Patients with AIDS and endstage cardiac, renal, and chronic obstructive pulmonary disease increasingly are being cared for in the palliative care setting. Patients with incurable neurologic diseases, Alzheimer's disease, and Huntington's disease also benefit from palliative care.

11. Is palliative care limited to adult patients?

The concepts of hospice and palliative care were derived from treating adults. However, children also develop incurable diseases, which may cause the entire family considerable distress. The philosophy of hospice and palliative care is eminently suitable in children. Although pediatric malignancies such as acute leukemias and Wilms' tumors are amenable to cure, other solid tumors such as neuroblastomas, hepatoblastomas, and brain tumors may be refractory and terminal. Children are prone to genetic life-limiting illnesses such as cystic fibrosis and other enzyme deficiencies. Until recently pain as a distressing physical symptom in children was largely ignored. However, pediatricians have quickly drawn upon the experience of palliative care and hospice physicians to treat children with life-threatening diseases. Some hospices accept children, and palliative care may become part of the pediatric curriculum.

12. Is death the endpoint for palliative care?

Inclusion of the patient's family in care is unique to the hospice component of palliative care. Loss of a family member to any disease, particularly cancer associated with great suffering, can perpetuate grief and bereavement. One member of the hospice palliative care team continues to follow the family for up to 1 year after the death of the patient. Bereavement service helps the family to cope with loss and prevents pathologic bereavement.

13. Who are the providers of palliative care, and what are their roles?

Members of the palliative care team come from diverse disciplines, but the approach to the patient is always a unified team approach focusing on the patient and the family. The team approach is both multidisciplinary and interdisciplinary. The team must never lose track of the patient. The team may be led by an oncologist or internist with experience in treating advanced diseases and complex symptoms. Nurses specially trained in taking care of advanced cancer patients and terminally ill patients are the key to continuity of care and symptom control. Social workers experienced in dealing with family dynamics and financial needs provide psychosocial support for coping with end-of-life issues. The grief and bereavement coordinator offers bereavement support after the patient's death. A case manager coordinates the inpatient, outpatient, hospice, home care services, discharge planning, and placement. The addition of a psychiatric nurse or physician team member may be an asset. Specially trained volunteers help the patient with day-to-day nonmedical needs and offer companionship to the patient and caregiver. Regardless of the religious background of the patient, clergy members can offer support.

14. Where is palliative care given?

Any location where the goal is to control symptoms and improve the quality of life is suitable for palliative care. Inpatient palliative care units, inpatient or home hospice, and subacute and extended care facilities may become suitable sites for palliative care.

15. Describe hospital-based palliative care.

The U.S. has only a handful of hospital-based palliative care programs to take care of patients with advanced cancer. A palliative care program may consist of a consultation service or a special ward staffed by specially trained palliative care team members. Services may include inpatient consultations, transfers and admissions to the palliative care unit, and complete assessment for taking over full palliative care or helping other physicians.

Two types of inpatient palliative care units can be established. One is an acute palliative care unit or tertiary palliative care unit. This unit controls physical symptoms and complications due to cancer and prepares patients to go home or to other facilities. Diagnostic and treatment procedures are carried out as for any acute care patient, so long as they are of palliative intent. The other type is a hospital-based hospice unit, to which patients who are nearing death are admitted for comfort care. Invasive procedures or treatments are rare.

16. How is palliative care given at home?

Two types of palliative services can be offered at home. One is the existing home care; nurses typically visit the home under the direction of the patient's physician. Another type, the home-based hospice, has become quite common. The goal is to keep the patient at home and to support the family. There is a 24-hour call service to deal with new problems or emergencies.

This program is coordinated by a hospice medical director with a hospice palliative care team. Its services are reimbursed by Medicare on a per diem basis limited to 6 months of care.

17. Can palliative care be given at outpatient clinics?

Outpatient palliative care clinics are not common in the U.S. A comprehensive hospital-based palliative care program may include an outpatient clinic, served by the entire palliative care team for follow-up care. New patients referred in consultation may require a comprehensive evaluation for symptom recognition. Follow-up patients may belong to hospice or nonhospice groups and may need evaluation of current symptoms, response to treatments, and identification of new problems. Depending on the severity of symptoms or performance status, patients may be seen once in 2 weeks or once a month. Outpatient evaluation and recommendations must be conveyed to the caregivers at home immediately. Some patients may visit the outpatient clinic for palliative care procedures such as paracentesis to relieve discomfort from recurring ascites. Blood transfusions given for symptom control can be carried out on an outpatient basis.

18. Can palliative care reach out to traditional extended care facilities such as nursing homes?

Many elderly patients with life-limiting illnesses reside in extended care facilities and will benefit greatly from symptom control by a palliative care approach. Hospice nurses may be called upon to help nursing home teams for patients nearing death, particularly in the area of pain management. Several sectarian extended care facilities run by religious or philantrophic foundations offer palliative care, even though it is not recognized as such.

19. Is it easy to establish a hospital-based palliative care program?

Ideally, every hospital with a comprehensive cancer care program should establish a palliative care program. The concept of *comprehensive cancer care* loses its meaning without palliative care. A medical oncologist or internist is needed to form and lead the palliative care team. Clear-cut policies and procedures required for eligibility criteria to admit patients to palliative care services must be in place. The hospital may expand its own home care services to include palliative care or establish its own home hospice program as another arm of palliative care.

The hospital may choose to establish an acute or tertiary palliative care unit model, inpatient hospice unit model, or both. Eventually a palliative care consultation service, palliative care inpatient unit, palliative care outpatient clinic, and homecare hospice may be integrated to serve the patient. Starting a new program may not be easy, but it is quite feasible once the concepts of palliative care become known to the hospital administrators. The first step is to form an interdisciplinary palliative care team consisting of hospital staff. The next step is education of medical and paramedical staff regarding hospice and palliative care concepts. The third step is to formulate written policies and procedures, which are readily available from existing guidelines from hospice and palliative care organizations. The community at large needs to be educated. It is a mistake to launch a palliative care program without educating the physicians in the community because numerous barriers still exist in the enrollment and referral of patients to hospice and palliative care.

20. What are the benefits of a palliative care program to the patients?

1. The patient becomes a team member along with a family member or caregiver.
2. A sense of security is provided to the patient by the existence of a nurse who can be reached by phone 24 hours a day.
3. Patients and family become better educated to make decisions on the end-of-life issues.
4. Patients enrolled in hospice become eligible for Medicare coverage, thus reducing the stress of the financial burden.
5. Spiritual support is provided to help comfort the patient.
6. Patients need not be admitted to the hospital; they can choose to die at home.

21. What are the benefits of a palliative care program to the family?

All decisions are made with the full knowledge of the patient and family. If a living will is made, one of the family members has the power of attorney for health care when the patient is incapable of making decisions. Support offered to the family by the palliative care program helps to prevent the overwhelming sensations of burden, helplessness, and burnout. Other benefits include:

1. Family members are taught how to take care of patients at home.
2. Family members are comforted to know that care is not compromised, even if the patient is dying at home or at the hospital.
3. Family members have a chance to become involved in support groups.
4. Other community agencies can be enrolled to help take care of the patient.
5. Family members are better prepared for grief and bereavement.

22. What are the benefits of a palliative care program to the hospital?

An increasing number of cancer patients are entering the advanced stages. As the community grows older, palliative care will be needed more than ever. A hospital with a palliative care unit now is well prepared for the future. Other benefits include:

1. The hospital establishing palliative care can stand out as a unique establishment and in the forefront of the community.
2. Innovation and new services for patients will result in increased patient activity.
3. The hospital may be able to secure more managed care contracts because palliative care is recognized as more cost-effective than other types of care.
4. Income generated from palliative care can rise because an increasing number of cancer patients are entering advanced stages.
5. The hospital can expect to attract philantrophic gifts.
6. The hospital can improve community relations because palliative care focuses primarily on the local community and home care.
7. The hospital can attempt to justify palliative services as part of a comprehensive cancer center.
8. The Health Care Financing Administration has announced the approval of a new diagnosis code for palliative care, which was included in the international classification of diseases.
9. Palliative home care/hospice and outpatient clinics can be established for patients discharged home from the hospital to ensure continuity of care.

23. What is ahead for palliative care?

Most advanced cancer is incurable, and other complex diseases have predictable progression associated with physical and emotional morbidity. Although hospitals have technology and expertise to take care of acute illness, most physicians and surgeons lack skills to care for terminally ill patients. In recognition of this deficiency, the American Board of Internal Medicine has mandated that every internist should become competent in palliative care to take care of terminally ill patients. Curricula increasingly are being developed in academic institutes to educate physicians in training. Finally, the American Society of Clinical Oncology has taken a stand to recognize palliative care as an integral part of cancer patient care.

BIBLIOGRAPHY

1. Bailes JS: Cost aspects of palliative cancer care. Semin Oncol 22:64–66, 1995.
2. Blackburn A: Care of the dying patients in hospital. Why care of the dying is still poor. BMJ 309:1579, 1994.
3. Didich J, Weick JK: The development of a palliative care program. Cleve Clin J Med 56:762–764, 1989.
4. Foley KM: Palliative Medicine, Pain Control, and Symptom Assessment in Caring for the Dying. Identification and Promotion of Physician Competency. Educational Research Document. 1996. Section III. Project of American Board of Internal Medicine.
5. Lindop E, Beach R, Read S: A composite model of palliative care for the UK. Int J Palliat Nurs 3:287–292, 1997.
6. MacDonald N: Cure and care: Interaction between cancer centers and palliative care units. REC results. Cancer Res 121:399–407, 1991.
7. Walsh D: Palliative care: Management of the patient with advanced cancer (review). Semin Oncol 21:100–106, 1994.
8. Woodruff RK, et al: Palliative care in a general teaching hospital. 2. Establishment of a service. Med J Austr 155:662–665, 1991.

2. ESSENTIALS OF PALLIATIVE CARE

Suresh K. *Joishy*, M.D., F.A.C.P.

1. Why should we discuss essentials?

The field of palliative medicine is vast. It encompasses treatment of a wide spectrum of complex diseases in their advanced stages. This chapter summarizes essential components of palliative medicine; details are provided in subsequent chapters. To help readers remember the information, each of the major topics is divided into about five essential items, many of which are further described by five subitems.

2. What is the first essential component of palliative care?

The need for a core group focusing on patient care.

3. Who are the core members of a palliative care team?

The core group includes (1) physicians, (2) nurses, (3) social workers, (4) dietitians, and (5) physical therapists. Other members of the team may include psychiatrists, psychologists, volunteers, and spiritual counselors.

4. What is the role of physicians?

1. He or she will become the team leader and assume the roles of a teacher and troubleshooter to help other team members.

2. The physician may serve as a consultant to help other physicians.

3. Physicians may choose to give palliative care as hospice coordinators or hospice directors for inpatient or home hospice only.

4. A physician serving in a hospital-based palliative care program may take care of inpatients and outpatients only.

5. What is the role of nurses?

1. Their role is probably the most important one because they spend most of their time in direct patient care.

2. Their role in the hospital setting and outpatient setting is equally important.

3. Some nurses may choose to take care of patients in homecare situations only.

4. Nurses increasingly are involved in providing palliative care in extended care facilities.

5. The nurse is responsible for giving tender loving care and education to the patient and family.

6. What is the role of social workers?

1. They assume a broad role in the palliative care setting.

2. Social workers can function as a liaison between patient and family and between health care team members and the patient.

3. Social workers understand the patient's financial needs better than other team members.

4. Social workers are indispensable in arranging family meetings.

5. The logistics of discharging a palliative care patient can be formidable. Social workers are adept at identifying the needs of patients and family for a safe discharge.

7. What is the role of physical therapists?

1. Assessment of palliative care patients for morbidity is paramount.

2. Helping the patient and teaching caregivers to help patients get out of bed and ambulate is important in preventing decubitus ulcers, muscle wasting, and hypercalcemia of malignancy.

3. Assessment of activities of daily living is an integral part of discharge planning.

4. For patients with limitations in activities of daily living, physical therapists can help patients find suitable, durable medical equipment such as bedside commodes, walking aids, and appropriate methods of exercise.

8. What is the role of the clergy?
1. Spiritual counseling is valuable even to patients who have no religious faith.
2. Enhancement of faith can serve as a coping mechanism and even be therapeutic for dying patients.
3. Chaplains can form a valuable bond between patients and other members of the team.
4. The presence of a clergy member at the death bed of the patient is soothing.
5. Spiritual care can reduce the family's grief and prevent pathologic bereavement after the patient dies.

9. What is the second essential component of palliative care?
Symptom recognition.

10. What are the major categories of symptoms that are recognized in palliative care patients on a daily basis?
The categories are (1) pain, (2) GI symptoms, (3) fatigue, (4) dyspnea, and (5) psychosocial issues.

11. What are the essential features of cancer pain management?
1. It is important to understand cancer pain as a distinct entity and multifaceted symptom.
2. Pain may be associated with or aggravated by other symptoms.
3. Patients may have more than one kind of pain.
4. Daily assessment of the intensity of pain and its response to treatment is difficult but must be carried out.
5. Misconceptions about pain and opioid therapy are still stumbling blocks in adequate pain control.

12. What are the common GI symptoms suffered by palliative care patients?
1. Loss of appetite, loss of taste, and gastroparesis are common in cancer patients, even with malignancies not involving the GI tract.
2. Oral problems such as mucositis, mouth ulcers, and candidiasis can be very painful and are common with immunosuppression, malnutrition, and prior radiotherapy.
3. Constipation is a major problem for patients on opioids unless treated diligently.
4. Nausea and vomiting with or without bowel obstruction may be multifactorial.
5. Abdominal and pelvic pain may result from organomegaly, obstruction, or invasion of viscera.

13. What is the role of fatigue in patients with advanced cancer?
1. Assessment of fatigue is difficult. Terms such as *weakness, tiredness, lack of energy,* and *asthenia* are not very specific.
2. Identifiable causes of fatigue may include anemia, hypoxia, malnutrition, and metabolic derangements, in which cases fatigue may be reversible.
3. Fatigue associated with progression of metastasis may be irreversible.
4. Fatigue may be closely associated with unresolved psychosocial issues, fears, depression, and anxiety.
5. Ability to carry out activities of daily living may be a good indicator of the degree of fatigue.

14. Why is dyspnea an important symptom in palliative care?
1. Dyspnea may be a common symptom in patients without pulmonary disease.
2. Acute or chronic dyspnea may indicate pulmonary complications: pneumonia, pleural effusions, aspiration, pulmonary embolism, and lymphangitic spread of tumor.

3. Anemia, fluid overload, and hypoxia may be reversible.

4. Terminal dyspnea is common in cancer patients who are actively dying.

5. Opioids such as morphine should always be considered in the treatment of severe dyspnea in cancer patients.

15. How do you recognize psychosocial issues that are affecting a patient's psychological symptoms?

1. One needs to identify if psychological—internal—symptoms are affecting the patient's social—external—behavior such as cognitive dysfunction and interpersonal relationships.

2. Anxiety, depression, insomnia, and delirium are common psychological symptoms in advanced cancer patients.

3. Physical symptoms may be associated with or aggravated by psychosocial symptoms, i.e., pain aggravated by anxiety, depression, sleeplessness.

4. Social issues such as financial pain or spiritual pain occasionally are identified as symptoms.

16. What is the third essential component of palliative care?

Patient evaluation.

17. What are the essentials of patient evaluation in palliative care?

The essentials are the (1) primary diagnosis, (2) extent of the disease, (3) previous therapies, (4) current problems (symptoms list), and (5) "do not resuscitate" (DNR) status.

18. Are the clinical diagnostic methods any different in palliative care?

1. Many patients with advanced cancer are too feeble to give a "medical student type" of clinical history. Therefore, history taking should be symptom-oriented, precise, and timely.

2. History taking should not cause or aggravate anxiety or depression in the patient.

3. Daily assessment of symptoms is required.

4. Diagnostic procedures should be minimal and noninvasive.

5. One must remember to identify associated paraneoplastic syndromes and other nonmalignant conditions.

19. What is the importance of extent of disease in patients who are already in advanced stages?

1. Locoregional metastasis, even to limited extent, can cause considerable problems, including dysphagia, dyspnea with mediastinal tumors, and severe chest wall pain in locoregional metastasis of lung and breast.

2. Soft tissue metastasis to lymph nodes and muscle tissues can cause local symptoms.

3. Organ metastasis to the liver and adrenal gland can be a source of considerable pain. Central nervous system metastasis can cause personality changes, seizures.

4. Serous membrane metastasis may result in severe symptoms due to malignant effusions such as pleural effusion and malignant ascites.

5. Skeletal metastasis is extremely common and may cause severe pain, fractures, and hypercalcemia.

20. How can cancer therapies cause current symptoms?

1. Symptoms may be related to organ loss due to surgery. Pain and obstructive symptoms may persist.

2. Radiotherapy to the pelvic region may cause severe mucositis with diarrhea or cystitis with bladder spasms. Head and neck radiotherapy may lead to symptoms of xerostomia.

3. Certain chemotherapeutic drugs such as vincristine and platinum compounds cause pain, tingling, numbness, and weakness due to peripheral neuropathy.

4. Patients with hormonal therapy for breast cancer (progesterones, tamoxifen) are at higher risk for deep vein thrombosis.

5. One should ask the patient about alternative therapies. (Patients do not reveal information unless asked.)

21. What current problems need to be identified in the judicious management of advanced, life-limiting cancers?

1. Identify symptoms related to cancer according to primary diagnosis, extent of the disease, and previous therapies.

2. Distinguish symptoms related to cancer and other associated diseases, e.g., a diabetic patient with cancer may have neuropathy unrelated to chemotherapy.

3. For pain assessment and disability, carefully assess metastatic complications.

4. List psychosocial problems next to physical symptoms.

5. Identify if there are problems with the patient's caregivers at home.

22. How do you establish DNR status?

1. Discussion must be carried out with every patient with life-threatening disease unless the patient is cognitively impaired.

2. Attitudes, knowledge, and communication skills of physicians are the most critical factors in establishing DNR status for a patient.

3. Misconceptions about DNR status abound in the medical community and society at large. Statewide education may help.

4. Physicians and the palliative care team must become culturally competent in discussing DNR with various ethnic groups.

5. The patient and family need to be thoroughly educated on the advantages and disadvantages of resuscitation, and they should never feel abandonment after DNR status is obtained.

23. What is the fourth essential component of palliative care?

Pain control.

24. What are the essentials of pain management?

The essentials include (1) pain classification and syndromes, (2) pain assessment methods, (3) full knowledge of opioid therapy, (4) full knowledge of adjuncts to opioids, and (5) nonpain symptoms affecting pain.

25. Why is it important to classify pain?

1. No two patients appear to suffer from the same pain to the same degree.

2. Pain is a subjective symptom, and pain classification attempts to define pain objectively.

3. To help determine treatment.

4. To help standardize communication about pain among health care professionals.

5. The International Association for Study of Pain publishes a manual that classifies pain as somatic, visceral, neuropathic, and mixed pain syndromes.

26. How do you assess pain in palliative care patients?

1. Pain needs to be assessed in its site, character, intensity, extent, relieving and aggravating factors, and temporal relationships.

2. Pick a simple tool to assess pain intensity, such as a numeric scale of 0 to 10. Avoid pain scales with too many questions, and avoid questions that cannot be answered objectively.

3. Pain assessment must be done daily and must be charted until pain is stabilized.

4. Caregivers at home need to be educated on pain assessment and charting.

5. Pain assessment should go hand-in-hand with dose adjustments of analgesics.

27. What are the essentials of opioid therapy?

1. Drug, dose, schedule, and route of commonly used opioids must be known.

2. Equianalgesic potency ratios between different opioids must be referred to using a chart or scale when switching from one opioid to another.

3. Morphine and hydromorphone can probably be used by every route available in the body: oral, sublingual, rectal, transdermal, intravenous, subcutaneous, epidural, and intrathecal. Equianalgesic potency must be known for different routes for the same opioid.

4. Preemptive action must be taken to control side effects.

5. Principles of around-the-clock and rescue dosing and use of adjunct drugs must be known.

28. What are the indications for using adjuncts with opioids?

1. Adjuncts may be used with opioids to control side effects.

2. Adjuncts may be used for specific pains not responding well to opioids.

3. When side effects of opioids become troublesome, an "opioid-sparing" adjunct may be used to reduce the dose of opioid and indirectly reduce the side effects.

4. Side effects of the adjuncts must not be forgotten.

6. Steroids as adjuncts are very useful in several pain syndromes.

29. What nonpain symptoms affect pain?

1. The pain threshold may be decreased or increased by associated symptoms.

2. Good morale, mood, and nutrition increase the pain threshold, which means that the patient has less pain.

3. Anxiety, depression, and fears decrease the pain threshold, which means that the patient has more pain.

4. The concept of "total pain" refers to any unmet needs of the patient that may aggravate pain (financial pain, spiritual pain).

5. Pain may not be controlled unless associated symptoms are relieved.

30. What is the fifth essential component of palliative care?

Noninvasive palliative therapy.

31. What are the essentials of noninvasive therapy in the management of palliative care patients?

The essentials include (1) pharmacotherapy, (2) radiotherapy, (3) physical therapy, (4) psychosocial issues, and (5) spiritual issues.

32. What is the role of pharmacotherapy in palliative care?

1. Pharmacotherapy is the mainstay of palliative care.

2. The role of the clinical pharmacologist needs to be better defined for the palliative care team.

3. Symptoms in cancer patients are complex and numerous. Always know the first and second line of drugs for the same symptoms.

4. Polypharmacy is common in palliative care. To reduce polypharmacy, consider drugs that can control more than one symptom ("portmanteau" medications).

5. Limitations of drug use in organ dysfunction and elderly patients must be taken into account.

33. What is the role of radiotherapy in helping advanced cancer patients?

1. Radiotherapy is one of the oldest methods of treatment for inoperable cancer and for local control.

2. Radiotherapy is used to control symptoms in palliative care.

3. Radiotherapy is excellent in controlling severe somatic pain due to skeletal metastasis.

4. Radiotherapy is useful in controlling central nervous system metastasis and cord compression.

5. Radiotherapy is useful in treating hemorrhage from tumors (e.g., hemoptysis, GI bleeding, and gynecologic bleeding).

34. Is physical therapy useful in treating advanced life-limiting diseases?

1. The role of physical therapy is underestimated in palliative care.

2. Activities of daily living diminish as cancer progresses. A physical therapist's help is extremely valuable in encouraging patients to exercise and to move around with or without the help of equipment such as a walker.

3. Physical therapy is useful to prevent residual damage due to central or peripheral nervous system diseases.

4. The physical therapist can help the family to create a safe home environment for the patient.

5. Physical therapists, speech therapists, and occupational therapists work closely to address the patient's needs and improve quality of life.

35. Who will provide and receive psychosocial support in palliative care?

1. The role of the social worker as a team member is well defined.

2. Psychosocial support must be provided by all members of the palliative care team.

3. Family members and friends of the patient need to be counseled to diminish stress and fears.

4. Caregivers at home may be supported by a hospice team.

5. Palliative care team members themselves, particularly those with close contact with patients, may need psychosocial support to prevent burnout.

36. How useful is spiritual counseling in palliative care?

1. The spiritual counselor, whether a clergy or nonclergy member, is integral to the palliative team.

2. Spirituality helps the patient understand self better.

3. Spirituality may help the patient think beyond self and cope with cancer better.

4. If the patient has strong beliefs, spiritual healing methods sought by the patient should not be criticized.

5. Spiritual counseling helps family members face death of the patient and reduces grief.

37. What is the sixth essential component of palliative care?

Invasive palliative therapy.

38. Are invasive therapies applied in contradiction to palliative care philosophy?

No. Invasive treatments are given to control complications of cancer and consequently control symptoms, which is the main goal of palliative care. Invasive palliative care therapy can be useful with (1) pleural effusions, (2) malignant ascites, (3) dysphagia, (4) deep vein thrombosis, and (5) pathologic fractures.

39. Name some characteristics of pleural effusions with dyspnea.

1. Temporary outpatient drainage of pleural effusions are of limited value because recurrence is common. Thoracentesis with chest tube insertion and postdrainage pleurodesis are very effective, and recurrence is uncommon.

2. Metastatic breast cancer is one of the most common causes of malignant pleural effusion.

3. If primary cancer is well known, it is futile to establish a diagnosis of malignant effusion by the presence of tumor cells. Some tumors may not shed cells, or cells get lysed by the time the fluid is sent to the lab.

4. Bilateral pleural effusions are not uncommon and drained one side at a time only.

40. How is malignant ascites managed in palliative care?

1. Abdominal carcinomatosis and metastatic breast cancer may lead to malignant ascites; chylous ascites may arise due to obstruction of the abdominal lymphatic system.

2. Patients tend to request frequent paracentesis, even without significant symptoms, because ascites is readily visible.

3. Generally, paracentesis should be conducted only if symptoms warrant: shortness of breath, inability to lie down and rest, or abdominal pain.

4. Paracentesis can be performed at an outpatient clinic, and patients can withstand large volumes of drainage.

5. Furosemide with spironolactone may help prevent recurrence or diminish ascites.

6. When ascites requires too frequent drainage, a permanent drainage tube may be considered and the patient trained to drain by himself at home, as needed.

41. What causes dysphagia in palliative care patients?

1. Dysphagia is a common symptom in palliative care.

2. Oropharyngeal lesions may cause odynophagia.

3. Esophageal motility problems may be caused by a paraneoplastic condition or central nervous system lesion.

4. Esophageal candidiasis, particularly associated with chemotherapy or radiotherapy, is a common problem.

5. Obstructive lesions or structures may be managed by stents or a feeding tube.

42. Is deep vein thrombosis (DVT) common in patients with advanced cancer?

1. Mucin-producing adenocarcinomas are a well-known risk factor for DVT.

2. In palliative care patients, the risk factors may be immobility and bedridden status, causing DVT rather than cancer per se.

3. Heparin followed by warfarin is the mainstay of treatment to prevent pulmonary embolism.

4. Low-molecular-weight heparin is a good choice if the patient wishes to be treated at home; treatment with warfarin follows.

5. Debilitated patients in palliative care have problems titrating with anticoagulants. In these situations, unless there is considerable swelling of the lower extremities or phlegmasia, an inferior vena caval filter is a good choice.

43. Describe characteristics of pathologic fractures in palliative care.

1. Skeletal metastasis is common in cancers, particularly of the lung, breast, and prostate.

2. Pathologic fractures should be considered serious because of risks of immobilization and poor quality of life.

3. Quick assessment by an orthopedic surgeon and radiotherapist is mandatory, and treatments of fixation and/or radiotherapy should be started immediately.

4. Vertebral metastasis with compression fracture and spinal cord compression is an emergency. Emergency evaluation with computed tomography or magnetic resonance imaging, high-dose steroids, and emergency radiotherapy are indicated.

5. Prophylactic pamidronate may be considered in widespread bone metastasis.

44. What is the seventh essential component of palliative care?

A family meeting.

45. What essential information is given by a palliative care physician during family meetings?

The physician (1) traces the clinical course of disease, (2) discusses current issues, (3) gives discharge planning, (4) provides prognostication about the future, and (5) discusses logistics and finances. Conducting a family meeting should be an important activity of all palliative care physicians. Family meetings are best conducted in a structured manner at a time chosen well ahead. The presence of the patient and as many family members as possible is coordinated by a social worker. All of the patient's medical information should be in place prior to the meeting.

46. What clinical information is given to the patient and the family??

1. Unless the patient objects, no information needs to be withheld from the family. Trace all the symptoms from the diagnosis until the meeting.

2. Explain normal and abnormal test results.
3. Describe the extent of the disease honestly. Show radiographs or draw diagrams.
4. Outline responses to previous therapies and explain the palliative care plan.
5. Answer all questions asked by the patient and the family.

47. What current issues are discussed with patients and family?
1. Enumerate outstanding and active symptoms.
2. Give prognostic factors for each symptom-related complication.
3. Discuss what response is predicted with treatment.
4. DNR should be discussed and making a living will encouraged.
5. The patient's goals are identified, and a plan of action is given.

48. How do you discuss prognosis and future in a family meeting?
1. Family members may pressure the physician to predict survival time. While the life-limiting nature of the illness should be discussed honestly, no numbers should be given. Taking care of end-of-life issues, finances, and making a will are encouraged.
2. End-of-life spiritual issues are identified and relayed to the chaplain.
3. The social worker will give further information on community resources.
4. If the patient still has unmet wishes or needs, see how far they can be met in a limited time.
5. Allay the patient's fears of being a burden to the family or fears that the family may become helpless.

49. How is discharge planning discussed with the family?
1. Explain how medical factors may determine the type of discharge: home with caregiver or with hospice help.
2. Discuss how caregiver status may determine the safety of a patient going home when performance status of the patient is poor.
3. Discuss the types of supportive care services available from health care professionals and the community.
4. Discuss medications and how to assess response and side effects in patients.
5. Discuss follow-up care.

50. What logistical and legal matters require discussion at a family meeting?
1. The nature of an advance directive/living will is discussed.
2. Health care insurance policies and benefits are discussed and need to be examined by the social worker.
3. A spokesperson for the entire family is chosen.
4. Power of attorney for health care of the patient is chosen.
5. Logistics of settling the patient at home or at a health care facility is discussed.

51. What is the eighth essential component of palliative care?
The discharge checklist.

52. For a good discharge, what are the items written down?
The items are (1) diet, (2) activity, (3) medications, (4) follow-up appointments, and (5) durable medical equipment.

53. What are the dietary concerns when the patient goes home?
1. Many palliative care patients may be on special diets.
2. Diet is a major problem in patients with anorexia.
3. Patients on tube feedings may require special education or equipment for going home.
4. Diet often is more of a concern to the family than to the patient because the family may fear that the patient may starve to death.
5. Simple and practical written information from a dietitian is invaluable.

54. What questions are asked by the patient and family about activity on discharge?

1. Most patients in palliative care are retired or disabled. Questions on work-related activity are rare. The physician may be required to fill out disability forms.

2. Patients taking opioids generally will continue to drive an automobile when pain is under control despite their knowledge of the dangers. Concerned family members may ask whether the patient should drive an automobile.

3. The physical therapist may give instructions on ambulating.

4. Questions about long-distance travel arise.

5. If patients need to travel long distances, they are advised to carry full medical information and telephone numbers of the nearest hospital in case of emergency.

55. How do you discharge patients with medications that were started in the hospital?

1. Polypharmacy is common in palliative care patients. Some patients are taking more than 10 drugs.

2. As far as possible, all parenteral medications should be switched to oral forms at least 24 hours before discharge to determine the patient's response.

3. A clearly written medication sheet describing drugs, doses, routes, schedules, purpose, and any ending dates must be given to the patient and explained by the discharging nurse.

4. Caregivers monitoring the patient's drugs are identified and educated.

5. Late discharges may cause problems to patients buying drugs from outside pharmacies. Availability of an adequate supply of opioids in the patient's pharmacy must be known.

56. What issues are involved in the follow-up of discharged patients?

1. If the patient was treated in a teaching hospital and had a prolonged stay with multiple problems, more than half a dozen physicians may have been involved in that patient's care.

2. Patients going home may not know when and who they will be seeing in follow-up.

3. Patients should be given a list of primary physicians and consulting physicians.

4. Patients should *not* be instructed to call after discharge and secure an appointment on their own.

5. Every patient leaving the hospital must have an appointment card to see a physician for follow-up. If the patient is in home hospice, the hospice coordinator should take care of follow-up.

57. What type of durable medical equipment may be required when the patient is discharged?

1. A hospital bed for patients requiring total nursing care at home.

2. Equipment to transfer the patient out of bed to a chair if the caregiver has difficulty lifting the patient.

3. A bedside commode.

4. Walking aids, a wheelchair, and specially designed chairs to sit in the tub or take a shower.

5. Cleaning and dressing materials, catheters, bags, and other similar equipment.

58. What is the ninth essential component of palliative care?

Discharge placements.

59. What types of placement facilities are suitable for palliative care patients?

Facilities include (1) home only, (2) home with hospice, (3) home health care, (4) a skilled nursing facility, and (5) extended care facilities.

60. Under what circumstances can palliative care patients be sent home without the need for professional help?

1. Any patient who can eat normally and ambulate within the house can be sent home.

2. The patient ideally should have the help of a family member or friend. If not, community resources such as Meals on Wheels may be sought.

3. Volunteers from the patient's church may visit and help the patient.
4. Arrangements need to be made so the patient can contact someone in case of an emergency.
5. Transportation to and from the clinic may be arranged.

61. Which palliative care patients will meet the criteria for discharge to home hospice?
　　1. Patient and family members accepting the hospice philosophy.
　　2. Patients expected to live less than 6 months.
　　3. Patients in whom DNR status has been established.
　　4. Patients having a caregiver at home.
　　5. Patients with health insurance accepting hospice care.

62. Which palliative care patients are best managed by a home health care agency?
　　1. Patients with symptoms requiring daily nursing visits.
　　2. Patients requiring parenteral therapies.
　　3. Patients who are not yet identified as DNR.
　　4. Patients with health insurance that favors home health care.
　　5. Recurrent hospitalizations can be reduced by enrolling the patient in home health care.

63. Which palliative care patients may require a skilled nursing facility?
　　1. Patients with symptoms requiring nursing care.
　　2. Patients with no caregiver at home or with a caregiver who is incapable of further management for a while.
　　3. Patients who may have a chance to return home.
　　4. Patients who need acute care nursing but have exhausted eligible days in a hospital.
　　5. Patients on treatments started in the hospital, such as intravenous antibiotic therapy, that may need to be continued for some time.

64. Which palliative care patients may be discharged to an extended care facility?
　　1. Patients who need 24-hour nursing observation.
　　2. Patients with no caregiver at home.
　　3. Dying patients can be discharged to an extended care facility that is capable of taking care of them.
　　4. Hospice may still follow the patient at the extended care facility.
　　5. This type of discharge should be the last resort.

BIBLIOGRAPHY

1. Bone RC (ed): Hospice and palliative care. D.M. XLI(12):780–842, 1995.
2. George RJD, Jennings AL: Palliative medicine. Postgrad Med J 69:429–494, 1993.
3. Hardy JR, et al: Prediction of survival in a hospital based continuing care unit. Eur J Cancer 30A:284–288, 1994.
4. Saunders C (ed): Hospice and Palliative Care. An Interdisciplinary Approach. London, Edward Arnold, 1990.
5. Storey P (ed): Primer of Palliative Care. Gainesville, FL, Academy of Hospice Physicians, 1994.
6. Weissman DE: Consultation in palliative care. Arch Intern Med 157:733–737, 1997.

3. THE INTERDISCIPLINARY TEAM

Charles G. Sasser, M.D.

1. Why is an interdisciplinary approach essential for the care of persons and families coping with life-limiting illness?

An elderly business executive is diagnosed with **lung cancer**. His **anger**, associated with the diagnosis, is complicated by unresolved **grief** over the death of his wife 2 years earlier. He begins to **drink heavily**, which aggravates ongoing **conflicts with his children**. Impatient to assume leadership of the family business, they threaten nursing home placement. This awakens suppressed **childhood fears** of abandonment, related to his parents' divorce and his father's departure when he was 6 years old. **Fears of guilt and punishment** arise, related to an earlier loss of interest in his religious community. All of this crystallizes into a **crisis of meaning** as he reviews past accomplishments and failures, and faces a future without obvious purpose.

Chronic, progressive, life-limiting illness is characterized by complex and multidimensional suffering. Each issue significantly contributes to the business executive's suffering, but only the first, his cancer, is potentially treatable with medical intervention. Therefore, multidimensional suffering is best addressed through the investment of an interdisciplinary team that includes non-medical as well as medical health care disciplines. Such a construct has been integral to the philosophy and structure of the hospice/palliative care movement from its modern inception.

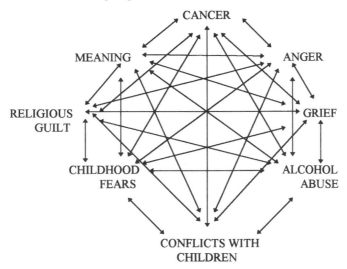

Multidimensional suffering of patients with advanced, life-limiting illness.

2. How does the hospice/palliative care interdisciplinary model of care for chronic, life-limiting illness relate to the acute health care model?

Central to any discussion about chronic, degenerative, and ultimately terminal illness is an understanding of the nature of suffering. Not surprisingly, because modern medical technology is primarily designed for cure, restoration, and survival, there is no language for suffering, no DSM code for chronic loss, no meaningful address of aging and death. Biomedicine does not distinguish between "pain" and "suffering," yet they are clearly different issues. As Cassell has pointed out, pain is what the body experiences, but suffering is the experience of "persons." Because a person is multidimensional and more than just a body, the threatened or actual loss of any dimension—the loss of a sense of intactness—causes suffering. Such a construct further suggests that the locus of suffering is actually the interpersonal space. Healing, the process of becoming "whole," involves the development or restoration of intactness in the web of relationships with self and others and may occur in the midst of steady functional decline, even at the end of life. The hospice/palliative care model both challenges and complements the acute care model by providing a structure that includes the exploration of suffering, healing, and the spaces between relationships.

3. What is the difference between multidisciplinary team (MDT) health care and care provided by a hospice/palliative interdisciplinary team (IDT)?

Multidisciplinary care is clearly hierarchical. Leadership is income and social-status derived, with participating medical members assuming both legal and moral responsibility for decisions and outcomes. For example, relationships among various medical specialties, nurses, social workers, and chaplains in an acute care setting would rarely be considered collaborative. Communication takes place predominantly in a sequential fashion through the medical record. Contributions by nonmedical disciplines are generally devalued despite overwhelming evidence that if the non-medical dimensions of suffering are not appreciated and addressed, suffering will not be relieved and healing will not take place. Furthermore, because of ever-lurking legal jeopardy, such tangential support by nonmedical participants does little to reduce the physician's sense of personal risk, loneliness, and isolation. Conversely, the hospice/palliative care IDT, when functioning optimally, becomes a single, dynamic organism in its response to the multidimensional needs of both patient and family. Leadership is shared, depending on the tasks at hand. Rather than "take over" the leadership or "go it alone" in the decision-making process because "you aren't exposed to the same legal risks that I am," the physician learns to separate authority from liability and enjoy the shared moral authority of the IDT. The dynamic is one of mutuality ("we're all in this together"), respect ("what you bring to the healing dynamic is just as important as what I bring"), and interdependence ("if participation by any of us is hindered, healing will be hindered").

4. What are the seven core functions of palliative care?

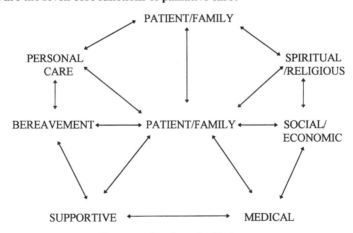

Seven core functions of palliative care.

1. Spiritual/Religious. This may be the most challenged of the disciplines because of preconceived notions and a general lack of distinction in our culture between religion and spirituality. The **spiritual specialist** demonstrates his or her gifts by the ability to recognize the universality of spiritual issues in the suffering experience; draw out the patient's spiritual issues and reframe them in a healing dynamic without interjecting his or her own agendas into the equation; clarify symptoms of spiritual/religious suffering to enhance patient, family, and team understanding;

provide spiritual counseling to the patient, family, and team; and actively participate in the plan of care to address and reduce suffering by all participants.

2. **Social/Economic.** Much more than a socioeconomic problem solver, the **social worker** is the team's resident anthropologist. His observational skills provide enhanced understanding of context—the uniqueness of each individual in a particular setting—as well as complexity—how the many parts relate to the whole. Sensitivity and openness to things as they are facilitate his ability to interpret and translate the patient and family for the team in empathic fashion. His counseling skills are often required for mediation and conflict reduction, as well for organizing and moderating family conferences.

3. **Medico-palliative.** The importance of the **physician** and **nurse** team members' symptomatology skills (physical pain and symptom control) cannot be stressed enough. For the patient to find meaning and healing in the illness experience, he must be able to step back from it somewhat, or "step out of his body" (interior distancing). But, if he is in physical pain, this kind of perspective is not possible because pain "nails him to his body." Excellent pain and symptom skills are essential to facilitating the healing experience. The physician and nurse team members also play a secondary role as educators of the patient's primary physician. It is important to be continually mindful that good palliative care is much more than mere symptomatology.

4. **Supportive.** The care of chronic and terminally ill people is exhausting and often lonely work, and the burden is usually placed on one or two family members. The interventions of trained **volunteers**— "the heart of hospice"—can dramatically reduce the physical and emotional stress of the family unit and often help to make the experience of death more of a healing process rather than a terrible tragedy.

5. **Bereavement. Grief counselors** do not usually enter the scene until the funeral, but sometimes their work begins earlier, especially when small children are present and families need assistance in preparing them for death. Nevertheless, they play an important ancillary role by participating in team discussions, advising the team about subtle grief issues, and becoming familiar with family as the patient's illness progresses. Of course, the principal responsibility of the grief counselor is to carefully and caringly monitor and facilitate grief work by survivors in the year following the death of a loved one. This is accomplished through mailings, individual counseling, and organized support groups.

6. **Personal Care.** When polled about what service people would pay for if they had to pay, the overwhelming response was for a **certified nursing assistant (CNA)** to give them a bath. There is something about the intimacy of bathing another person that provides incredible opportunity for the sharing of one's deepest, innermost secrets. CNAs are often the most knowledgeable about family dynamics and the most effective listeners on the team. Their supportive role, as death approaches, becomes indispensable.

7. **Patient/Family.** Note that the chart places the patient and family in the center as both the focus and the locus of care, as well as in the outer circle as members of the team. This is to remind professional team members about the two insights essential to the interdisciplinary frame of reference: in the healing dynamic, the distinction between giving/receiving and teaching/learning becomes blurred. Here resides the potential for *self-healing* for all participants.

5. What are the interactions of the IDT with patient and family?

Fortunately, the flaws in the radical autonomy model of doctor/patient relationships, a model prevalent through the 1990s, have been exposed as prescriptions for physician abandonment and tyranny of the individual. An "enhanced autonomy" model, proposed by Quill and Brody, is relationship-centered and allows for wider circles of participation by patient, family, and the IDT in the decision making process. This model is mutually empowering and consonant with fundamental shifts toward an understanding of individuals within the context of community. At the same time, Dame Cecily Saunders' earliest exhortation, "Let the patient be your teacher," rings as true as ever. Robert Coles expands this idea with a remarkable observation: "Hearing themselves teach you, through their narration, patients will learn the lessons a good instructor learns only when he becomes a willing student, eager to be taught." Good interdisciplinary care of people with life-limiting illness is largely a self-learning enterprise. According to Mount, "After physical symptoms are controlled, facilitating the discovery of meaning is the most important role health care professionals can play. Our role is not to impose our view of meaning on others but to act as vessels, drawing theirs out."

6. How can a physician member of the IDT maintain viable communication with other IDT members?

In theory, the primary physician is an essential member of the IDT. Unfortunately, and in part because the time and location of IDT meetings are inconvenient to medical practice, direct participation by the patient's physician in team meetings is rare. It thus becomes the role of various team members to serve, as they do for the patient and family, as surrogates and advocates for the patient's physician. When conflicts develop between the primary physician and team members over the goals of care, the relationship may become strained. Nevertheless, recognizing and addressing this responsibility, through enhanced communication, requires significant literary and diplomatic skills by team members. Photocopied or faxed handwritten notes, designed to meet third party requirements, are inappropriate. Telephone communication by nurses or medical directors is time-costly and usually occurs to address a relational crisis, leaving little opportunity for affirmation of the primary physician in her difficult position of having to depend on the skills of strangers to make difficult therapeutic decisions. Nevertheless, the key is communication. Whether written (i.e., typed) or verbal, the communication must be organized and succinct, in the physician's own language (biomedical), the tone respectful and framed with affirmation. (Of course, these five characteristics apply equally well to all communication in the optimally functioning IDT).

7. What are the essential issues to be addressed in a successful IDT meeting?

- **Who is this person we are called to help?** New patient discussions should begin with a word picture of the person and family in the context of their particular environment, an anthropological perspective or "mini-ethnography." Great narrative and orational (storytelling) skill is needed here to keep the presentation tight. Input by the different disciplines, though inefficient, provides "flesh" to the story. The presentation is successful if empathy is generated. Periodic patient reviews must be even tighter, although someone on the team must continue to represent the patient's voice and remind the team about the individual under discussion, who is the focus of concern. Perhaps the greatest challenge to effective team care is to prevent the reason for care (the patient) from being cast into the mass grave of countless disease nomenclatures and failing body parts.
- **What are the specific challenges and opportunities to which our skills may be applied?** This is the problem list, the hub for assigning duties, establishing goals that can be monitored and measured, and constructing the treatment plan. Although the problem list is itself problematic (see question 10), its use as a documenting tool is firmly entrenched in the current mindset and reimbursement mechanisms.
- **What do I need to know to do *my* job?** Here the distinction between multidisciplinary teams and interdisciplinary teams is most evident. Members of the MDT carve out their individual responsibilities and communicate their contributions after the fact and through the medical record; the IDT meets, discusses, agrees, and initiates action prospectively. The meeting is central, the roles of each participant are highly interdependent, and the whole is greater than the sum of its parts. Thus, individual team members are always aware that their interventions, although very important, are only a part of a much larger design. The question is always: What is it that *we* need to know?
- **What information should be relayed to persons not in attendance?** The most important recipients of IDT meeting activity are the patient and family. Central to the meeting is a common understanding of the multidimensional situation, from the team's perspective, and a mutually agreed upon strategy of involvement. For all others, including absent team members, the primary physician, consulting physicians, supportive professionals, pharmacists,

therapists, and invested third parties and focused medical reviewers, a single written summary must suffice. One brief statement (or form) must include changes in the clinical condition, response to therapeutic interventions, current spiritual and psychosocial dynamics, medication adjustments to be recommended, and assignment of specific communication tasks, all in a tone that is conciliatory, hopeful, positive, affirming, and understandable. Although daunting and requiring some skill, such a statement is not impossible to construct (although, to be honest, none of the forms I collected from various hospices around the country, including my own, met the above requirements). Recent encounters with the legal profession over issues of pain and symptom control have served to remind me how the threat of litigation helps crystallize the function of documentation. Stated positively, if you were accused of successfully reducing pain and suffering in the terminally ill, would there be sufficient evidence to convict?

8. What are the common obstacles to optimal IDT function?

- **Third-party documentation vs. in-depth discussion of complex multi-layered issues.** There will always be some tension between the need to transcribe, in narrative form, complex patient care situations with carefully considered options for intervention, and the need to document with a series of checks, for reimbursement purposes, that something has been done.
- **Language issues.** Often unrecognized is the manner in which specialty language—the mysterious jargon of each discipline—shifts the balance of power and authority in that direction. This is most commonly employed (unconsciously) by doctors and nurses, but social workers and chaplains may also be guilty. Often needed is the presence of a "language policeman." This role can be played by anyone with sensitivity, but it is easiest for a lay person with a stronger sense of self who is not afraid to say, "I don't understand. Would you explain that in words I can understand?" This is not "dumbing down." This is paying respect to the most important reason for team meetings: the enhancement of understanding equally among all present.
- **Patient care issues vs. personal agenda issues.** In every telling of another's story, there are ghosts. The ghosts represent the parts of our personal past, culture, pain, and story that we unconsciously insert into someone else's story. Clarifying "who's story is this?" requires trust and the willingness to be vulnerable.

9. How do you gauge the efficiency vs. the efficacy of the IDT?

Efficiency is a simple mathematical term relating to the ratio of outputs to inputs. The greater the ratio of outputs per input, the greater the efficiency. The emphasis here is on keeping the input, whether it be an investment of time, energy, or money, at its lowest. Efficacy, on the other hand, places emphasis on the quality of the desired output: what it is, exactly, that we are trying to achieve. In short, the rationale underlying the existence of the IDT is that a room full of highly paid professionals, engaged in an intense 20-minute discussion about one patient/family situation, is terribly inefficient but highly efficacious if the results are understanding, empathy, and concerted action.

10. How applicable is the problem-oriented approach, with its tendency to dissect patients and families into a list of potentially solvable problems, to patient care in the IDT setting?

According to Monroe et al., "Care imitates language;" that is, we tend to relate to people the same way we write and talk about them. Thus, when we see them in terms of diagnosis (the leukemic), diseased organs (the kidney failure patient), emotional problems (the hysteric), or socioeconomics (the financial disaster), we will relate to them only at that level and fail to see them in "whole person" terms. The risk is great that we will fail to appreciate the multidimensional nature of their suffering or fail to identify the dormant seeds of healing potential that require nurture. Most documents currently used by IDTs to communicate patient and family care activities are problem oriented and, thus, fragmenting. Narrative descriptions are inefficient and too complex for third party review, but essential to maintaining whole person perspectives.

11. How can the IDT meeting be made more efficacious?

- At bedside, each team member, depending on the circumstance, may be called on to fill the role of another discipline. Role confusion at team meeting, however, fosters loosely associated and disorganized discussion. Although the contribution each member makes by sharing observations from his or her own perspective is invaluable to the fleshing out process, the provision of scientific information should be confined to the authority of his or her own specialty. Such disciplined communication greatly tightens the flow of pertinent information and significantly reduces superfluity and redundancy.

- Team members *must* be cognizant of the difference between authoritative and authoritarian presentations. This requires a healthy self-awareness, sensitivity to various agendas in tension, acknowledgment of interdependence, and respect for the legitimacy and healing authority of each participating discipline.

- Most effective is a sensitive and self-assured moderator who can identify, before the start of the meeting, those discussions that will require the most time and those patients who will need less input. That moderator then considers the overall time allotted and plans the agenda accordingly.

- Some conflicts that are voiced in IDT meetings, either among team members or between a team member and patient or family, need more extensive discussion and are better dealt with in another setting. A moderator who can deftly defer such discussions without bruising fragile egos is a gem and should be rewarded handsomely (if not in cash, then at least in accolades and affirmation).

- Continuing education in effective IDT purpose, conduct, and function is essential. Problematic and conflict-laden patient care situations may be re-presented in an educational format that emphasizes process over personalities, asks "what can we learn from this" and reaffirms the difficult challenges of the palliative care enterprise.

12. How does the IDT manage ethical issues?

Ethical conflicts are inherent in end-of-life care in general and in interdisciplinary care in particular. Not the least of these are the conflict-of-interest issues that arise from the fact that one agency may serve as both health care provider and fiscal intermediary. Thus, all members of the team should have some interest in practical approaches to the resolution of ethical conflicts, at least with reference to their own discipline. The social worker, for example, is usually the most knowledgeable about the patients' rights issues; the physician, about withholding vs. withdrawal of death-prolonging interventions. The assistance of an outside ethicist to address particularly sticky situations should rarely be necessary but can be very educational.

13. Is there any way in which the IDT, with all its cumbersome inefficiency, can ever survive in the new millennium?

The gradual replacement of 17th century Newtonian science by the quantum model is leading to the emergence of new realities pertinent to interdisciplinary care. The flaws in the modern constructs of efficiency, predictability, and control are increasingly apparent as an enhanced appreciation of complexity, complementarity, and uncertainty, all central to quantum theory, unfolds. In particular, the Newtonian idea of entropy—the mechanistic view of life and the universe as a clock winding down—is gradually being replaced by the quantum idea of autopoeisis—the capability of living organisms to, over time, display self-organization and self-renewal. (This construct validates the hospice experience of personal growth and development in the midst of ongoing physical decline.) An autopoietic structure such as an IDT might be considered a portfolio of skills or a bundle of competencies (rather than a collection of optimally functioning units), and has the inherent potential for self-reference. This means that no matter what type or how powerful outside pressures may be, as long as the IDT is clear about its mission and purpose, change and adaptation can occur without loss of integrity. Quantum thinking would also encourage us to accept the reality that chaos—a good name for the state of health care these days—is here to stay but not all bad. This is why it is so important to hold onto, in the constant swirl of change, the original vision about the centrality of the IDT in end-of-life care.

BIBLIOGRAPHY

1. Cassell EJ: The Nature of Suffering and the Goals of Medicine. New York, Oxford University Press, 1991.
2. Coles R: The Call of Stories: Teaching and Moral Imagination. Boston, Houghton Mifflin, 1989.
3. Kleinman A: The Illness Narratives: Suffering, Healing and the Human Condition. New York, Basic Books, 1988.
4. Monroe WF, Holleman WF, Hollema MC: Is There a Person in This Case? Lit Med 11:1, 45–63, 1992.
5. Mount B: Beyond Physical and Psychosocial Care. Presented at the International Hospice Institute Conference. Estes Park, CO, June 10, 1990. Tape available from Rollin' Recordings, 208 River Ranch Rd, Boerne, TX 28006; 210-537-5494.
6. O'Murchu D: Quantum Theology. New York, Crossroad Publishing, 1997.
7. Quill T, Brody H: Physician recommendations and patient autonomy: Finding a balance between physician power and patient choice. Ann Intern Med 125:763–768, 1996.
8. Wheatley MJ: Leadership and the New Science: Learning about Organization from an Orderly Universe. San Francisco, Berret-Koehler Publishers, 1992.

4. THE ESSENCE OF PALLIATIVE CARE NURSING

Sharon Bean Heidecker, B.S.N., CRNH

1. What distinguishes oncology nursing from registered nursing?

Nurses graduate from nursing programs with generalized knowledge to allow them to practice safely. They must sit for national nursing boards and obtain an acceptable score to earn the title "registered nurse" (RN). RNs may then begin to work in areas of specific interest to obtain specialized knowledge.

Oncology nursing requires further education and training to learn the specific demands and needs of caring for patients with cancer. Some of this specific knowledge pertains to cancer treatments such as chemotherapy, radiation, blood stem cell transplantation, and bone marrow transplant. Training also includes management of psychosocial issues faced by the patient and/or family. Also, RNs may sit for oncology nursing certification after meeting criteria related to years in nursing and specific hours of oncology nursing experience.

The credential of Oncology Certified Nurse (OCN) acknowledges that the RN possesses an identified level of knowledge in this area. Certification must be renewed every four years by re-examination. The examination is constantly updated. After the year 2000, all new candidates must possess at least a bachelor's degree in nursing. RNs can also join the Oncology Nursing Society, which promotes excellence in this field.

2. Are there subdivisions in oncology nursing?

There are 30 special interest groups recognized within the Oncology Nursing Society. Some examples of these are: advanced nursing research, bone marrow transplant, chemotherapy, ethics, hospice, and spiritual care.

3. How does palliative nursing differ from oncology nursing?

In palliative nursing, all efforts are directed toward decreasing symptomatology and increasing quality of life. The patient has arrived at a place in the disease continuum where cure is not possible; therefore, comfort becomes paramount.

Both oncology nurses and palliative care nurses may deal with some similar components of patient care. Oncology nurses may care for patients receiving chemotherapy or radiation to cure their cancer. Palliative care nurses may also care for patients receiving chemotherapy or radiation, but the intent of those treatments is to shrink a tumor's size to control symptoms such as pain or obstruction.

Oncology nursing usually involves much more invasive treatment than does palliative nursing. Part of oncology nursing care is aimed at patients receiving treatments in an attempt to eradicate or cure cancer. Many of these treatments may create side effects and symptoms of distress such as fatigue, nausea, vomiting, etc. Treatment side effects are *not* acceptable in palliative nursing.

4. How are hospice nursing and palliative nursing similar?

Both hospice nursing and palliative nursing focus on symptom management to increase quality of life. Each area uses an interdisciplinary team to afford the patient expertise in critical areas such as pain control, symptom management, psychosocial issues, and spiritual issues. A patient and his or her caregivers are viewed as a unit of care by the team. The interdisciplinary team approach is based on the concept that no one person can meet all of the needs of the dying patient. In any life-threatening or serious illness, both patient and caregivers require empathy and support.

5. How does hospice nursing differ from palliative nursing?

One of the major differences can be length of life expectancy of patients in hospice nursing. Currently, a physician must certify that a patient has a life expectancy of 6 months or less to qualify for a hospice program. A palliative care patient may be beyond cure, as is a hospice patient, but has a longer life expectancy (≥ 1 year).

Treatment options may also differ. For example, surgical intervention to alleviate a symptom may be perfectly appropriate for a patient with a life expectancy of a year or more, but totally inappropriate for a patient with less than 6 months to live. Patients further along the disease continuum usually lack the physical and/or emotional stamina to withstand highly invasive procedures. Also, these procedures may not produce equivalent effects of palliation at different points along the disease continuum.

6. Is there a lack of education in nursing curricula pertaining to hospice and palliative care?

YES! Nursing students receive instruction on death and the dying patient. However, this is very different from learning about the palliation of symptoms. Nursing students should be placed in palliative care clinics or hospices to learn firsthand about patient needs and the team approach. ALL nurses WILL care for patients who have need for palliation, although the patient may not be labeled as such. It is important to understand the processes of treating symptoms when cure is no longer an option. There also needs to be more emphasis on communication, ethical and legal issues, and grief and bereavement concerns in nursing curricula. This lack of education in palliative care is also acutely felt in the medical school curricula in the training of physicians.

7. Can palliative care and hospice nurses be certified?

YES! After meeting eligibility criteria with years worked in the field and as an RN, a nurse may sit for certification in hospice and palliative care. A nurse need not have completed a bachelor's degree, but must possess the title of RN. Upon successful completion of the exam, the RN may place the initials "CRNH" (certified registered nurse of hospice) after their name. Passing the exam demonstrates a level of expertise in hospice and palliative care nursing. The Hospice and Palliative Care Nurses Association promotes excellence in the field.

8. Is hospice and palliative care nursing just for cancer patients?

NO! This approach can be utilized for any end-of-life disease process—cancerous, neuromuscular, pulmonary, or cardiac. It can even be utilized for patients experiencing dementia such as that induced by Alzheimer's disease.

9. Is there a role for the nurse practitioner (NP) in hospice and palliative care?

According to Stedman's Medical Dictionary, a nurse practitioner is defined as "a registered nurse with at least a master's degree in nursing and advanced education in the primary care of particular groups of clients. An NP is capable of independent practice in a variety of settings." NPs must sit for certification in their specialty after their education process is complete. Some of these specialties include adult health, acute care, pediatrics, and family health. Currently, there are no specific programs in existence that train nurses only in the specialty of palliation. However, there are nurse practitioners who have sought specialized knowledge in this area and are already in practice. This role is in its infancy and is being defined and developed. Now is the perfect time for those who have an interest in this role to speak up and take action to assist in its creation.

Nurse practitioners in advanced clinical practice must possess a master's degree in nursing. Required skills include knowledge of advanced pathophysiology, physical assessment, medications, and diagnostics. Excellent psychosocial skills are also crucial. Research, education, and the leadership role pertaining to management and consultation are also stressed in a master's program.

The nurse practitioner can function in vital capacities in the hospice and palliative care role. With advanced skills and knowledge, the NP could act as a valuable resource to an interdisciplinary team by visiting patients, taking the history, performing physicals, and suggesting changes in care to the attending physician and supporting families. This nurse could also be utilized to rotate on-call schedules with the palliative care physicians, thus serving as a support. Research has demonstrated that NPs are cost-effective and provide excellent care. Medicare, Medicaid, and private insurance companies now provide reimbursement for NP services. It only seems logical to utilize NPs with advanced knowledge of end-of-life issues to provide palliative care.

10. Is the nurse an advocate for the patient, the family, or the physician?

WOW, the million dollar question! The nurse is always concerned with patient advocacy. However, in palliative care and hospice nursing, the patient and family are viewed as a unit of care and all needs must be considered. At times, it is important to advocate for the immediate needs of the patient—for example, if a patient is too ill to safely remain alone at any time. Family members must be instructed that it is necessary to obtain a 24-hour caregiver. This may mean significant life changes for them, but the patient's needs must be considered first. At other times, it is necessary for the nurse to advocate for a caregiver's needs. Sometimes patients demand that one specific person care for them at all times. That may be possible if a patient's life expectancy is extremely limited to hours or days. However, it is virtually impossible for one person to render 24-hour care for an individual over a significant period of time and remain emotionally healthy. All caregivers require respite, although even the caregiver may not recognize this need. It is the nurse's responsibility to advocate for the caregiver in this situation. Sometimes caregivers feel that they cannot refuse the demands of a loved one because that person is so ill. The guilt they feel can be overwhelming. But the dying individual also needs to recognize that their illness does not give them the right to cause someone else physical, emotional, or spiritual harm.

The nurse may also act as the physician's advocate. It is not unusual for a nurse to call the physician and request certain medications or treatments for a patient and thus function as a patient advocate. However, patients sometimes refuse medications or treatments that are necessary for their comfort because they feel the physician is "just ordering another pill," or because they want a medication or treatment that the physician will not order for good reason. It is the nurse's responsibility to advocate for that physician.

All of this means that the situation often gets very sticky! A good sense of yourself and a great sense of humor helps!

11. In what situation does the nurse become a buffer between the patient and family?

The nurse can act as an excellent buffer by promoting a sense of trust among the patient, the family, and herself. Palliative care and hospice care afford the nurse an excellent opportunity to initiate this at the onset of care. It should always be explained at this time that the patient and family are viewed as a unit of care and that "everyone counts." This helps the patient *and* the family to utilize the nurse as a person to discuss feelings, frustrations, and situations. It tends to de-escalate tensions so that major problems are less likely to occur.

12. How can a nurse become a buffer between the doctor and the patient?

At times the situation can become very tense if persons are very demanding or the physician is experiencing emotional stress. I have seen physicians, as well as nurses, experience increased emotional turmoil when the situation "hits close to home." We are all human and the caring, nurturing, helping qualities that draw us into the field of medicine/nursing sometimes mean that we will identify with people and hurt for them. If the nurse can allow herself and the physician the right to verbalize some of this, it helps to relieve stress and promote clearer thinking. When patients are demanding, the nurse can buffer the situation by acting as a middle-man by asking questions of the physician and the patient and relaying the information.

13. What are the strategies adopted by palliative care and hospice nurses in comforting the patient?

Comfort can mean different things to different patients. It can even have a different meaning to the same patient at different times. The most important strategy is to first assess what actions would serve the patient's need for comfort.

Active listening is the best method of accomplishing this goal. What is the patient saying? What is their body language saying? What is the patient *not* saying—but is the real message coming across loud and clear? Only after ascertaining what the real need is can the nurse attempt to meet it. Active listening, while allowing the patient to verbalize whatever emotions they may be experiencing, is sometimes all that is needed. We have all experienced verbalizing about a situation and feeling relief. The presence and attention of the person who allowed us to talk brought the gift of comfort.

Touch can also be used to bring great comfort to patients. Sometimes a hug, holding a hand, or a light touch on the shoulder lets that person know they are not alone. In our hospice home care, the home health aides are valuable members of the team. They render gentle, personal care, such as baths and grooming. The very tasks they must perform demand some form of intimacy and touch. We have found that even those patients most reluctant to agree to an aide won't give them up after the first few visits! I believe it is because the patients are comforted by the attention and the touch of the aide.

Another strategy used is prayer. Some patients ask for prayer and sometimes nurses will offer it if its seems appropriate. The nurse must be comfortable with the concept. It is important to remember that it is the PATIENT'S spirituality that is important to his or her comfort. We must never force our spirituality or belief system on the patient.

14. What part does control play in the patient's comfort and plan of care?

Control is most crucial to patients who are facing major physical changes from illness to death. Keep in mind that the patient realizes he is gradually losing control over all things. At the end of the illness is death and an end to everything familiar.

We should tell our patients from the beginning that they are active members in their plan of care. They have the right to refuse any procedure or treatment. At times, nurses can experience great discomfort when patients refuse medications or procedures that we **know** will bring them **physical** comfort. But, we must examine why the patient makes these choices.

There are two areas that seem to be major issues with many patients. One is pain control. Some patients who are well controlled on pain medications will deliberately reduce their dosage and once again experience pain. **Why**? Because, for whatever reason—increased alertness, the belief that increased medication means deterioration, or even the fact that the pain reminds them that they are alive—being uncomfortable brings them emotional or psychological comfort, which is more important to them than physical comfort. We must always respect the patient's autonomy.

The other area of control is the need for Foley catheters or adult incontinence briefs. Many patients resist these because they represent a loss of independence and dignity. This is especially hard on caregivers who must constantly take the patient to the bathroom or change clothing and bed linens. We need to lend support to help caregivers "ride out" this difficult time, while at the same time respecting the patient's wishes.

15. What are the difficulties faced by the palliative care or hospice nurse when death occurs suddenly?

Some of the difficulties may be related to the cause of the terminal event. In some advanced cancers, there is danger of hemorrhage or "bleeding out." This is a very stressful event for families as well as for team members. The nurse **must** prepare the family if this event is a possibility. Some of the strategies used for this emphasize that it is not a painful event for the patient, using dark towels so that the blood is not so apparent and directing that the nurse or physician be called if the event begins to occur. Other sudden death scenarios may occur with aneurysms or embolisms, sudden congestive heart failure, or pulmonary edema. These can be overwhelming events that begin a cascade of emotions that cannot be stopped.

There are also bereavement issues when a patient has a serious illness but death is not imminent. We must remember that families usually have an "idea" or scenario of what the disease progression and death will be like. Families often expect that a patient will experience progressively worse symptoms, that these symptoms will be reasonably controlled, and that there will be time to say goodbye, and they hope that death will be peaceful. They prepare for the death, but it is considered to be an event that will occur sometime in the future.

If events unfold as expected, families have time to deal with some grief issues before death occurs. This is called anticipatory grief. It does not mean that all of their grief work is completed before the patient's death. But, when a patient dies suddenly or unexpectedly (even with a terminal diagnosis), families can be thrown into the same type of grief reactions experienced as when persons are killed in accidents. Shock and disbelief dominate their reactions. Even team members are not exempt. Families usually need a little extra support with these deaths as do members of the interdisciplinary team who were closely involved.

16. How do hospice nurses handle the time of death of the patient?
Because the nurse works so closely with the patient and family, death is not usually a surprise. Many signs and symptoms point to deterioration and it is the nurse's responsibility to educate the caregivers about the dying process. In an in-patient hospice unit, there would be nurses on the floor at all times. In homecare, nurses are often not present at the actual time of death, but are called when the patient has already died. Unless the family requests differently, the nurse visits and lends emotional support, provides personal care for the patient, and notifies the physician of the death. Sometimes families call the funeral director, but the nurse will also do this if requested. The nurse may also take part in spiritual rituals at this time as many families will request a visit from clergy to recite prayers. Opioids, and other drugs prescribed earlier to the deceased patient, are usually disposed of by the nurse, but this also depends on the policy of the agency or unit.

The nurse continues to lend emotional support until the family has left the unit or until the body has been transported by the funeral director. A difficult time for many families is when the body is being carried out of the home. The nurse can lend much support at this time and does not leave until the family is ready. It is always stressed that there will be bereavement follow-up. This usually continues for 13 months after the death. Hospice team members often attend funeral services or memorial services for patients.

17. What are the difficulties faced by nurses when they know a patient should be DNR, but the physician is reluctant to discuss the issue with the patient?
Ideally, it should be the physician who broaches this issue. When this does not occur, patients face uncertainty. They rely on the physician to speak openly and honestly. They may continue with more aggressive treatment because they feel that this is what the physician wants and that it is in their best interest. These emotional issues then become nursing problems that are difficult to solve. When a nurse attempts to speak to the patient about deterioration and the choices that are available, it is not uncommon to hear, "But my doctor has never said this!" Psychologically, the patient may label the nurse as "the bad guy" and trust is eroded. It also supports a sense of denial and the patient cannot prepare properly for the end of life.

18. Should DNR be a nursing decision?
I say, "**No!**"
I personally believe that the patient has the right to choose or refuse DNR status. This may make them inappropriate for a palliative care or hospice program, especially if they choose aggressive treatment. This should be explained to them at the appropriate times, so that the patient can make their best personal decision. We all have personal opinions, but we truly cannot answer for another unless we have been given that right—Power of Attorney for Healthcare. It is easier when a patient has a living will or speaks forthrightly—"I don't want any heroics!" Unfortunately, this does not happen all the time.

I believe that physicians and nurses can help the patient decide this issue by presenting the facts in a realistic manner. There should **never** be any coercion! It should also be known that this is sometimes an ethical issue when patients and families "want everything done," and the outcome is grim. Who decides that? Communicating with the patient and the family in a family meeting and coming to a consensus usually helps.

19. What are the day-to-day frustrations felt by nurses?

Some of the frustrations involve the setting. For example, palliative care or inpatient hospice nurses would most likely work alongside their peers and not experience as much isolation as would a homecare hospice nurse. However, there may be problems with understaffing or a large number of patients. You must have a good ratio of nurses to patients to give comprehensive care. Depending on the setting, there may even be problems with logistics and administration at the institutional facility.

Time is an issue for the homecare nurse. She may be required to work 8, 10, or 12 hours a day, depending on patient care time, paperwork time, and travel time to each patient setting. The day may constantly change and grow longer if problems arise that require additional time to be resolved.

On-call hours are also frustrating for many nurses. It is difficult to work full days, be up all night answering the beeper or making visits, and then work the next day. On-call varies, of course, and some nights are quiet.

Paperwork is always an issue among homecare nurses. It isn't just the daily charting of notes. It also involves recertification of patients, discharge charts, and patient summaries. Many times it falls on the homecare nurse to contact insurance case managers for updates and approval of visits.

Last, but not least, physicians can sometimes be the cause of frustration. Some physicians are not as aware of palliation as others and will refuse certain medications or treatments. Some physicians do not like the nurse to be the one to suggest anything! It is frustrating to know that a patient is suffering and the physician refuses to order the treatment/medication that will ease that suffering. This scenario is occurring less frequently as more physicians become familiar with palliative care.

20. Do family members become stressed and get angry with the nurse?

It is not uncommon for family members to grow weary and fatigued, which reduces their capacity to cope. Thus, they feel out of control and fearful or frustrated. Because the nurse is usually the member of the team closest to the patient and the family, anger is often directed that way. At times a family may have a legitimate complaint—perhaps they called about a problem and the nurse or the physician did not return the call in a reasonable amount of time. If an error has occurred, the nurse should look for ways to reconcile the situation. At other times, through no fault of the nurse, he or she is bombarded with all of the anger and frustration that the family is feeling. The best course of action is to remain calm and to allow the family members to vent their feelings. There is a difference between normal anger and abusive behavior. If a situation escalates out of control, and safety is compromised, the nurse should leave immediately. Also, another member of the palliative care or hospice team may join in the resolution of any conflict perceived or real.

21. Nurses spend the most time with patients and yet many patients wait for the doctor to tell them their daily progress. Why?

I believe this occurs with some patients because the physician is viewed as the ultimate authority. I have experienced this many times in hospice. The nurses are excellent patient educators and the patients trust and believe them. But many times, patients seem to view the physician as the final word. When they hear it from the doctor's mouth, it takes on a new reality.

22. What can a nurse do if the physician cannot deal with the patient at times of greatest need?

The nurse advocates for the patient's needs to the physician. If the physician does not respond to repeated requests for symptom control and patient comfort, the nurse should explore other options with the patient and family. Perhaps a family meeting with the physician is in order. If the physician refuses and calls are still unheeded, it may be time to explore the option of the patient choosing a new physician. This option is never offered routinely. Most physicians **do** meet patients' needs. The nurse should never damage the physician-patient relationship. Likewise, we must not allow a patient to suffer if a physician is not fulfilling his or her role.

23. Can a patient feel abandoned by a nurse or physician?

Yes! Sometimes these feelings are legitimate. Sometimes they arise out of fear or loneliness. Physicians, nurses, and the entire interdisciplinary team should always maintain an atmosphere of trust. To accomplish this we need to be sensitive, open, and empathetic. We need to keep promises. If the nurse tells the patient that he will receive a phone call the next day, that phone call should be placed. If trust is breached too many times, that relationship will suffer and the patient will feel abandoned.

There are also times when a patient or family expect attention beyond reason. Patients may begin to refuse visits if a particular nurse cannot visit because of illness or vacation. Taking vacation days or sick days does not constitute abandonment. We all need time away from patient care to renew ourselves. And such time off is an excellent opportunity to demonstrate the workings of the interdisciplinary team. I have found that preparing a patient and family *before* taking time off works wonders.

24. Are hospice care and palliative care stressful?

Hospice and palliative care nursing can be very stressful. Nurses are continually faced with end-of-life issues and loss. It is natural to identify in some respect with patients. There are also occupational, environmental, and individual factors that enter into considering the stress level of nurses. Some of the factors associated with increased stress and a higher rate of burnout are: younger staff, poor social support, unresolved personal grief experiences, and poor support from the workplace.

25. What can be done to help nurses deal with stress and prevent burnout?

1. **Recognize that newly hired nurses require an adequate orientation to hospice or palliative care nursing**. There are different goals to be met and it can be extremely stressful to feel confused over what the real issues are. Once nurses are oriented, it is also important to provide back-up support for on-call issues or questions. It is frightening to feel all alone when unsure of the "rightness" of the answer to a patient's question or symptom.

2. **Allow nurses to participate in program changes**. Management often decides an issue and announce changes that will be implemented. Allowing the staff to participate in decision making will empower them and provide a sense of control.

3. **Make team building an absolute priority**. Remember, the interdisciplinary team exists because no one person can meet all of the needs of the patient and family. All team members should be treated with respect and a trusting atmosphere must be maintained. There is no room for superiority on the team. Patient care will suffer and stress levels will be high if the team is dysfunctional. Some hospitals or agencies sponsor retreats or special in-services for staff to build and promote trust and equality among the team. Issues that are significantly affecting the team must be addressed. Some of these issues might be severe personality conflicts, failure to share pertinent information about patients and families, or excessive absenteeism of any one member because of illness or other commitments.

4. **Give the staff positive feedback**. Families will often send letters of thanks to individual nurses. They will also return survey questionnaires and mention certain nurses and their contributions. Management should always bring these to the nurse's attention. Voice mail, notes, or face-to-face communication should also be used to give encouragement in demanding situations.

5. **Schedule regular support meetings for nurses to allow verbalization of anger, frustration, or grief**. Memorial services and stress management in-services are a MUST! Ensure that there is a chaplain or counselor available for the staff to utilize on an individual basis.

6. **Provide educational and professional development opportunities**. Palliative care, as well as hospice, is a growing field with exciting new developments. Conferences, in-services, and certifications allow nurses to gain new skills and knowledge and demonstrate expertise.

26. Is it always possible to make positive differences in a patient's care?

No. We must revisit patient autonomy again on this issue. As caregivers, we are always interested in helping and making positive differences. But patients do not always allow us to "help" them. We also should not feel that our perceptions are always correct. Patients will sometimes choose to experience pain, eat things that make them deathly ill, and refuse assistance when they can barely move. Life experiences and genetics influence how we perceive and react to life.

With some patients, I believe we make a difference, but we may not perceive this. I learned a valuable lesson from a patient several years ago. She never followed through on any of my attempts to help her. Each visit was uncomfortable for me because I felt like an intruder. One day I said to her, "I know you just wish I would leave you alone, but I really need to clean your tracheostomy tube." When I returned to her, she had written—"I may not show it but I appreciate everything you do." What an eye opener! She never changed, but I learned that I had made a positive difference.

There are some patients, however, who will not allow any kind of positive experience into their lives. This *does not* mean that the nurse or physician has failed.

27. Do you ever use self-disclosure when working with patients and families?

Absolutely! But the nurse must discern the appropriateness of the information to be disclosed and the motivation behind it. Because we are in a therapeutic relationship, we must always remember that our goal is to support the patient and family. They should feel OUR support and not be placed in the position of supporting the nurse. But there are times when sharing a similar experience can truly assist someone in their grief or searching.

Because the nurses are so intimately involved with patients and their families, there tends to be a relationship formed where more information may be shared. Nurses are usually asked if they are married . . . if they have children . . . if they have ever experienced caring for a loved one who is dying . . . etc. If a family member is inappropriate in the information they are requesting, it is wise to share as little information as possible. At other times, the nurse may share information more deeply with a patient/family member than with a friend. I can give a personal example of this.

A few years ago, I was assigned as primary nurse to a young woman with a somewhat rare form of cancer. She was the same age as me, and she had three children the same genders and ages as my own. At every visit, our relationship grew a little deeper and she began sharing some experiences of her life that she needed to discuss. When asked about my family, I shared that I was married and had four children, but had lost a daughter when she was 8 years old. She asked a few more questions about my daughter and then spoke of other issues. Many weeks later, I made a routine visit and the house was empty except for her and me. After the routine questions and an assessment, she asked me to stay for some coffee and to talk. What transpired then was difficult for me, but also, extremely meaningful.

She had been thinking of all the significant people she was leaving behind and was attempting to find ways that would help them after she died. Because I had lost a child, she had many questions for me pertaining to the loss that her own mother would be experiencing soon. "What did it feel like?" "Did the hurt get better?" "What helped me through the most difficult times after my daughter's death?" All of her questions were appropriate and she asked me because I could give her "real" answers. So, I answered her questions about my own experience with honesty, and I promised that I would visit her mother for bereavement. I drove back to the office for some emotional support before visiting my next patient, thus utilizing the team for my needs.

I felt that I had done the right thing in answering her questions. She never questioned me again in this manner and died within a few weeks. I never knew what she actually said or did for her mother, but I'm sure she followed through on something. When I made my bereavement visit to the parents, I had the opportunity for some time alone with her mother. She played a video of her daughter and shared with me her feelings about her daughter from a mother's grieving heart. I had to smile to myself because her daughter had used all of my sharing to gain insight into what her mother would be experiencing, then shared with her mother that I had lost a child. Her mother immediately connected with this and was able to open up more about her difficult loss.

In this case, specific self-disclosure was appropriate. I might not share so specifically with everyone. Remember, self-disclosure is a *tool* to aid and assist our patients!

28. What can hospice and palliative care nursing mean to the nurse?
This field has allowed me to use all of my education, skills, personal knowledge, and spirituality for the good of my patients and their families. The patient and family must be viewed holistically. This alone calls for continuous personal and professional growth.

Although it can sometimes be stressful and demanding, it is also tremendously rewarding to walk with a patient and family to the end. Every patient and family is different. All have a story. Experiencing the joys and sorrows of everyday life with them is humbling, as we will all face death someday. I have learned to search for what is truly important to me and make each day count. Most patients and families express gratitude to the nurses and to the other team members who care for them. I would like to express my gratitude for all of the "gifts" they have given to me.

29. What information resources are available to the nurse interested in palliative care?
The nurse may call or write:

Hospice and Palliative Nurses Association
Medical Center East, Suite 375
211 N. Whitfield Street
Pittsburgh, PA 15206-3031
    Phone: 412-361-2470
    Fax: 412-361-2425
    E-Mail: hnafan@usa.pipeline.com
    http//www.rOxane.com/HNA

Oncology Nursing Society
National Office
501 Holiday Drive
Pittsburgh, PA 15220-2749
    Phone: 412-921-7373
    Fax: 412-921-7373
    E-Mail: customer.service@ons.org

Palliative Care Letter
Roxane Laboratories, Inc.
P. O. Box 16532
Columbus, Ohio 43216
    Phone: 614-276-4000
    Fax: 614-276-8061

Other resources:

Marketing Services
American Nurses Credentialing Center
P. O. Box 2244
Waldorf, MD 20602
    Phone: 800-284-2378

American Academy of Nurse Practitioners
Capital Station, LBJ Building
P. O. Box 12846
Austin, TX 78711
    Phone: 512-442-4262

National Certification Board of Pediatric Nurse Practitioners/Nurses
416 Hungerford Drive
Suite 222
Rockville, MD 20850-4127
   Phone: 301-340-8213

BIBLIOGRAPHY

1. Bottorff J, Gogeg M, Engelberg-Lotzkar M: Comforting: Exploring the work of cancer nurses. J Adv Nurs 22:1077–1084, 1995.
2. Cummings I: The interdisciplinary team. In Boyle B, Hanks G, MacDonald N (eds): Oxford Textbook of Palliative Medicine. Oxford, Oxford University Press, 1998, pp 19–30.
3. Jodrell N: Nurse education. In Boyle B, Hanks G, MacDonald N (eds): Oxford Textbook of Palliative Medicine. Oxford, Oxford University Press, 1998, pp 1201–1208.
4. Koesters E: Hospice Care. In Hickey J, Gulmette R, Venegoni S (eds): Advanced Practice Nursing: Changing Roles and Clinical Applications. Philadelphia, J.B. Lippincott, 1996, pp 327–333.
5. Nelson ME: Client advocacy. In Snyder M, Mirr M (eds): Advanced Practice Nursing: A Guide to Professional Development. New York, Springer, 1995, pp 103–113.
6. Stedman's Concise Medical Dictionary for the Health Professions, 3rd ed. Baltimore, Williams & Wilkins, 1997.
7. Taylor B, Glass N, McFarlane J, Stirling C: Palliative nurses perceptions of the nature and effects of their work. Int J Palliat Nurs 3:253–258, 1997.
8. Weggel JM: Palliative care: New challenges for advanced practice nursing. The Hospice Journal 12:43–56, 1997.

5. SOCIAL WORK AND PALLIATIVE CARE

Mary Raymer, M.S.W., A.C.S.W.

1. What is the definition of social work?

Social work is the professional practice of helping individuals, families, groups, or communities enhance or restore their capacity for optimal social, emotional, and psychological health. Social work achieves this goal through counseling, referral, and advocacy and by working to enhance the environment.

2. What are the key values of the social work profession?

Professional social workers embrace the values of service, social justice, the dignity and worth of the individual, the right to self-determination, the importance of human relationships, integrity, and competence.

3. Are there specific educational requirements to call oneself a social worker or are any helping professionals appropriately called social workers?

Professional social workers are trained professionals who have a bachelor's, master's, or doctorate in social work. Social workers practice in a variety of settings in addition to palliative care, but the training of social workers is very specific and places special emphasis on understanding the milieu of the person in his or her situation, including psychological, social, and interpersonal components. All states license or otherwise regulate social work.

4. At what point is it appropriate to refer to social work?

Social workers should be a consistent component on the palliative care team. When cure is no longer possible, a variety of psychosocial stressors rise to the surface for all individuals and their family members. Addressing these issues through problem-solving, counseling or psychotherapy, resource management, and active advocacy helps to significantly alleviate depression, anxiety, and feelings of isolation and abandonment.

5. Are there specific goals that are consistent standards for social workers in palliative care?

There are five primary goals that palliative care social workers are seeking to achieve:
1. Enhancing the responsiveness of the environment
2. Stimulating internal and psychological coping skills of the individual and his or her family
3. Screening for psychopathology
4. Enhancing the self-worth of the family system as well as the individual
5. Providing specific symptom relief

6. Do social workers play a role in physical symptom control?

Specific techniques such as relaxation skills, imagery, and deep breathing help significantly with pain and nausea for many individuals living with an incurable illness. The provision of specific tools that the individual can learn and practice has the added benefit of helping the individual feel more in control of the situation, which then reduces feelings of helplessness and anxiety. Counseling to alleviate depression, anxiety, and other distressing symptoms that exacerbate somatic distress often produces dramatic results in reported physical comfort levels. Palliative care recognizes this complex interplay between the physical and the emotional and seeks to treat the "whole" person. Any professional intervention that reduces stress and tension will most likely assist with the physical aspects of symptom control.

7. Is there a role for social workers with their colleagues on palliative care teams?

Social workers believe that they have an ethical responsibility to their colleagues. The National Association of Social Workers' Code of Ethics clearly mandates a commitment to respect and support professional colleagues. On an interdisciplinary care team, social workers often identify team stress or breakdown on certain cases and work to alleviate that stress and to assist their colleagues. Enhancing the responsiveness of the environment for the patients they serve includes facilitating the best teamwork possible. Social workers also have an ethical responsibility to educate their team members about the specific beliefs, values, spirituality, and cultural mores of the individuals and families being served. This information is crucial to providing effective palliative care, and without this knowledge we may inadvertently create more distress for family systems. Individuals and families coping with serious illness, death, and grief need to know that the palliative care team is tuned into their needs and honors and respects their strengths and their right to make choices that are right for them.

8. Why do social workers ask people so many questions?

Social workers commonly hear this question, and often it is not worded quite this delicately. Social workers on a palliative care team are responsible for an initial psychosocial history and assessment. This crucial clinical assessment tool is the basis for planning social work interventions. The psychosocial assessment addresses the individual and his or her family systems' emotional and social needs. To obtain a clear picture of the people served, social workers ask questions regarding family history, social history, physical history, support systems, current needs (including financial and legal), strengths, and beliefs. Generally, when people suggest that social workers are asking too many questions of the patient or family on the first or second visit, it is because the purpose of a psychosocial assessment has not been clearly explained. This is a tool that provides social workers with the information necessary to help address the family systems' needs and to identify potential problematic arenas. It also provides other team members with crucial knowledge that will help them understand certain coping mechanisms or reactions, thereby helping empower them to help the family more effectively. Strengths of the individual and family are also identified and subsequently built on to help them cope and find meaning in their current situation.

9. Is grief counseling a part of the social workers' role in palliative care?

Grief counseling is a large part of the social workers' role with individuals and families. The individuals and families served in palliative care are coping with numerous difficult and painful losses. Social workers provide information about the kinds of feelings that are normal, and provide support, active listening, and problem-solving to help people take care of unfinished business, express their feelings, and often, to search for their own personal meanings. Complicated grief as a result of alcoholism or unresolved previous losses requires more intensive therapeutic approaches. In these cases, social workers would employ psychotherapeutic techniques to help alleviate the distress.

10. Do social workers make home visits? What is their interaction with caregivers of palliative care patients at home?

Depending on the program, most social workers make home visits. Social work services are covered under skilled home care and hospice benefits. To assess someone in his or her own environment is the ideal for a social worker. Generally, social workers can pick up an even stronger sense of the person and family there than in an in-patient setting. The home setting is where many people are most comfortable because they feel more in control. The social worker tunes into the family dynamics and the caregivers' stress levels as well those of the patient. Examples of interventions with caregivers may include facilitation of anticipatory grief, short-term therapeutic counseling to alleviate depression, stress management techniques, facilitation of resource referrals and respite care, education about a variety of psychosocial issues, and provision of emotional support. Common subjects addressed to social workers include what feelings are "normal," how to bring up certain topics, how to handle conflict, what to do about substance abuse issues, and how to help children.

11. What are the psychosocial emergencies encountered by social workers when on call after working hours?

There are numerous issues that social workers are called in for after hours. Some common reasons include an agitated patient or caregiver, family disputes, concerns about suicide potential, or impending death. The social workers' role is to assess the situation, provide crisis counseling and problem solving to resolve the situation, and to alert appropriate team members. In the event of an impending death, social workers will assist the family in whatever way the family requires. Because every family is different, intervention may vary from helping with final arrangements to facilitating memory sharing to quietly being with the family and supporting their ability to be with the person who is dying.

12. In these times of shrinking health care dollars, how can a social worker help family members facing financial difficulties?

Resource management is another key role of social work. Social workers are knowledgeable about community services and programs that can ease financial strain for families in need. Palliative care patients frequently express a great deal of anxiety and guilt about their fear of using up family resources. Addressing these concerns makes a significant contribution to comfort levels. Social workers will assess the financial concerns and needs, develop a plan in concert with the family, and continue to monitor the process of resolution. Locating resources, filling out paperwork, and educating families regarding their options are all helpful interventions that social work may provide.

13. What is the interaction of the social worker with clergy?

Social workers are trained to view a person in that person's environment. That environment usually includes spiritual and religious needs. Palliative care patients are frequently searching for ultimate meaning in their lives; thus, addressing spiritual questions and needs is a crucial component of effective pain control. If the person does not already have his or her own resource, social workers may link them up with the appropriate spiritual caregiver at the patient's request. Spiritual interventions, whether traditionally religious or otherwise, must be consistent with the beliefs, values, and desires of the patient. Because spiritual care and religious care are not necessarily synonymous, social workers generally explore the spiritual/religious arena by addressing the patient's spiritual concerns, beliefs, and existing support and identifying any additional support desired. Palliative care teams cannot assume that, just because a patient turns down clergy or states that he does not have a clergy or faith, there are not serious spiritual concerns. Common issues are feelings of abandonment by God, guilt, and punishment issues, fear of "ceasing to be," and feelings of alienation. All of these concerns may and do exacerbate pain, agitation, and depression.

14. What are the situations for which a nurse or a physician calls a social worker when the patient dies in the hospital?

Social workers may assist by helping the family with final arrangements and other final details. They also provide emotional support for the family and staff and crisis intervention for more difficult family situations such as a family member who states suicidal intention. Along with other team members, they encourage families to take their time with their loved one's body and validate family needs and rights to say good-bye in the manner they choose.

15. How can a social worker help resolve day-to-day ethical issues?

An individual's right to self-determination is a primary value of the profession of social work; therefore, it is a common role of social work to discuss the patient's wishes regarding choices at the end of life. It is also the social worker's role to advocate for and educate appropriate family (or even team) members regarding these wishes if there are any conflicts, questions, or disputes. Taking care of these issues is both a difficult and empowering process. In many instances, patients feel a sense of taking charge, which helps them cope with their feelings of loss of control. Discussing these issues also facilitates the anticipatory grief process. Like many issues in social work, taking care of more concrete issues opens the door to help people cope with the more abstract emotional processes. Social workers may discuss and facilitate advance directives including clarification of code issues where appropriate, durable power of attorney, and every day ethical dilemmas. For example, if a palliative care patient stops eating, family members may have difficulty accepting that not eating may actually make their loved one more comfortable due to fatigue levels and other factors. Social workers may facilitate a family conference to explain or clarify this process and to help them sort out feelings and get answers the family needs from the appropriate member of the palliative care team.

16. Are there organizations available to provide more information to or about social workers in palliative care?

The National Hospice Organization in Arlington, VA, has a section devoted to hospice social work and provides information, support, and education for social workers providing palliative care. Other groups that would be helpful include the National Association of Social Workers in Washington, DC, and the association of Oncology Social Work in Baltimore, MD.

BIBLIOGRAPHY

1. Barker RL: Social Work Dictionary, 3rd ed. Washington, DC, NASW Press, 1995.
2. Compton B, Compton G: Social Work Processes. Pacific Grove, CA, Brooks Cole Publishing Co., 1989.
3. Fish NM: Hospice: Terminal Illness, Teamwork, and the Quality of Life. In Kerson TS (ed): Social Work in Health Settings: Practice in Context. New York, Haworth Press, 1989.
4. Garfield C: Psychosocial Care of the Dying Patient. New York, McGraw-Hill, 1978.
5. Hepworth D, Larsen J: Direct Social Work Practice: Theories & Skills. Pacific Grove, CA, Brooks Cole Publishing Co., 1993.
6. Proffitt LJ: Hospice. In Minahan A (ed): Encyclopedia of Social Work, 18th ed. Silver Spring, MD, National Association of Social Workers, 1987.
7. Richman JM: Hospice. In Edwards RL (ed): Encyclopedia of Social Work, 19th ed. Washington, DC, NASW Press, 1995.

6. SPIRITUAL CARE: CONSOLING, COMFORTING, AND COUNSELING

Rev. Stephen Rosendahl

1. What is the role of the chaplain, clergy, or religious representative in palliative care?

The chaplain's primary role is to provide emotional and spiritual support to the patient and family. The chaplain can provide reassurance that, whatever may happen, the patient and family will not be left alone. The chaplain can help the palliative care team sort out spiritual and religious issues and relationships that may have an impact on other interventions of the palliative care team. The chaplain can serve as a liaison with a patient's clergy and describe to him and the family the goals of palliative care. The chaplain also can be the liaison with the palliative care team so that the patient and family are aware of everyone's role on the team.

2. What is the difference between a chaplain and parish clergy?

The College of Chaplains is the main certifying group for health care chaplains in the United States. Chaplains certified by the college have gone through an extensive education, training, and certifying process. Parish clergy have varied educational and experiential backgrounds. The parish clergy can bring to the team a wealth of information concerning the patient. The chaplain and parish clergy can tap into the various support networks provided by churches and the local religious community. More information about chaplains can be obtained by writing to the following address:

Association of Professional Chaplains
1701 E. Woodfield Rd. Suite 311
Schaumburg, IL 60173
847-240-1014; fax 847-240-1015

3. What basic information is needed for an initial spiritual assessment?

A number of initial assessment forms are available. Ask your local hospice group what it uses. The following information is also valuable:

1. Is the person involved with a religious group, and if so, which group?
2. How involved is the patient in the group?
3. How does the patient describe his or her own spirituality?
4. How does the patient feel about spirituality at this time? Is it helping, or is it getting in the way?
5. Are there any particular spiritual needs, resources, or rituals that would help the patient at this time?
6. Is there a particular person from the patient's religious tradition who would be welcome on a regular basis or only for crisis events?
7. What are the patient's beliefs about life, death, and pain?

4. When should I call the chaplain or clergy?

Most chaplains and clergy are available any time of the day or night, especially at crisis times. Depending on the kinds of issues with which one is dealing, the chaplain may be called early for consultation or to draw attention to specific palliative care issues. The chaplain can be consulted when support is needed by the palliative care team, patient, or family.

5. What is spirituality?

One of many definitions for spirituality describes it as that which gives meaning to your own life. It is a sense of transcendence and how you relate it to yourself. It is the way you process information about yourself and the world around you and then organize it and use it as the foundation for how you will be and how you will live. It may have a sense of a higher being, separate and different, or it may not. Spirituality differs from religion in that religion describes an organized and institutionalized pattern of doctrines and rituals in which you participate by yourself or with others.

6. What is suffering?

Suffering means different things to different people. It can apply to living with unrelieved physical, social, emotional, or spiritual pain. Some people attach spiritual meaning to unrelieved pain. It can be seen as something the person must or deserves to experience because the person has done something bad, or it can be seen as a path to healing. Sharing the ideas of forgiveness and being human can help people work through these issues and thus be more open to measures that will relieve pain and discomfort.

7. What sort of spiritually related concerns do people with terminal diagnoses talk about?

The answer to this is as varied as the cultures and the patients themselves. For many their first concern is their family's welfare. Others think about their beliefs about life and death and suffering. No one wants to deal with unrelieved pain, be it physical or emotional. Many find it easier to come to grips with physical pain than emotional and spiritual pain. Some make funeral plans so that their family will not have to deal with these issues at the time of death.

8. What spiritual concerns are most common?

A wide range of issues can have spiritual overtones. Many suggest that every aspect of life has spiritual threads. Questions such as the following are routinely voiced:
- How could God let this happen to me?
- Why is God doing this to me? I must have done something really terrible for this to happen.
- Why is God punishing me?
- I can't believe there is a God if this could happen.
- I used to feel so close to God, but now I just don't know anymore.

It is a mistake to assume that everybody will ask these questions. Some people do not—either because of denial or because they have already worked through these questions. Some people seem as if they can never find a way to make peace with these issues.

9. What kind of psychosocial-spiritual issues do persons in need of palliative care have?

For many patients, the need for palliative care triggers a time when life's meaning, purpose, and values are challenged. People begin to look at what has shaped their living and formulate those events, feelings, and thoughts that will help give meaning to their end. Many persons review their lives. They often retell the same story as a way of coming to terms with what the event meant to them then and what it means now. They may still need to make peace with it emotionally, psychologically, and spiritually. The story may be told as a way of sharing who they were in their lives. It may be told as a way of ensuring that the legacy they wish to leave is heard and remembered.

Dying persons may have unfinished business. They may want to mend an estranged relationship. They may have losses that were never fully grieved. They may need to process these memories and come to terms with what they mean. They may still be evaluating and critiquing the paths they have chosen and the ones they did not travel.

10. What do people need to do spiritually as they anticipate death?

People need to come to terms with their belief system. Although people may be part of a tradition that has a well-formulated doctrine, the ways that they have appropriated it into their lives will be as unique as their fingerprints. Many people will be processing the way that they saw themselves in relationship to the world, the universe, to other people, and to God. Others may spend little, if any, time on these considerations.

For some people their spirituality and their beliefs have been a constant companion that has grown and changed with them throughout life. Then, when confronted with the potential for life's end, their spirituality is like an old friend with whom they merely spend more time. Their spirituality is up-to-date. It knows what to say. It is comfortable with any question, even the ones for which there are no ready answers.

11. With whom do patients talk about spiritual issues?

Many people will talk to whomever is with them when they learn their life is ending. They may feel a particularly strong bond with their health care professionals and therefore will turn to them. All issues, medical and spiritual, are rolled into one issue with which they must now deal. There is no separation of one issue from the other.

12. Is there a simple answer or procedure the health care provider can offer?

Health care professionals often are uncomfortable with spiritual issues because they don't have simple answers. Medically, we can offer a change of medicine or another test, but questions about God and life and death are not so easily addressed. Health care workers who are not at ease with their own sense of spirituality and life's boundaries will have trouble supporting those in palliative care as fully as possible.

13. I'm uncomfortable talking about spiritual matters. What do I do?

Refer the patient to the chaplain, minister, priest, rabbi, or spiritual leader of the patient's tradition. It is also helpful to attempt to recognize what is making you uncomfortable—the patient's distress facing death or your lack of background to talk about spiritual concerns. These are different concerns that need to be dealt with differently.

14. How do I work with persons whose beliefs are different than mine?

We first need to be secure in our own beliefs. We need to know how our beliefs shape us, to serve as a foundation for working with others who see things differently. Secondly, we need to be open to what our patients believe, because their beliefs are important to them, have shaped them, and will be among the resource they will use to deal with their present situation. Thirdly, we need to listen to how these beliefs are helping or hindering them. When we listen carefully, we can help them look at their beliefs for further support. We also can help them to reevaluate their beliefs and relate them to their present needs.

15. How can I help someone who is dealing with spiritual questions?

Remember that there are no right or wrong, good or bad, emotions. Also remember that this is a time of many emotions, which will affect the patient psychologically, socially, and spiritually. The process of spirituality is often as important as any answer patients may find within a book or themselves, i.e., the process of asking and exploring what one feels, thinks, and believes is the critical need. Patients need affirmation that asking and exploring hard questions is OK. What we may think or believe may be important for them, but one ought to be careful about offering answers too quickly. When requested of us, our thoughts and ideas can be helpful if offered as pieces of a puzzle that is unique to the patient.

16. What should I remember that will help me deal with the complexity of end-of-life issues?

Remember that emotional and spiritual issues are very individualized and extremely fluid. What can seem to be solved one day may seem as if it never had been discussed the following day. Everyone will interact with these issues differently. Some will talk, and some will retreat into silent introspection. It is important to have a working knowledge of loss and grief, which Elizabeth Kubler-Ross described as including denial, anger, bargaining, depression, and acceptance. A common mistake is to see these as linear steps. They are not.

17. What do I say to someone who says, "Why me?"

We need to assess at what level these words are voiced. They have a number of components. They can be an expression of the emotions the person is feeling, from anger to frustration.They also can be an expression of the patient's spirituality and understanding of God. The expressed question may seem to conflict with how the person states his or her belief system. For many the question is a step toward accommodating themselves to their new situation.

The first strategy is to listen and to help patients reflect upon their feelings and conflict. Once they have achieved some emotional relief, they may be willing to discuss what they believe and how it is helping or not helping them. Depending on your relationship with a patient, you may be able to help point out conflicts they had not recognized and help them find providers of internal support and comfort. Perhaps the most comforting thing we can offer is the affirmation that questions at all levels are acceptable and that we do not have an immediate answer.

18. How can I help someone who seems stuck in denial? Is there a risk that I can make them more depressed by bringing up end-of-life issues?

Someone stuck in denial cannot be forced to deal with anything other than that which they choose. The word *denial* is often misleading. A person who is not seeming to deal with the issues may not have the energy to do so. Denial merely may be the way the person gains the time he needs to regain internal strength to confront his new reality. Perhaps another word to use is *postponement*. Once we've heard bad news, we can't, at least at some level, deny it. We can, however, postpone dealing with it and the changes it will bring. The only person we can change is ourselves. However, patients sometimes invite us into their journey of change when they are ready. Most people will eventually deal with what they need to when they need to. Quite a few will speak hopefully of healing even as they are making funeral plans.

19. Are spiritual needs and acceptance issues affected by sex, age, and educational or socioeconomic levels?

Although spiritual concerns generally remain individual, there are differences according to the above factors. We are just beginning to understand the differences between how men and women deal with life issues and crises. Men often will deal with these issues silently and by keeping busy. Women will more often want to talk about it. Certainly age plays a role in the impact of the illness on life, but as important is how the person viewed life and his or her own spirituality. It is important to have a working knowledge of the developmental stages of life and a realization that we continue to grow and change even in our adult years. Some people work at their spirituality throughout their lives. Although educational level can bring changes in spirituality, educational level does not of necessity indicate a person's spirituality. Different cultures and religions may have their own ways of dealing with end-of-life journeys and expectations.

20. At what point is spiritual counseling important? Are there any barriers to spiritual counseling?

Spiritual counseling works best when initiated by the person in need of such support and guidance. We can be most helpful when the patients are ready to ask questions and voice concerns about their beliefs. The spiritual counselor should approach the issues gently, with patience, and with an understanding that the process is a journey of discovery. Often the biggest barriers for the patient are past experiences that were not conducive to a spiritual journey. For example, the patient may have attempted to raise these issues with individuals holding strong negative beliefs about spirituality, and the response was resistance, even hostility. Additionally, some patients may believe certain stereotypes about roles various people play in health care. One is that chaplains and clergy are the bearers of bad news. Even on general rounds, I occasionally see fear and apprehension on the faces of patients as I introduce myself as the chaplain. Until I can reassure them that their physician has not sent me to deliver a bad diagnosis and that I merely stopped to introduce myself and see how they were doing, their fears will influence our interaction and relationship, and whatever needs they may have had before meeting me will remain unvoiced and unmet.

BIBLIOGRAPHY

1. Carlton R: Breath of life. Caregiver Journal 8:37–42, 1991.
2. Harvey T: Who is the chaplain anyway? Philosophy and integration of hospice chaplaincy. Am J Hospice Palliative Care 13:41–43, 1996.
3. Highfield MF: Spiritual health of oncology patients. Nurse and patient perspectives. Cancer Nurs 15:1–8, 1992.
4. Kubler-Ross E: On Death and Dying. New York, NY, MacMillan Publishing, 1969.
5. Mossi JP: The request of the dying for pastoral care. Journal of Pastoral Care 50:107–110, 1996.
6. O'Conner T, McCarroll-Butler P, Gadowsky S, O'Neill K, et al: Making the most and making sense: Ethnographic research on spirituality in palliative care. Journal of Pastoral Care 51:13–24, 1997.
7. Peay P: A good death. Common Boundary 5:32–41, 1997.
8. Purdy W: Theological reflection on the ethics of pain control among the terminally ill. Journal of Pastoral Care 46:13–18, 1992.
9. Reisz FH Jr: A dying person is a living person: A pastoral theology for ministry to the dying. Journal of Pastoral Care 46:184–192, 1992.
10. Simmonds AL: Pastoral perspectives in intensive care: Experiences of doctors and nurses with dying patients. Journal of Pastoral Care 3:271–282, 1997.
11. Slater GR: When God hides: Therapy for life's impasses. Journal of Pastoral Care 51:79–90, 1997.
12. Wangerin W Jr: Mourning into Dancing. Grand Rapids, MI, Zondervan, 1992.

7. HOSPICE

Christine Duelge, C.R.N.H.

1. What is hospice?

In medieval times, a hospice was a resting place for travelers on a long journey. Over the past 20 years, Americans have embraced the hospice concept as a compassionate way of caring for terminally ill patients. Hospice is a philosophy and concept of care that celebrates life and neither hastens nor prolongs death. To the patients and families coping with life-limiting illnesses, hospice offers an effective alternative to there being "nothing else to do" and an opportunity to live fully in the time that remains. Hospice works with respect and reverence for individual values and offers compassion and support. When patients, their families, and physicians agree that death is inevitable, comfort is the goal. Hospice allows death with dignity.

Hospice allows patients and families to make choices about how they want to live the last days of their life. Hospice provides this care with a unique interdisciplinary team (IDT) approach that coordinates a program of palliative and supportive services in both the home and inpatient settings. The patient and family are seen as part of this IDT and the focus of care. The team addresses all aspects of care, with the goal being to meet the physical, psychological, social, and spiritual needs of the patient and family.

Hospice care is provided to terminally ill patients at any age with any diagnosis.

2. When was modern day hospice established?

The Irish Sisters of Charity established St. Joseph's Hospice at London in 1905. However, the best known contemporary hospice is St. Christopher's in London, which was started by Dame Cicely Saunders, M.D., in 1967. This hospice focuses on aggressive symptom management rather than aggressive curative care of patients with life-limiting illnesses.

In the United States the beginning of hospice care is identified with the opening of Hospice of Connecticut at New Haven in 1974. Hospices at this time were usually staffed by volunteers and were driven by nurses and social workers.

In 1983 the Medicare Hospice Benefit was created by the Tax Equity Fiscal Responsibility Act. This opened the door for physician involvement, development of standards of care, stringent admission rules, and development of a wide variety of hospice programs. Pain control standards and pain initiatives were just being developed.

Starting about 1995, protocols for admission and pain and symptom management began to be developed. The scope of care widened to include noncancer patients, and the guidelines were less stringent. Programs for palliative care and inpatient units were established, and the business end of hospice care started to unfold.

The future of hospice is uncertain in light of Medicare/Medicaid reform and corporate business involvement in the reimbursement of the services provided by hospices. Palliative care medicine has become a specialty in the United States, and there are now specific requirements for board certification.

Although the face of hospices may change, the heart of hospice and the care it provides for terminally ill patients and their families are not likely to. Hospice care has not changed since medieval times.

3. What types of diagnoses make patients suitable for hospice care?

Patients admitted to hospice care have only weeks or months to live. The Medicare guidelines state that life expectancy is 6 months or less. Patients and families have chosen to stop aggressive curative treatment or there is no curative treatment left to try. Diagnoses mostly have been cancer, but the need for hospice care for noncancer diagnoses has become apparent. The

National Hospice Organization (NHO) and Medicare have developed guidelines to assist in determining prognosis in noncancer diagnoses. These guidelines are helpful because it is difficult to determine a prognosis in noncancer patients.

4. What are the eligibility criteria for admission to hospice?

The guidelines mention several different markers for hospice care. They talk about weeks or months of survival. The usual determination, 6 months or less, is then qualified by saying that predicted survival is to the best of the physician's knowledge if the disease progresses as expected. Rather than timeframes, which are at best a guess, demonstrating disease progression, including comorbid factors, is the best way to determine why and when a patient is appropriate for hospice care.

Several questions need to be addressed. It is important first to determine whether the terminal diagnosis is cancer. The NHO guidelines and the Medicare guidelines have several markers for each disease process. The guidelines are very specific and will assist with the final determination of a patient's appropriateness for hospice care. However, a few simple questions can help in the beginning stages of a hospice referral.

5. What are the questions that need to be addressed during the assessment of a patient's eligibility for hospice?

1. Has aggressive curative treatment been tried and failed?
2. Are any further treatment options left for aggressive curative treatment?
3. Does the patient or family want to stop aggressive curative treatment?
4. Is the patient or family expressing concerns that further treatment is decreasing the quality of life that is left?
5. What are the comorbid factors affecting the primary diagnosis?
6. Is the patient or family asking about hospice care?
7. What are the wishes of the patient or family for end-of-life care: do not resuscitate, living will, medical power of attorney?

6. What is an IDT?

In hospice care, an IDT is an interdisciplinary team of professionals and nonprofessionals who determine the plan that best meets the needs and desires of the patient and family. Team members can be paid staff or volunteers in any mix as long as the core services required by Medicare are provided. Team members include a coordinator or director, medical director, nurses, physicians, clergy, social workers, dietitians, pharmacists, other therapists, home health aides, and volunteers. The patient, family, and friends are also an important part of the team and may participate in IDT meetings.

7. How is the initial assessment of the patient and family carried out by the IDT?

Which discipline makes each of the assessments may differ from hospice to hospice, but the disciplines that are represented are usually the same.

The admissions assessment starts with the referral or admissions department. Clinical medical information, labs, radiographs, scans, and hospital or office records are shared by the referring physician. This information is reviewed according to the guidelines with the admissions team. The referring physician must sign an initial plan of care and certification of terminal illness. The medical director must agree with the terminal diagnosis and sign the certification of terminal illness. At the time of admission the medical authorization for treatment will be signed. These orders will describe medications, treatments, frequency of visits by the team, and durable medical equipment. A physical assessment by the medical director may be needed if he or she is to assume the patient's care in the hospice program.

At this time the patient is determined to be appropriate for hospice care. The patient and family are then approached about their choice to have hospice care. Services are explained and paperwork is signed to start care. Paperwork includes consent of care, rights and responsibilities, and a determination of goals for care. The paperwork can be done by any member of the team.

A nursing assessment will be provided within 24 hours of admission to determine the patient's physical status. The assessment will cover medication use and equipment needs. The hospice nurse will explore psychosocial needs that may be affecting physical problems, such as financial or caregiver issues. Like all nurses, hospice nurses work under the direction of physicians, but their level of expertise in symptom management allows them to diagnose and treat a variety of anticipated problems with greater independence. With standing orders and protocols to assist them, hospice nurses can prevent crises in many situations related to the patient and family care. They are the managers of the team and, with the team to assist, provide quality end-of-life care in an holistic manner that considers physical, psychosocial, and spiritual needs. They will determine when referrals to other disciplines within the team are necessary. The initial assessment may be done by an admissions nurse, and the patient's care is transferred to a primary nurse for the duration of hospice care.

A social worker will assess the family dynamics, coping skills, financial status, and identify high-risk families who will need referral to other team members. Resolution of the concerns identified by the social worker allows the family and patient to focus on quality-of-life issues. The hospice social worker helps the patient and family to access community resources related to but not limited to the patient's illness. The social workers will assist with the development of advance directives, legal problems, management of bills and insurance, and emotional and spiritual support. It has been found that unresolved psychosocial problems are an important factor in unrelieved physical symptoms, which is another reason that the hospice IDT approach works so well.

The spiritual needs of patients and families are assessed on admission. Spiritual or religious beliefs affect what types of treatment a patient or family will allow and how well it will work. As with the psychosocial assessment, cultural and other belief systems have an impact on the physical care.

Volunteers are at the heart of hospice care. They make an important difference so many times in the delivery of the hospice plan of care. They are unique due to the amount of training and continuing education required of them to become part of the IDT. An assessment is done on admission to determine what needs the volunteer can meet for the patient or family. Hospice volunteers can participate in all aspects of patient and family care, from hands-on physical care to spiritual and emotional support.

Bereavement care is an important part of hospice care that is not only unique to hospice but is required by Medicare as part of the IDT plan of care. The assessment of bereavement needs starts on admission and includes a determination of which caregivers will be followed after the patient's death.

8. When can hospice referrals be made?

Any time during the course of a disease that has led to a limited life expectancy. A referral does not mean that the patient is automatically admitted. At the time of the referral, the guidelines will assist in determining if the patient is appropriate for hospice care. The patient and family may decide they do not want hospice care.

Referrals are made as early as the time of diagnosis as a treatment option or as late as hours before a death to assist the family with bereavement. However, patients and families benefit most when referrals are made early. Early referrals allow the hospice team to assist with better physical symptom management and preparation for death.

9. Who can initiate a referral to hospice?

Anyone. However, a physician is needed to certify that the illness has a terminal prognosis of weeks or months. Referrals by patients, families, or other professionals are usually for information about hospice services or assistance in evaluating the patient's appropriateness for care. The hospice staff will assist in obtaining a formal referral if it is determined to be appropriate and wanted. The staff also can direct care to the appropriate agency if hospice care cannot be provided.

10. What is the role of the referring physician in implementing hospice care?

To certify that the patient has a terminal diagnosis. The same or another physician manages patient care with the hospice team. The referring physician may be a specialist, and the patient may have a primary physician who will manage hospice care. If the referring physician does not want to manage care and there is no primary physician, the hospice medical director can be requested to manage the patient's care. This usually requires the referring physician to discuss the patient directly with the medical director. The medical director may want to see the patient before assuming care.

11. Who develops the plan of care?

The plan of care is determined during the IDT meeting. The plan is then presented to the patient and family, who are part of the team and not controlled by it. The physician is kept informed formally; written reports are sent by the IDT if the physician is unable to attend meetings.

12. What patient-related factors are barriers to hospice care?

Hospice care is a choice; it can be refused. Patients may meet the criteria for hospice care but not want if for a variety of reasons:

1. Patients and families may be unaware of what services hospice can provide. This information can be provided by local hospices, state hospice organizations, or the National Hospice Helpline at (800) 658-8898. In addition, many hospices have a staff member dedicated to the education of health care consumers related to hospice services.

2. They may want to pursue aggressive treatment for cure even if the chance of cure is small.

3. The patient or family may be in denial that the illness is terminal. Even if they acknowledge that the disease is terminal, they may believe that being under hospice care will take all hope from the patient and thereby cause the patient to die sooner.

4. Patients and families may believe that hospice care is only for the very end of life and therefore do not need it yet.

5. Patients and families with home health care may choose to remain with those services because they feel a change is not beneficial or may be too disruptive to them.

6. There can be misinformation about the cost of care. Families and patients are often concerned that their money will be used quickly and are fearful of programs with which they are not familiar.

13. How can patients' and families' misconceptions about hospice care be alleviated?

Patients or families often have wrong information about what hospice care is, but if they get the accurate information they may change their minds and even wonder why they waited so long to get quality end-of-life care. They are relieved to find out that with hospice care many of their financial problems are resolved because a number of services are paid for by the hospice program. The quality of symptom management, support, and education about the disease and dying process are always a plus for care with dignity. Patients are often relieved to find that the care continues for their family long after their death.

14. What physician-related factors are barriers to hospice referral?

1. Lack of knowledge regarding hospice services.

2. Many physicians seem reluctant to refer patients to hospice, perhaps because they perceive referral as an admission of failure. Because physicians are trained to be curative in their thinking, they often will offer more treatment instead of confronting the patient and family with the news of a life-limiting prognosis. Physicians need to recognize that death is not failure, to fight disease rather than death, and to recognize when quality of life rather than longevity should be addressed.

3. Perceived loss of control. There may be misinformation about who will care for patients receiving hospice care. If desired, primary physicians can play a vital role in the care of patients referred to hospice. The physician becomes part of the IDT and remains actively involved in the patient's care.

4. Potential fear of death. Physicians may have unresolved personal or professional feelings related to past experiences with death. This could delay or hinder a hospice referral.

5. In light of the guidelines established by Medicare, physicians may believe a referral is too early or not appropriate.

15. What happens if the physician does not want to make a hospice referral?

The hospice team will help the patient and family explore the reasons a referral has been requested but not made. If the patient is appropriate according to hospice guidelines and the physician does not want to make the referral, the hospice team will help the patient and family explore other options. The medical director can talk to the physician to clarify any questions the physician may have.

16. How can you make a hospice referral go smoothly?

Plan ahead!

Referrals made when the patient and family are in crisis should be the exception rather than the rule. If a patient and family have time to adjust to the idea of hospice care and have time to start a plan of hospice care, they are more likely to have a better end-of-life experience. They will have time to learn to trust the different way of addressing their problems and will be more willing to call the hospice team for help instead of the physician or ambulance. Emergency room visits and hospitalizations can be decreased. When needs such as additional equipment and medications can be arranged calmly, the quality of end-of-life care improves.

Whether the patient is at home or in the hospital at the time of the referral, keeping all interested caregivers involved and well informed makes the referral and admission process progress more smoothly. All persons involved in care are then able to ask questions and understand the goals of the plan of care. Open and honest communication about the disease, its progression, and outcome are key factors in an easy transition into hospice care.

The presence of the physician assures the patient and family that they are not being abandoned and left to die alone.

More time in hospice before death allows for the hospice team to anticipate caregiver and patient needs to make the death as peaceful for everyone as possible.

As soon as the patient and caregivers decide they want hospice care, arrangements can be made for medications, equipment, team member visits, home health aides, and volunteers. Allowing time for a smooth transition from hospital, home health, or having no services helps to make the plan of care work and allows for trust and security to develop into the belief that care needs will be met.

17. How is the plan of care for the patient and family determined by the IDT?

An initial plan of care (POC) must be established before services can be started. The member of the team who makes the initial assessment consults with at least one other member of the team to start the POC.

Members of the IDT perform a complete assessment of the patient and caregivers after admission. With the patient and caregivers, the goals for care are determined and implemented. The POC is signed by all members of the IDT. The POC will cover the scope and frequency of services that best meet patient and caregiver needs.

The POC will cover related and nonrelated services as well as palliative and curative services. The POC will be reviewed as the patient's and family's needs change or with each review prior to rectification periods.

18. Define "caregiver" in hospice care.

The caregiver can be a family member, significant other, friend, or paid caregiver. The primary caregiver may provide but is not required to provide the care or even live with the patient. However, the caregiver must be willing to work with the IDT to determine what care is needed and how it will be provided.

19. Can patients who live alone and have no primary caregiver receive hospice care?

Yes. Patients may stay in their own home until they can no longer care for themselves or do not wish to be alone. Then the prearranged plan to provide their care will be implemented. Patients may have chosen to hire sitters, seek nursing home placement, or, if available, enter the inpatient hospice unit.

20. What are the key elements of the NHO guidelines?

The NHO guidelines were established as parameters to help hospices assess noncancer diagnosis prognosis. They outline specific requirements for each diagnosis that assist in determining the end stage or terminal phase of the disease. Guidelines have been established for:

1. Heart disease
2. Pulmonary disease
3. Dementia
4. HIV disease
5. Liver disease
6. Renal disease
7. Stroke and coma
8. Amyotrophic lateral sclerosis

There is a category classified as *General Guidelines for Determining Prognosis* that can assist with other diseases that are not classified specifically.

The guidelines evaluate type, strength and consistency of evidence, performance status scales, functional assessment classifications, and typical course of disease. The guidelines contain worksheets for each disease and detailed descriptions of indicators for prognosis.

21. What are the key elements of the Medicare guidelines?

Medicare took the NHO guidelines and revised them. Some of the indicators in each of the disease categories should be present along with comorbid factors to verify the terminal illness. Documentation of the reasons for admission and continued care is important for reimbursement.

There are benefit periods for recertification under the Hospice Medicare Benefit. These have changed since the Balanced Budget Act in 1997. Under the benefit, patients must be recertified with documentation of the terminal illness. This occurs after the initial certification, first at 90 days, then at the second 90 days, followed by an unlimited number of 60-day periods. Physician certification/recertification must be made at the beginning of each period. The initial certification should be completed by the medical director of the hospice and the patient's attending/referring physician. The purpose of the certification and recertification is to document the patient has a medical prognosis with a life expectancy of 6 months or less if the illness runs its normal course.

Patients must sign an election statement for hospice care for the hospice to be reimbursed by Medicare. This statement informs the patient and family of services covered and not covered by the hospice. It explains patients' responsibility for seeking approval from the hospice for all treatments not covered in the plan of care. Patients are responsible for bills incurred in treatments and services not included in the plan of care and those provided by physicians or facilities not contracted by the hospice.

22. What are the levels of care and sites in which hospice care is provided?

There are four levels of hospice care:

1. Routine homecare (RHC) is provided in the patient's place of residence, which most often is the patient's or caregiver's home. Hospices may have contracts to provide care in nursing homes and personal care homes. Here the IDT works with the staff to provide quality end-of-life care.

Hospices give care in freestanding inpatient facilities or hospitals with units designated for terminal care. These inpatient units or hospice houses are for short stays at the end of life.

2. Continuous homecare (CHC) is for crisis management of medical symptoms, which predominantly need nursing management, in the patient's place of residence.

3. Respite care (RC) for caregiver relief is provided in a skilled nursing facility or a nursing facility.

4. General inpatient care (GIC) is for acute symptom management that cannot be controlled in the patient's residence. This care is provided in hospitals or inpatient hospice facilities.

Patients can move from one level of care to another at any time depending on their needs. Regardless of where care is provided, the care and services are the same and are managed by the IDT.

23. How is hospice paid for?

Medicare Part A and Medicaid have a hospice benefit that reimburses the hospice for care. This benefit is paid at a per diem rate, which allows the hospice to manage patient and caregiver needs at the end of life more effectively. Per-per diem means the hospice gets a daily rate for care. The rate depends on the level of service provided. Routine homecare is reimbursed at a different rate than inpatient respite or acute care. There is also a separate rate for continuous care provided in the home. Most private insurance companies, health maintenance organizations, and managed care organizations have hospice benefits that reimburse for hospice care, which may be at a per diem rate or fee for service.

Medicare/Medicaid benefits pay for medication, durable medical equipment, treatments related to the terminal diagnosis, nursing visits, home health aide visits, social worker visits, and bereavement care. Private insurance companies may negotiate with the hospice for services provided, but the hospice's IDT plan of care should provide the same level, quality, and scope of care to all patients and families regardless of ability to pay.

If there is no outside payment source, hospices may provide free care or bill for services depending on their status as for-profit or not-for-profit. Hospices that provide free or reduced payment care are often able to do this because they have received donations from the community, grants, private donors, or fundraisers.

24. When is continuous care provided?

According to the Medicare guidelines, continuous care is provided when the care needed by the patient is given by the IDT at least 8 out of every 24 hours. The care can be given at any time during which a patient is with the hospice program. The patient may be nearing the end of life or simply have a caregiver who is unable to provide the needed nursing care. The care is usually short-term and more than half of the time must be provided by a registered nurse or licensed practical nurse. During the remaining time, care can be provided by a certified nursing assistant.

25. What is respite care?

Respite is defined as a rest or relief. Respite care is provided to give the caregiver a break from the care of the patient. Primary caregivers are often elderly and have their own health problems, or they may be adults who juggling their own families and careers. Respite care can be provided at any time throughout hospice care, and it usually lasts no more than 5 days. The care can be provided in a skilled nursing facility, hospital, inpatient hospice, or a nursing home. The plan of care will be continued by the IDT.

26. How are tests or treatments ordered by the physician paid for?

The physician is responsible for coordinating care with the hospice team. This ensures that the POC is understood and followed by all of the team members.

If the treatment is part of the POC, it will be approved by the hospice team and paid for by the hospice program. If the patient has private insurance, payment may need to be negotiated. The hospice team will help the patient determine what is part of the POC. If the treatment is not part of the POC determined by the hospice team, the patient will have several options:

1. If the treatment is not related to the life-limiting illness, payment would be coded as not related and the patient's prior payment source would pay for treatment separate from hospice care.

2. If the treatment/services are outside the hospice team POC but related to the terminal illness, patients can terminate or revoke their hospice care or pay for treatment/services themselves. At that time, the prior payment source would begin payment as before hospice care.

27. Is a hospice patient required to see a physician on a regular basis?

Physician visits continue as necessary to maintain continuity and ensure optimal end-of-life care. The only time a visit may be required is when certification/recertification that the illness is terminal is needed. These visits allow the hospice interdisciplinary team to assess the patient's disease progression and determine if the patient continues to meet the guidelines for hospice care.

28. Can a hospice patient go to the physician's office or outpatient clinic?

Yes. If there are problems with transportation or scheduling, the hospice team will assist. Continued contact with the primary physician is encouraged to provide security and continuity of care for the patient and family.

29. Under what circumstances can the hospice patient be admitted and treated in the hospital for acute emergencies?

Admissions may be for:

1. Pain control
2. Medication adjustment
3. Observation
4. Symptom control
5. Patients whose caregiver is not willing to permit needed care in the residence.

During hospitalization, the IDT will work with the physician to continue the POC and assist with return to routine home care.

30. Why would a patient who already has home health care need hospice care?

Because hospice care is specifically provided for patients with terminal illnesses, the hospice interdisciplinary team can use its expertise in symptom management to provide excellent control of physical problems that could cause the death to be painful. The hospice team's knowledge of psychosocial and spiritual needs surrounding the dying process is seen as an equally important issue to ensure that the death is peaceful for the patient and family.

While other programs may address some of these issues individually, the hospice team approach makes the management of the dying process unique and maintains a high level of success for the death to be an acceptable end to life's journey.

31. Can hospice care and home health care be provided simultaneously?

No, because some of the services may be duplicated. The patient and family have the option to choose which service best meets their needs. Some other types of in-home care services may be continued, and the hospice interdisciplinary team, especially the social worker, can help the patient and family to investigate what services will continue and which will be replaced by the hospice team.

32. How is hospice different from home health care in the United States?

Hospice care is limited to patients with terminal illness. Its goals are for palliative care, especially providing comfort at the end of life. Hospice care is guided by quality, not length, of life. It is team-directed, and the patient/family is part of the team. Home health care requires the patient to need skilled services. End-of-life care is itself a unique skill, which encourages emphasis on more than just physical care needs.

Hospice Compared with Home Health Care in the United States

HOSPICE CARE	HOME HEALTH CARE
Hospice is a philosophy of care.	Home health care is a method of delivering care.
Patient has been diagnosed with a terminal illness.	Patient has a specific need.
Focus is on comfort and care, not cure.	Focus is on rehabilitation and cure.
Education focuses on the normal dying process.	Education focuses on disease process.
Holistic approach involving nurses, physicians, social workers, chaplains, volunteers.	Nursing tasks are the primary focus; other therapies are involved as needed.
Patient and family considered a unit of care.	Care is client-oriented.
Nurses specialize in pain and symptom management.	Nursing is task-oriented.
Emphasis is placed on providing emotional support.	Emotional support is not usually required.
Staff available 24 hours a day.	24-hour call, if available, is only for nursing care.
Respite care available.	
Care continues throughout end of life.	Patient discharged when need no longer exists.
Bereavement counseling offered.	Bereavement counseling not available.
Written bereavement care plan necessary.	No care plan needed; family not followed after death.

33. Under what circumstances would hospice care be discontinued?
- When, according to the guidelines, the patient is no longer terminally ill.
- When the patient moves out of the hospice's service area.
- When the safety of the hospice staff is questioned and all options to correct the problem have been pursued.
- When a patient moves into a nursing home with which the hospice does not have a contract and a contract cannot be obtained.

34. Who can terminate hospice care?
Revocation of hospice care can occur only if the patient chooses to discontinue hospice care. Patients can do this at anytime for any reason. They must sign a statement indicating their wish to revoke and why. Thereafter, the regular Medicare/Medicaid or private insurance benefits will be reinstated.

35. What happens if the patient is noncompliant?
Noncompliance may also discontinue hospice benefits. Patients could be considered non-compliant if they:
- Seek aggressive curative treatment for their terminal illness.
- Seek treatment/services in a facility that does not have a contract with the hospice.
- Seek treatment/services that are not in the POC or not preapproved by the IDT.

If a noncompliant patient chooses not to revoke, the patient will become responsible for all charges, because neither Medicare/Medicaid nor the hospice will pay.

36. Can patients stay in hospice longer than the usual 6 months?
Patients can remain under hospice care as long as they continue to meet the criteria that determine that their illness is terminal and progressive.

37. How is the plan of care carried out by each member of the IDT on a day-to-day basis?
Once the plan of care is determined, team members will visit according to patient and family needs. They will manage day-to-day problems as they arise and work together to prevent crises and meet team goals.

38. How is the plan of care carried out by hospice nurses?
Hospice nurses are licensed and trained in all the same basic nursing skills as home health nurses, but they must have extra training in symptom management and emotional support of patients and families. Their nursing assessment is holistic and specific to end-of-life care. A national certification exam has been developed, which has helped to ensure that the quality of hospice nursing will continue to improve. The hospice nurse manages the patient's care and integrates the hospice IDT plan of care to best meet patient and family needs. Nursing visits are determined by patient and family need, not by what will be reimbursed by Medicare, Medicaid, private insurance, or inability to pay. This allows the nurse to meet individual needs of each patient according to the IDT.

39. How is the plan of care carried out by social workers?
Hospice social workers may be addressing similar needs as home health social workers. However, the focus of the care is different. Because there are end-of-life issues, the need for social workers is greater. They not only assist with financial, legal, and social concerns but are trained to provide emotional support to patients and families with grief and end-of-life issues. Hospice social workers continue to visit patients and families throughout their hospice care. They are part of the primary team providing care and, with the primary nurse, direct the plan of care with the assistance of the IDT.

40. How is the plan of care carried out by health aides and homemakers?
Just like home health aides, hospice health aides and homemakers provide physical care and homemaker services. However, as part of the IDT, they have input into the plan of care. They are

trained not only in how to meet physical needs but to provide emotional support. Because they may be spending the most time in the home, their insights into physical and psychosocial needs are invaluable to the IDT. Medicare has specific requirements for their continuing education to ensure quality end-of-life care.

41. How is the plan of care carried out by volunteers?

Hospice volunteers, as part of the IDT, meet special needs for patients, families, and the hospice program. They are required to document visits and hours just like the rest of the team. They attend IDT meetings and contribute to the plan of care. In contrast, home health care does not require the use of volunteers in the services it provides to its patients. Other facts about volunteers include:

1. The hospice Medicare benefit requires that a minimum of 5% of the hours of services provided by the hospice to patients and families be given by hospice volunteers.

2. Hospice volunteer services are provided to every patient/family after an assessment of their specific needs.

3. Hospice programs have guidelines they follow in accepting volunteers to provide care for patients/families.

4. Hospice volunteers provide a variety of hands-on care and support services, which may include visiting patients and families, running errands, offering transportation for appointments, preparing meals, providing respite care, sharing hobbies or other interests, sharing their professional skill, participating in the hospice program's office work, directing special projects for patients/caregivers, and helping with fundraising efforts for the hospice program.

42. What are the common problems addressed by the on-call nurse?

1. Symptom management, which can involve pain, nausea, vomiting, constipation, diarrhea, shortness of breath, anxiety, and insomnia. These problems usually can be addressed with the standing orders and protocols.

2. Family or caregiver fears or questions, which is where the on-call nurse's expertise really comes into play. The nurse is able to listen and reassure patients/families to avoid a crisis. These calls may be more time-consuming and require more frequent visits than those related to physical problems.

3. Deaths or impending deaths.

4. Unforeseen events, including increasing symptoms, new symptoms, or the caregiver's inability to provide care.

43. How does the on-call nurse manage emergency situations at night?

The role of on-call hospice nurses differs from that of on-call home health nurses in part because they have access to protocols and standing orders, which gives them more autonomy and allows them to implement orders under the direction of a physician's plan of care more efficiently. The scope of their practice permits them to provide care without unnecessary emergency room visits or hospitalizations. Call nurses, like primary nurses, manage the plan of care established by the IDT. They focus on physical and emotional needs. They are free to make after-hour visits for assessments and can reach other team members as needed to assist with after-hours problems. The willingness of the after-hours team to go to the patient again assures quality end-of-life care in the environment chosen by the patient or family. As part of the IDT, they are always updated on changes in patient/family status and provide input into IDT meetings.

44. How can the medical community help hospice maintain its high level of service?

By understanding the guidelines that determine a patient is appropriate for hospice care and by referring patients. The physician who has referred a patient is encouraged to work with the IDT for additional treatment and services. This ensures that continuity and high quality of care will be provided.

Physicians can support hospice by being part of the medical advisory board. These board members can develop protocols, standing orders, educational programs, and standards of care.

45. How can the community help the hospice best serve patients with life-limiting illnesses?
Volunteering and participating in community education are key to a hospice's continued growth and its ability to provide quality care. Individuals can be members of a community advisory board, which develops and fosters the goals of the hospice in the community.

Through fundraising efforts the community can ensure that the hospice remains financially able to meet the varying needs of the patients and families it serves.

RESOURCES

Academy of Hospice Nurses
32478 Dunford Road
Farmington Hills, MI 48334
(303) 432-5482

American Academy of Hospice and Palliative Medicine
P.O. Box 14288
Gainesville, FL 32604-2288
(352) 377-8900
general E-mail: ahp@ahp.org
Web site: http://www.ahp.org

American Cancer Society
1599 Clifton Road, N.E.
Atlanta, GA 30329
1-800-227-2345

Hospice Education Institute
Five Essex Square
P.O. Box 713
Essex, CT 06426
Hotline: 1-800-331-1620
(203) 767-1620 ("Hospice Link")

Hospice Nurses Association, National Office
5512 Northumberland Street
Pittsburgh, PA 15217
(412) 687-3231

National Cancer Institute
Cancer Information Services
P.O. Box 24128
Baltimore, MD 21227
1-800-422-6237

National Hospice Organization
1901 N. Moore St. Suite 901
Arlington, VA 22209
1-800-658-8898
(703) 243-5900

ACKNOWLEDGMENT

The author gratefully acknowledges the cooperation of the Albany Community Hospice Interdisciplinary Team, Albany, Georgia.

BIBLIOGRAPHY

1. Boon T: Don't forget the hospice option. RN February 1998.
2. Byock I: Dying Well, Peace and Possibilities at the End of Life. New York, Riverhead Books, 1997.
3. Miller KE, Miller MM, Single N: Barriers to hospice care: Family physicians' perceptions. Hospice Journal 12(4):1997.
4. National Hospice Organization: Hospice: A Special Way of Caring. Channing L. Bete Co., 1997.
5. National Hospice Organization: Hospice Under Medicare. Channing L. Bete Co., 1998.
6. National Hospice Organization: Medical Guidelines for Determining Prognosis in Selected Non-Cancer Diseases. 2nd ed. 1996.
7. Palmetto Government Benefits Administration: Medicare advisory. Hospice 97–13, 1997.
8. Saunders C: The hospice: Its meaning to patients and their physicians. Hosp Pract 1981.

8. SYMPTOM RECOGNITION

Suresh K. Joishy, M.D., F.A.C.P.

1. Why is symptom recognition important?

The foundation of palliative care is symptom control. The strength of this foundation depends on the knowledge and experience of the palliative care team members in recognizing the symptoms.

In palliative care, each symptom becomes its own distinct disease entity with its own etiology, pathogenesis, prognostic factors, and response to treatment. "Cure" equals effective symptom elimination. Unfortunately, in advanced cancer patients with incurable and progressive disease, one can only hope for good symptom control rather than complete symptom resolution.

Quality of life in cancer patients must be equated foremost with symptom control. When symptoms are severe enough to affect the activities of daily living (ADL) such as eating, sleeping, ambulation, and bowel and bladder elimination, quality of life is certainly affected. Therefore, it is necessary to address symptom recognition first.

The spectrum of symptoms experienced by patients with life-limiting illness is so wide that no two patients have identical needs. The physician must treat each patient with respect and humility. Dogmatic beliefs that specific treatments will eliminate specific symptoms are untenable. At the same time, there are a sufficient number of treatments in the palliative care armamentarium that the physician should never believe that "nothing can be done." There is always something the physician can offer to keep the patient comfortable. Palliative care is unceasing until symptoms are controlled.

2. What is meant by "the vicious circle of symptoms"?

Symptoms causing distress and suffering create the basic "vicious circle." However, symptoms in advanced cancer patients enter into not one, but multiple vicious circles. For example, cancer pain can cause considerable suffering, provoking depression, anxiety, and loss of sleep and affecting activities of daily living such as eating and getting out of bed. Each of these factors may affect pain and its response to treatment. Dramatic changes may occur in all other symptoms once pain is controlled: the patient may emerge as a totally rejuvenated person. Again, pain may not be relieved unless the symptoms of anxiety, depression, and sleeplessness are addressed. The swiftness with which the palliative care physician and team members are able to break these cycles depends on their ability to recognize the interplay of these complex symptoms.

3. What is the etiology of physical symptoms?

The etiologies of physical symptoms are as complex as symptoms and just as numerous.

A single physical symptom with a single etiology. This simple situation is uncommon, e.g., a single skeletal metastasis causing a focus of somatic pain. Even in this situation, pain may depend on associated etiologies such as the site of metastasis in weight bearing or mobile bone, the size of the lesion, and whether or not the periosteum is affected.

Multiple physical symptoms with a single etiology. Liver metastasis can cause abdominal pain, nausea, vomiting, fever, and the discomfort of an enlarged abdomen caused by ascites.

A single physical symptom with multiple etiologies. Nausea or vomiting may be caused by metabolic conditions, organic lesions, or central stimulation of vomiting centers. Pain has an ever greater number of etiologies.

Iatrogenic symptoms
- *Polypharmacy* is inevitable in palliative care because patients are multi-symptomatic. Unfortunately, each drug has its own toxic profile, causing side effects. A classic example is the nausea, sedation, and constipation caused by morphine.
- *Post-surgical pain.* The chest wall pain of thoracotomy is one type of neuropathic pain that can be quite severe.

- *Radiotherapy induced.* These include xerostomia with mouth ulcers, skin reactions, fibrosis, mucositis, and cystitis. Nausea and fatigue are also common.
- *Chemotherapy induced.* These include peripheral neuropathy. Mucositis with oral ulcers can also be painful.

Physical symptoms of unknown etiologies. Despite high-tech diagnostic tools, one may never find the causes for some physical symptoms, such as fatigue, dyspnea, gastroparesis, and anorexia.

4. What is the etiology of psychosocial symptoms?

These symptoms fit into multiple symptom complexes with multiple etiologies and enter into the vicious cycle of interacting with and perpetuating physical symptoms. The most common symptoms are those that arise from fear of cancer, uncertainties about the end of life, and losses in life control, independence, job, and finances.

5. Is there any meaningful way to classify cancer symptoms?

- **Symptoms directly related to cancer.** Usually these symptoms are local or regional and result from inflammation, infection, pressure, or obstruction of adjacent viscera.
- **Related to metastasis.** These symptoms occur in areas other than the organ of involvement, having their effects at metastatic sites. These include CNS metastasis cord compression and pathologic fracture.
- **Related to paraneoplastic syndromes.**
  Organic symptoms: Neuropathies, myopathies, and deep vein thrombosis.
  Symptoms of metabolic and endocrine syndromes: Hypercalcemia, hyponatremia, Cushing's disease, and carcinoids.
- **Symptoms unrelated to cancer.** A large number of patients are elderly and may have been suffering from several chronic symptoms related to arthritis, diabetes mellitus, and heart disease. These symptoms may be aggravated or compounded by cancer symptoms.
- **Undifferentiated symptoms.** Some cancers defy histologic classification and are called undifferentiated cancers. Similarly, modern science still cannot classify some of the symptoms of cancer. This is not to say that undifferentiated cancers have undifferentiated symptoms. Any advanced cancer may be associated with undifferentiated symptoms. A symptom may be considered undifferentiated when its etiology is unclear, when the patient is unable to describe it well, and when the predicted response to treatment does not occur. Severe asthenia is variously described as fatigue or lack of energy. Cachexia of malignancy and symptoms of multi-organ failure can probably be considered undifferentiated.

6. Are there symptoms common to all cancers?

Certainly. Several symptoms are known to occur even before cancer is diagnosed, and these may continue during the entire course of illness. The following symptoms need to reflect or refer to the organ of involvement:

- Anorexia
- Altered or reduced ability to taste
- Nausea/vomiting
- Anxiety/depression
- Postural hypotension with fixed heart rate

7. Are the symptoms of non-malignant, life-limiting illness different from those experienced with cancer?

Because of different age groups, more years of chronicity, and debility, the progression of symptoms may be less rapid than those that occur with cancer. Symptoms generally tend to reflect the organ of involvement more so than with cancers. Of course, non-malignant conditions do not involve metastasis and related complications. Often, patients with non-malignant diseases are less worried about dying even if their suffering is the same. However, AIDS patients may suffer more than cancer patients.

- **Acquired immune deficiency syndrome (AIDS).** Younger patients experiencing symptoms of multi-organ involvement, poor coping mechanisms, and social stigma suffer greatly. Gastrointestinal and respiratory symptoms caused by infections are common in all AIDS patients. Symptoms are often refractory; hiccups may be observed more frequently in AIDS patients. When AIDS patients develop secondary malignancies such as lymphoma, Kaposi's sarcoma, and CNS tumors, their symptoms are more compounded than those of patients with non-AIDS malignancies. AIDS is certainly the disease that poses the most challenges to a palliative care team.
- **Neurodegenerative diseases.** Symptoms are generally neurologic and related to immobility as a result of sequelae. The patients are younger. Patients afflicted with Huntington's disease or ALS suffer from organ dysfunctions caused by a loss of neurologic supply. These dysfunctions include urinary incontinence, respiratory distress, muscle paralysis, and dysphagia. Pain may occur because of stiffness and contractures. Patients suffering from neurodegenerative diseases will require intensive physical therapy as well as occupational therapy to control symptoms, whereas pharmacotherapy is the mainstay of palliative care for cancer patients. Older patients with Alzheimer's disease fall into the palliative care domain.
- **End-stage cardiac, renal, and pulmonary disease.** Although fatigue is common in all these diseases, as in cancer, symptoms usually reflect failure of respective organs because of functional or metabolic derangements.

8. Do acute symptoms differ from chronic symptoms in life-limiting illness?

Palliative care patients already have chronic symptoms. Any increase in these symptoms probably reflects disease progression rather than an acute event. Similarly, new symptoms may also reflect disease progression or new sites of the same disease. Acuity and chronicity lose meaning, and treatments may not differ as acute symptoms are expected to remain chronic for the limited span of life.

9. Can symptoms help to prognosticate patient survival?

Traditionally, oncologists prognosticate by cancer staging, i.e., stages I–IV. This method is useless in palliative care because most patients are in stage III or IV. Sometimes a patient may even be beyond stage IV, having complex symptomatology and complications.

It is ironic that oncologists use symptoms to prognosticate only one group of cancers out of more than 200! In both Hodgkin's and non-Hodgkin's lymphoma, fever, chills, night sweats, and fatigue are considered when staging. The suffix "B," used in conjunction with the staging number, indicates a poor response to treatment. If this principle is applied, almost all of the patients receiving palliative care belong to the "B" staging group.

Experience has shown that symptoms can still assist the palliative care physician when prognosticating survival, albeit in its limited duration. The following factors predict a poor prognosis.

- Multiple symptoms
- Interdependent symptoms (psychosocial with physical symptoms)
- Symptoms immobilizing the patient (pathologic fractures, cord compression)
- Refractory or inadequately controlled symptoms (dyspnea with lymphangitic spread in the lungs)
- Unmet spiritual needs or spiritual pain
- Late entry into palliative care
- Symptoms of multiple metastasis to non-osseous organs

10. How are symptoms recognized if the patient is unable to provide a thorough history?

Some physicians frequently record in the patient's chart, "patient is a poor historian." I wonder how they would obtain history from a child! Information can always be obtained from a caregiver or a family member. Even if that person is not present, they may only be a telephone call away.

When patients are feeble and unable to talk, or unable to put their thoughts together because of severe symptoms, it is sufficient to ask questions that can be answered with "yes" or "no" responses. The effectiveness of this depends on the skill of the physician when dealing with palliative care patients. A detailed history can be obtained when the patient's severe symptoms are stabilized. Sometimes a nurse or social worker is able to glean more information from a patient than can the physician; thus, their help must be sought.

11. What is the author's classification of symptoms for palliative care?
This author has classified symptoms in palliative care by taking into account the following variables:
  • The patient's coping mechanisms
  • The patient's performance status
  • The site of care of the symptomatic patient
  • End of life and actively dying status
Level I: Patients are treated in an ambulatory care setting, and their coping mechanisms are adequate enough for ADL, which reflects quality of life. Their most common symptoms are pain, anxiety, depression, and loneliness, and they respond well to treatment at this level.
Level II: Coping mechanisms are failing. Patients are developing symptoms caused by new complications and disease progression. These may include hypercalcemia, pathologic fracture, and bowel obstruction. Patients require hospitalizations for palliative medical and surgical treatments.
Level III: Performance status is worsening, and patients are moving toward complete disability and becoming bedridden. Symptoms are progressing despite adequate medical and surgical treatment.
Level IV: Patient are terminal. They have attained an ECOG performance status-4, irrespective of symptoms. They are hospice eligible and have a limited life expectancy. These patients may require respite care in the hospice of a hospital.
An algorithm of the levels of palliative care is presented on the facing page.

12. What is the relationship between spirituality and symptoms?
It is a grave mistake to reduce human beings solely to body and mind. Spirituality, associated either with religion or independent of religion, gains meaning for the dying patient. Patients ponder the purpose of their existence, try to put life into order in the face of losses, and worry about the burdens their family members will have to face.

13. What is the relationship between medical ethics and symptoms?
Nowhere else in the field of medicine is the triad of medical ethics as applicable as it is in palliative care.
Beneficence: Do good. Any measure to control symptoms means doing good to a suffering patient with advanced cancer.
Non-maleficence: Prevent harm. While intended to control symptoms, no palliative care measure should cause other symptoms such as side effects. If a patient is started on morphine, it is imperative to anticipate the side effects of nausea and constipation and to take concomitant preemptive measures.
Autonomy: Respect the patient's wish. No palliative care is provided without full knowledge of the patient as long as their cognitive functions are intact. This principle applies to simple measures, such as administration of a single drug, as well as to profound measures, such as declaring a patient DNR (do not resuscitate). In palliative care, even when family conflicts arise, it is important to ask, "What is/was the patient's wish?"
Euthanasia: This book will not debate euthanasia. However, the subject of euthanasia is often contemplated by the patient or caregivers because of their inability to control symptoms and the subsequent increasing intensity of suffering. This situation should not arise when good palliative care is being provided. Control of refractory symptoms is possible with terminal sedation, an ethically acceptable option (see Chapter 24, Question 26).

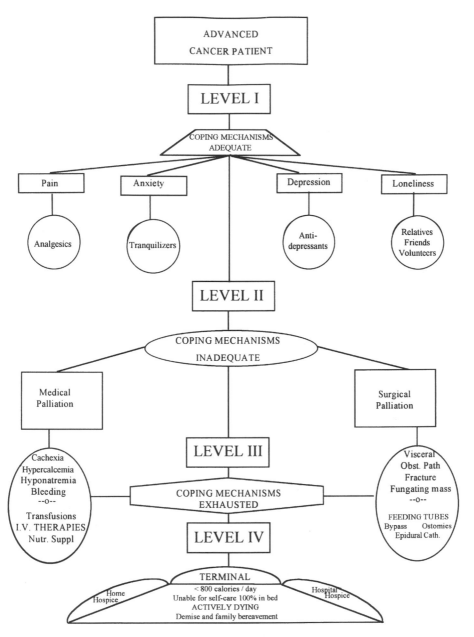

Algorithm in the palliative care of advanced cancer patients: levels of care.

BIBLIOGRAPHY

1. Bruera E, et al: The Edmonton Symptom Assessment System (ESAS): A simple method for assessment of palliative care patients. J Palliat Care 7:6–9, 1991.
2. Donnelly S, Walsh D: The symptoms of advanced cancer. Semin Oncol 22(suppl 3):67–72, 1995.
3. Hatcliffe Dawe R: How patients see symptoms. Palliative care assessment. Nurs Times 92:61–63, 1995.
4. Strause L, et al: A severity index designed as an indicator of acuity in palliative care. J Palliat Care 9:11–15, 1993.

9. APPROACH TO SYMPTOM CONTROL

Suresh K. Joishy, M.D., F.A.C.P.

1. What is the traditional approach to symptom control?

The traditional approach to symptom control focuses on obtaining a diagnosis first, via a series of steps including detailed history taking, thorough physical examination, and laboratory and radiographic investigations. Even when the patient presents acute symptoms in an emergency room, the patient will suffer until the diagnosis is achieved. Surgeons generally do not give analgesics for acute abdominal pain until the diagnosis is established lest "control of symptoms mask the diagnosis." It is not unusual for the patient to undergo an exhausting battery of tests while enduring persisting symptoms. There is a rush to cure the disease but not to control the symptoms.

2. Is the traditional approach to symptom control suitable for palliative care?

No. The traditional approach is suitable for patients whose disease is expected to be cured in a short period of time. The traditional approach defies logic by treating life-limiting illness with the same steps as those applied to curable diseases. Until recently, this attitude was the major stumbling block in introducing palliative care to the United States. The palliative care approach to symptom control is not "cure" but "care."

3. What are the barriers to good palliative care in the traditional approach to symptom control?

History taking via the traditional approach is thorough and redundant enough to exhaust any patient. A patient in palliative care with advanced cancer symptoms may be too feeble to speak. Traditional approaches confound efforts to connect physical symptoms with psychosocial factors. The spiritual approach is unheard of. Another major difference between the traditional approach and the palliative approach is that with the traditional approach, the physician is responsible for symptom control, with very little input from other health care professionals. Conversely, in palliative care, the entire team participates in symptom control.

4. What are the cornerstones of the palliative care approach to symptom control?

The interdisciplinary team approach is the hallmark of palliative care. Physical, emotional, spiritual, social, and ethical factors affecting symptom control are addressed by the team, which includes the patient and their family. Patient autonomy is respected in all decisions. DNR orders are invariably accepted, without affecting patient care.

5. What is the status of patients referred to palliative care?

Patients referred to palliative care have been diagnosed as having incurable diseases, mainly advanced-stage cancer. They have endured numerous tests and many futile treatments. The patients are usually referred to palliative care as a last resort.

Palliative care patients are usually accompanied by tired and distressed family members. These patients and their families are often poorly informed regarding their prognosis. They have misconceptions about hospice and palliative care, and unmet spiritual needs are common. Symptoms abound in these patients, often accompanied by associated fears, anxiety, and depression. The empathy and care given by the palliative care team is invaluable.

6. How are symptoms assessed?

When symptoms are uncontrolled, palliative care patients are in great distress. Thus, the palliative care team should assess symptoms quickly, and without expecting the patient to provide an elaborate history; they may be too feeble to do so. Focus on symptoms when taking the patient's history, and perform a brief physical examination.

When acute symptoms are addressed and the patient is stabilized, a comprehensive assessment is performed regarding the primary diagnosis, the extent of the disease, and previously provided therapies. Document any current problems. The interdisciplinary team then meets to discuss the patient, and a treatment plan is formulated.

7. What are the components of the interdisciplinary team approach to symptom control?

A problem-solving approach by the physician is complemented by first-rate patient care by the nursing staff. A social worker supports the patients and their family members regarding the non-medical issues that they face. Unmet spiritual needs are addressed by the spiritual counselor of the team. A physical therapist will help the patient with activities of daily living. A dietitian is consulted for nutritional support, and volunteers visit with patients and their families, providing company, cheer, and help with day-to-day chores.

8. What are the multimodal therapies applied in palliative care?

Any modality of therapy is applicable in palliative care, assuming it is directed toward symptom control, and assuming that side effects or complications do not compromise the patient's quality of life. Conventional multimodal therapies include pharmacotherapy, surgical procedures, and radiotherapy. Other multimodal therapies are supplied by the palliative care team members— social workers, a physical therapist, and a spiritual counselor. Interventional pain management specialists may help provide pain relief for patients by utilizing epidural, intrathecal devices. Psychiatrists may help with psychopharmacology and behavioral therapies.

Alternative therapies are not sought by palliative care physicians, but neither are they objected to. For example, acupuncture may be helpful, in limited situations, to some patients. Aromatherapy is becoming more popular for lifting patient mood and morale. Certainly, music therapy has proved to soothe patients who are in pain.

9. How is pharmacotherapy applied differently in palliative care?

The basic principles of pharmacotherapy remain the same. However, certain important concerns are more vigorously taken into account. Palliative care patients cannot afford to suffer from the side effects of drugs. Palliative care patients do not have the time to wait for assessment of responses by trial and error. If one drug is ineffective, a second-line drug should be readily available.

Chosen drugs must be versatile enough to be administered by many routes. Although the oral route is always preferred, debilitated patients frequently have dysphagia. Thus, the chosen drug should also be available in sublingual and rectal forms. If some drugs are not commercially available for rectal use, pharmacists should be willing to formulate suppositories. When the oral, sublingual, and rectal routes are not possible, drugs should be found that can be administered subcutaneously. Unfortunately, there are very few transdermal preparations. Drugs should be simple enough to be used at home by caregivers. The side-effect profile should be such that patient reactions to the drug do not cause family members to panic.

To reduce polypharmacy, the inventory should contain "portmanteau" drugs, i.e., one drug capable of controlling more than one symptom. For example, haloperidol can help a confused patient who is also nauseated. Dexamethasone is capable of controlling several symptoms simultaneously. Cost of drugs must not be forgotten, as patients have chronic symptoms.

BIBLIOGRAPHY

1. Bruera E, et al: The Edmonton Symptom Assessment System (ESAS): A simple method for assessment of palliative care patients. J Palliat Care 7:6–9, 1991.
2. Donnelly S, Walsh D: The symptoms of advanced cancer. Semin Oncol 22(suppl 3):67–72, 1995.
3. Hatcliffe Dowe R: How patients see symptoms. Palliative care assessment. Nurs Times 92:61–63, 1995.
4. Strause L, et al: A severity index designed as an indicator of acuity in palliative care. J Palliat Care 9:11–15, 1993.

10. A PRACTICAL APPROACH TO NAUSEA AND VOMITING

Jane M. Griffiths, M.D., C.C.F.P.

1. What is nausea?

Nausea is an unpleasant wave-like sensation usually felt in the back of the throat and in the upper abdomen. It is characterized by a loss of stomach tone and the gradual retrograde movement of the contents of the upper gut. This results in the contents of the upper gut being dumped into the stomach. Nausea is often accompanied by autonomic symptoms such as pallor, sweating, tachycardia, and salivation.

2. What is vomiting?

Vomiting is the forceful retrograde expulsion of stomach contents. This is different from regurgitation, which is a much more passive event. Usually, but not necessarily, vomiting is accompanied by nausea.

3. What is the prevalence of nausea and vomiting?

Nausea and vomiting are common complaints among the terminally ill. The National Hospice Study data, analyzed by Reuben and Mor in 1986, showed that 63% of patients with advanced cancer experience nausea and vomiting during their last 8 weeks of life. It seems to be more frequent in women and in younger individuals, as well as in those with stomach or breast cancer.

4. Why are nausea and vomiting important symptoms in palliative care?

Because they are common. In most cases, nausea is eminently treatable; however, persistent nausea may become a demoralizing problem that severely compromises a patient's quality of life.

5. What is the vomiting center?

Identified in 1949, the vomiting center is a small area in the brain stem. These early studies identified this area as the part of the brain that, when stimulated, precipitates emesis or vomiting. It is considered to be the final common pathway in the complex chain of events that culminates in the sensation of nausea and the act of vomiting. Anatomically, the vomiting center lies close to several other brain stem structures also involved in the coordination of vomiting. These include the salivary, vasomotor, and respiratory centers, as well as several cranial nerve nuclei.

6. What causes nausea and vomiting?

The causes of nausea and vomiting can be categorized into four groups. Each group is distinct from the others in the ways in which the various stimuli are detected and identified by the vomiting center.

1. **Visceral** causes such as organ distention, irritation, or obstruction constitute an important group. Examples include the direct effect of irritating substances on the lining of the stomach, gastric outlet and small bowel obstruction, hepatomegaly with stretching of the liver capsule, biliary or genitourinary disease, constipation, and oropharyngeal infection or inflammation. These messages are transmitted via the vagus and splanchnic nerves to the vomiting center.

2. **Chemical** imbalances in the blood stream or in the cerebral spinal fluid (CSF) are detected by the chemoreceptor trigger zone (CTZ), a region located in the floor of the fourth ventricle of the brain. The CTZ has a deficient blood brain barrier; thus, both blood and CSF have access to this area. The detection of an abnormality in the blood or the CSF will trigger the CTZ to stimulate the vomiting center. Examples of these abnormalities include hypercalcemia, uremia, chemotherapy, and the central effects of drugs such as opioids, digoxin, and estrogen.

3. **Central nervous system** causes can be classified into two subgroups. Psychological and cerebral causes such as severe pain, anxiety, or fear constitute the first subgroup. The second subgroup includes such causes as raised intracranial pressure or the direct effect of a local tumor on the brain. These central nervous system (CNS) causes are relayed directly to the vomiting center and trigger it.

4. **Vestibular** causes include motion or positional stimuli that stimulate the vestibular mechanism in the brain, which then triggers the vomiting center. Examples of these causes include roller-coaster rides, space travel, and travel by boat. This group would also include ototoxic drugs and tumors involving the vestibular apparatus in the brain (acoustic neuroma).

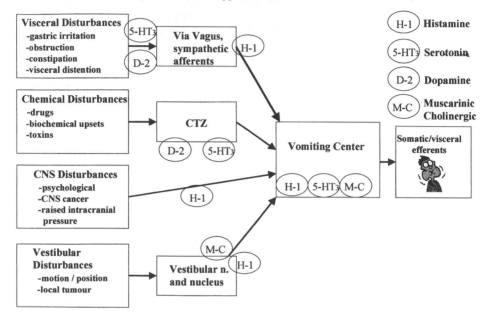

Pathways and neurotransmitters involved in nausea and vomiting.

7. Why is it important to classify the causes?

In general, each event that causes nausea and vomiting initiates a message that is transmitted to the vomiting center along a different neural pathway according to the category of causes to which that event belongs. By choosing the correct antiemetic, the neural pathway involved can be blocked. Classifying the causes of nausea and vomiting is key to determining the correct first-line antiemetic.

8. What is the clinical approach to determining the cause of the nausea and vomiting?

When taking the history it is important to know the tumor histology. (Hypercalcemia is common in tumors of epithelial origin such as breast and bronchus, as well as in myeloma.) The tumor spread and previous treatment are important to ask about when looking for clues to intra-abdominal disease or previous surgery. The medication history is also important. Ask about the timing of the nausea and associated symptoms. Large volume vomiting may suggest nausea due to gastric stasis or outflow obstruction caused by drugs or disease. The associated symptoms of drowsiness and confusion may point to hypercalcemia. The examination should include a careful exam of the oropharynx, abdomen, and neurologic system. One may consider a few key investigations such as serum creatinine, urea nitrogen, electrolytes, and calcium. Plain radiographs of the abdomen in flat and upright positions are useful in ascertaining visceral causes. In the more imminently terminal patient, empiric therapy is always more appropriate.

9. How does the neural message get transmitted to the vomiting center?

Neurotransmitters are chemicals that act on specific receptors to facilitate the transmission of messages between nerves (see figure in question 6). The main neurotransmitters (and the receptors they act upon) involved in nausea and vomiting are histamine (H_1 receptors), dopamine (D_2 receptors), acetylcholine (muscarinic-cholinergic receptors), and serotonin ($5-HT_3$ receptors).

10. How do antiemetic agents work?

Antiemetics block or antagonize the specific neurotransmitters that facilitate transmission of messages that trigger the vomiting center.

Commonly Used Antiemetics

DRUG	ACTION	DOSE AND ROUTE
Haloperidol	Antidopaminergic	0.5–5 mg po, sc, im q 4–8 h prn
Prochlorperazine	Antidopaminergic, weak antihistamine	5–20 mg po, pr, im, iv q 4–6 h prn
Scopolamine	Anticholinergic	0.3–0.6 mg po, sc q 4–8 h prn
Cyclizine	Antihistamine	25–50 mg po, sc, im q 8 h prn
Dimenhydrinate	Antihistamine, weak anticholinergic	50–100 mg po, pr, im iv q 4–6 h prn
Metoclopramide	Prokinetic, weak antidopaminergic	5–10 mg po, sc, im, iv t.i.d.–q.i.d. $^1/_2$ h ac and hs
Domperidone	Prokinetic, weak antidopaminergic	5–20 mg po t.i.d.–q.i.d. $^1/_2$ h ac and hs
Lorazepam	Anxiolytic	0.5–2 mg po, sl, iv q 6–8 h prn
Ondansetron	Antiserotonergic	8 mg po, iv q 8–12 h prn

11. Which drugs are good for visceral causes of nausea and vomiting?

There are many causes of nausea within this category for which a specific diagnosis can be made and a specific therapy can follow (e.g., radiotherapy for esophageal obstruction or an antiviral agent for herpes stomatitis).

Prokinetic drugs are good choices for nausea caused by gastric or small bowel stasis. Because they are antidopaminergic they can also have an effect at the CTZ and thereby help biochemically-mediated nausea. Metoclopramide may be given orally or subcutaneously, but may lead to extrapyramidal side effects. Domperidone lacks extrapyramidal side effects but is recommended for oral administration only.

The neurotransmitter serotonin is probably responsible for activating the vagal and splanchnic nerves, which then activate the vomiting center. Perhaps antiserotonin agents will someday have a role in these situations, but currently this role is not clear. The vagal pathway is mediated through acetylcholine and histamine. As anticholinergic agents seem to have a higher side effect profile, an antihistamine may be a better choice for the visceral causes that would not be helped by a prokinetic.

Bowel obstruction is a common cause of nausea and vomiting in the terminal cancer patient. In those who are not candidates for surgery, this condition has traditionally been treated conservatively by intravenous hydration and nasogastric suction. An alternate approach involving only subcutaneous medications can also be considered. A treatment regimen involving the delivery of subcutaneous analgesia, antiemetics, and antispasmodic agents is generally implemented. For example, subcutaneous morphine or hydromorphone for analgesia and cyclizine 100–150 mg/day and/or haloperidol 2–10 mg/day as an antiemetic, and scopolamine 1.2–2.4 mg/day as an antispasmodic, antisecretory, and sedating agent. If the intestinal obstruction is incomplete, a prokinetic agent such as metoclopramide 60–240 mg/day will be useful. If this approach fails to achieve symptom control, other measures such as the use of the drug octreotide, nasogastric suction, venting gastrostomy, or hypodermoclysis may have to be considered.

12. Which drugs are good choices for biochemical causes of nausea and vomiting?

The main neurotransmitter present at the CTZ is dopamine. Therefore, antidopaminergics are the logical choice in these situations. The antidopaminergic class of drugs includes the phenothiazines such as chlorpromazine, methotrimeprazine, and prochlorperazine, the butyrophenones such as haloperidol, and droperidol, and the prokinetic agents such as metoclopramide. The antidopamine agents have side effects that include extrapyramidal reactions (akathisia, dystonic reactions, and parkinsonism), hypotension, and sedation. These reactions are usually rare in the adult terminally ill patient. The phenothiazines have greater sedative/hypotensive properties and are less likely to cause extrapyramidal reaction, whereas the butyrophenones have less sedative/hypotensive effect and are more likely to cause an extrapyramidal reaction. Of these two drugs, haloperidol is much less sedating. Methotrimeprazine is an interesting antiemetic in that it has anxiolytic, analgesic, and antiemetic properties.

Prokinetic agents, while antidopaminergic, also have a role outside of the brain. These agents are particularly useful when nausea and vomiting are due to delayed gastric emptying, gastroparesis, or partial bowel obstruction because they normalize upper gastrointestinal motility.

Serotonin antagonists are the newest class of antiemetic agents. Most of the literature involving these drugs has analyzed them in the setting of chemotherapy-induced emesis and not in the palliative care setting. They may be very useful drugs but there are no recommendations for their use in terminal nausea and vomiting.

Hypercalcemia is a specific biochemical upset that produces a clinical situation characterized by nausea, confusion, and dehydration. This must be recognized and can be specifically treated with hydration and bisphosphonates.

13. Which drugs are good choices for CNS causes of nausea and vomiting?

When psychological causes such as anxiety and depression are implicated, the logical step would be to treat these problems. This means treating nausea with antiemetics and psychotropic drugs. An example of a commonly used anxiolytic is lorazepam, 0.5–2 mg orally every 8 hours as required. There are many psychotropic drugs that are useful antiemetics, the most obvious being the phenothiazines, which are powerful sedative and anxiolytic agents. Methotrimeprazine is special because it is an anxiolytic, sedative, and analgesic and has antiemetic properties, too. Amitriptyline has anticholinergic and antihistamine properties and is also a weak antidopaminergic. Thus, although it may not be a first line antiemetic, when it is used to treat neuropathic pain or depression, it will certainly also have antiemetic action. There are many nonpharmacologic approaches that are applicable in these circumstances, and these are described in questions 18 and 19. The nausea caused by increased intracranial pressure can be treated with steroids if appropriate for the clinical situation.

14. Which drugs are good choices for vestibular causes of nausea and vomiting?

The vestibular system contains histamine and acetylcholine receptors. Thus, an antihistamine is the logical choice of drug, particularly an antihistamine with anticholinergic side effects. The most common antihistamines used are cyclizine and dimenhydrinate. Cyclizine is less sedating than dimenhydrinate and can be given subcutaneously. Dimenhydrinate is available in a suppository formulation. Anticholinergics can also be used alone. The most common anticholinergic used is scopolamine, which can be given subcutaneously or orally. There is also a transdermal formulation of scopolamine, but its availability has been problematic because of concerns of unpredictable absorption.

The side effects of anticholinergics include sedation, dry mouth, constipation, confusion, increased intraocular pressure, and urinary retention. The side effects of antihistamines include sedation, dry mouth, and constipation.

15. What are the principles to keep in mind when choosing a drug?

The best drug choice is based on the working diagnosis and the knowledge of the neural pathway involved. If possible, treatment should address the underlying cause, while recognizing and considering the life expectancy of the patient. Bear in mind possible side effects, and try to choose the antiemetic(s) specific for the neural pathway to be blocked. In this way, unnecessary side effects are avoided.

The goal is to use the lowest effective dose within the standard dose range that will provide relief. When determining the dose it is important to keep in mind the changing metabolic function of the patient and the other drugs with which the antiemetic may interact.

16. Is there an all-purpose antiemetic?

The vomiting center in the brain triggers the sensation of nausea and the act of vomiting. This is an extremely complex pathway involving cortical areas of the brain, several different brain stem functions, and sympathetic and parasympathetic components of the autonomic nervous system. This is much too complex a step to consider interrupting with a single, all-purpose antiemetic. There are drugs that have all of the properties important in antiemesis (anticholinergic, antihistaminic, and antidopaminergic properties), but in choosing these drugs the trade-off is accepting the unnecessary side effects. It makes more sense to choose a drug that is specific for the neural pathway needing to be blocked.

17. Can adjusting the current drug regimen help relieve nausea and vomiting?

It may help a great deal. In fact, in some cases, that may be all that is required. As patients become more and more ill, there will inevitably be changes in their body weight and their metabolic function. They may become cachectic (a decrease in lean body mass) and require a smaller dose of a drug. As body systems slowly shut down, the hepatic and renal clearance of drugs become less efficient and serum levels may rise to toxic amounts. It is very important to consider these changes when updating a nauseated patient's drug regimen. Weigh the possible benefits against the risks and side effects frequently, and discontinue any medication that is no longer worthwhile. Hormone replacement therapy, antianginal medication, antihypertensive medication, or other drugs that are either prophylactic or designed for long-term gain may be easily discontinued. Gastric inflammation caused by nonsteroidal anti-inflammatory drugs (NSAIDs) is a common cause of nausea. A change to a less irritating NSAID may help. A concurrent prescription of an H_2 blocking agent or a cytoprotective agent may also be useful. It may be wise to consider changing the dosing schedule or the route of administration of various drugs if either of these can be implicated in the patient's nausea.

18. What nonpharmacologic measures can help ease nausea?

A clear liquid diet is helpful until symptoms begin to resolve. Avoid sweet, spicy, very salty, or fatty foods, as well as foods with strong odors. Food can be served cold or at room temperature. This will help to limit the odor.

Other odors must be kept to a minimum also. These include odors from the commode, from malignant cutaneous wounds, or from any other source found in the hospital or home. Fresh air and/or good ventilation will help ease the sensation of nausea. By keeping the patient in a sitting or semireclining position, by avoiding circumstances that have previously conditioned the feeling of nausea, and by providing distractions, the caregiver will be able to help make the patient even more comfortable.

Relaxation techniques, guided meditation, and massage therapy can also be very therapeutic.

19. How is nausea managed when fear and anxiety are the major complaints?

This situation requires a slightly different approach, although many of the measures applicable to other situations can also be helpful. The focus of therapy must be on using anxiolytics and on techniques such as hypnosis, guided imagery, and relaxation or massage therapy. A short course of cognitive or behavioral therapy specifically addressing the patient's fears will enhance these techniques.

20. Is radiation-induced nausea treated differently?

Palliative radiation may be a cause of nausea and vomiting depending on the dose, site, and timing of the radiotherapy. It is generally self-limited and will abate 1–2 weeks after the radiation treatment. When the radiation field involves the bowel, the therapy is likely to cause nausea. This is probably due to serotonin release from cells in the lining of the bowel, which then influences the chemoreceptor trigger zone and/or sets the vagus nerve firing, which then stimulates the vomiting center. Head and neck irradiation is also likely to cause nausea. It is probable that changes in the nervous system secondary to the radiation somehow influence the vomiting center directly. It may be that radiation causes pressure effects within the CNS, thus generating nausea. Both ibuprofen and corticosteroids have been shown to be useful for treating this type of nausea. Another rational choice of drug would be an antidopaminergic (such as haloperidol 0.5–2 mg po b.i.d.) or, as the literature suggests, an antiserotonergic such as ondansetron may become a future treatment of choice.

21. What are the routes of administration to consider when administering antiemetics?
The oral route is the simplest and most practical route to administer antiemetics. If the patient is vomiting frequently, this will not be feasible and an alternate route will have to be established. For patients at home, the rectal route may be preferred if the chosen antiemetic is available or can be prepared in suppository form by a pharmacist. Prochlorperazine, dimenhydrinate, and chlorpromazine are readily available in suppository form. The subcutaneous route is also an alternative. Prochlorperazine and chlorpromazine cause significant subcutaneous irritation when used this way, but hyoscine, cyclizine, haloperidol, metoclopramide, and methotrimeprazine are regularly administered subcutaneously.

22. What can you do when nothing else is working?
Most antiemetic doses are fairly flexible. When the antiemetic is not producing the desired effect, increase the dose. When this approach does not work, reassess the patient to consider other possible causes. A second antiemetic of a different class may be added if a different cause is suspected. Only 25–30% of patients will require two different antiemetics, and even fewer may require three. An example of a common and rational combination of drugs may be cyclizine, haloperidol, and metoclopramide, or dimenhydrinate, prochlorperazine, and scopolamine. Once this point is reached and the patient is still nauseated, many clinicians may consider adding a steroid to the regimen. Little is known about how steroids work for nausea, although they seem to be of some use. They are presumed to work either because of prostaglandin inhibition or because of their effect on cell permeability. They are generally not used alone but as adjuncts to other antiemetics.

23. What are the most common pitfalls to avoid?
All symptoms can be exacerbated by psychological, spiritual, or social distress. These can be easy to miss unless a total care approach is employed that keeps the caregivers open to identifying these problems. If such stresses are missed, even the most carefully chosen drug can be rendered useless. When these issues are identified, a plan including the nonpharmacologic, environmental, supportive, and pharmacologic modalities can be instituted.
Failure to recognize the importance of reviewing the drug regimen is another frequent mistake. Often, many useful changes can be made that can prevent, improve, or relieve a patient's nausea. For examples, see question 17.
When opiate use is initiated, constipation may result unless a bowel regimen is initiated at the same time. If this is overlooked, the constipation may cause nausea, which is often blamed on the opiate and leads to unnecessary changes to the analgesic plan. In fact, nausea due to opiates tends to fade over time just as seasickness will fade as one eventually becomes accustomed to the motion of the boat.

24. Can all nausea and vomiting be successfully treated?
With the right approach, complete success can be gained in over 90% of patients. Remember to establish the probable cause, consider the neural pathways, neurotransmitters, and receptors involved, select the class of antiemetics that antagonizes those neurotransmitters/receptors, then select the most potent from that group, keeping in mind the side effects.

BIBLIOGRAPHY

1. Allan SG: Emesis in the patient with advanced cancer. Palliat Med 2:89–100, 1988.
2. Allan SG: Nausea and vomiting. In Doyle D, Hanks GWC, MacDonald N (eds): Oxford Textbook of Palliative Medicine. Oxford, Oxford University Press, 1993, pp 282–290.
3. Leslie RA, Shah Y, Thejomayen M, Murphy KM: The neuropharmacology of emesis: The role of receptors in neuromodulation of nausea and vomiting. Can J Physiol Pharmacol 68:279–288, 1990.
4. Lichter J: Which antiemetic? J Palliat Care 9:42–50, 1993.
5. Regnard C, Comiskey M: Nausea and vomiting in advanced cancer—a flow diagram. Palliat Med 6:146–151, 1992.
6. Reuben DB, Mor V: Nausea and vomiting in terminal cancer patients. Arch Intern Med 146:2021–2023, 1986.
7. Rousseau P: Antiemetic therapy in adults with terminal disease: A brief review. Am J Hospice Care 12:13–18, 1995.
8. Rousseau P: Nonpain symptom management in terminal care. Clin Geriatr Med 12:313–327, 1996.
9. Twycross RG, Lack SA: Nausea and vomiting. In Control of Alimentary Symptoms in Far Advanced Cancer. Edinburgh, Churchill Livingstone, 1986, pp 117–165.
10. Young RW: Mechanisms and treatment in radiation induced nausea and vomiting. In Davis CJ, Lake-Bakaar GV, Grahame-Smith DG (eds): Nausea and Vomiting: Mechanisms and Treatment. Berlin, Springer-Verlag, 1986, pp 94–109.

11. THE NATURE OF CANCER PAIN

Suresh K. Joishy, M.D., F.A.C.P.

1. Why is cancer pain so special?

Cancer pain defies definition. It is as complex as cancer itself. Despite a large number of major tomes written on pain, cancer pain remains an enigma to the medical professionals. Can you imagine having a medical specialist just for a single symptom, such as nausea, fatigue, or constipation? No. Specialties are based on diseases of organ systems. Not so when it comes to pain. Pain is the only symptom for which two specialty boards exist in the United States. In the United States and many other countries, anesthesiologists assume the role of pain specialists.

Nature probably designed pain as a warning signal so that primitive humans would know something was wrong when they were injured. So how did pain become a part of modern life? Hardly a day goes by without someone reporting a simple headache or gas pain! Conversely, many people are devastated by migraine headaches and rheumatoid arthritis. One of the first questions cancer patients usually ask after diagnosis is, "Am I going to have pain?" What will your answer be?

2. What factors must be considered in addressing cancer pain?

Dr. Cicely Saunders was the first to bring to the world's attention how medical science failed to control cancer pain in the terminally ill. The hospice movement she initiated proved that science must be combined with compassion and care of both patient and family to control symptoms. Any physician embarking on pain control in cancer patients must remember these principles of palliative care.

The nature of cancer pain is such that it is not an isolated symptom. The pain threshold and response to pain therapy largely depend on patient-related factors rather than the potency of analgesics. Simple patient-related factors include mood, morale, and energy level. Profound patient-related factors include spiritual beliefs and religious faith. One may argue that this is true for any symptom, although pain always stands out as the most dynamic process. Classifying acute and chronic pain in palliative care patients is futile. When the patient complains of pain, it is pain.

3. How is cancer pain defined?

There is no standard taxonomy to define cancer pain. The best definition is given by the International Association for the Study of Pain. "Pain is an unpleasant sensory and emotional experience associated with actual or potential tissue damage or described in terms of such damage." It is important to remember that pain has both **physical** components and **emotional** attributes and unless both are addressed vigorously, pain may never be relieved adequately.

4. What is meant by "total" pain?

Pain is not an isolated symptom. It is affected by other symptoms, compounding the patient's suffering. The sum of all the following interactions is called "total" pain.

Physical: Cancer and noncancer
Emotional: Anxiety and depression
Social: Isolation and abandonment
Spiritual: Agonizing search for meaning and purpose
Financial: Fear of burdening the family

5. Do all cancer patients suffer from pain?

Not all, but most (75%) will before the end of their journey. Many patients suffer from more than one pain: 20% have one pain; 80% have two or more pains; and 33% have four or more pains.

6. What are the top ten pains suffered by advanced cancer patients?
   1. Bone pain
   2. Nerve compression
   3. Visceral pain
   4. Soft tissue pain
   5. Muscle spasm, which may be secondary to bone pain
   6. Chronic postoperative pain
   7. Peripheral neuropathy, which may be related to surgery or chemotherapy and is considered treatment-related
   8. Low back pain
   9. Capsulitis of the shoulder
   10. Constipation

The first four pains are directly related to cancer. The last three pains may be related to debility.

7. Is cancer pain site-specific like migraine or arthritis?
   No, cancer pain may be in a local area, a metastatic area, or referred away from the site.
   1. **Head:** Metastatic tumors to brain, bone metastasis to skull bones and base of skull, primary brain tumor
   2. **Orbit:** Retro-orbital, tumor invasion, proptosis
   3. **Oropharyngeal:** Severe mucositis, candida, herpes virus, radiation
   4. **Neck:** Lymph node metastasis, head and neck tumors, postradical neck
   5. **Chest wall:** Posthoracotomy, pleural metastasis, apical lung, pancoast tumor, brachial plexopathy
   6. **Upper abdomen:** Liver metastasis, pancreatic, splenomegaly
   7. **Lower abdomen and pelvis:** Retroperitoneal, gynecologic tumors, bowel obstruction
   8. **Spine:** Cervical, thoracic, or lumbar vertebral metastasis
   9. **Upper limbs:** Neuropathy, lymphedema
   10. **Lower limbs:** Neuropathies, lymphedema, deep venous thrombosis, vasculitis

8. What is the etiology of pain in advanced cancer patients?
   1. **Direct tumor involvement (70%)**
      • Invasion of bone
      • Invasion of compression of neural structures
      • Obstruction of hollow viscus or ductal system of solid viscus
      • Vascular obstruction or invasion
      • Mucous membrane ulceration or involvement
   2. **Cancer-induced syndromes (< 10%)**
      • Paraneoplastic syndromes
      • Pain associated with debility (e.g., pressure sores, constipation, rectal or bladder spasm)
      • Other (e.g., postoperative herpetic neuralgia)
   3. **Diagnostic or therapeutic procedures (20%)**
      • Procedure-related pain (e.g,. bone marrow aspiration or biopsy, lumbar puncture)
      • Acute postoperative pain or postsurgical syndromes (e.g., postmastectomy, postthoracotomy, postamputation syndrome)
      • Postradiation (e.g., injury to nerve plexus or spinal cord, mucositis, enteritis)
      • Postchemotherapy (e.g., mucositis, peripheral neuropathy, aseptic necrosis)
   4. **Pain unrelated to the malignancy or its treatment (< 10%)**

9. What factors alter a patient's perception of pain on a day-to-day basis?
   In addition to the status of the cancer, the patient's mood and morale and the meaning of pain to the patient are important in pain perception. These factors should be considered for day-to-day assessment of pain.

10. What emotional factors are known to lower the pain threshold and intensify pain?

Anxiety, depression, fear, anger, boredom, isolation, and social abandonment are known to lower the pain threshold and intensify pain. These factors must be kept in mind in day-to-day pain assessment.

11. What emotional factors increase pain threshold and diminish pain?

Relief of associated symptoms, good sleep and rest, mood elevation, relief of anxiety and depression, empathy, and understanding are known to increase the pain threshold and diminish pain. These factors should be considered as important as analgesics for relieving pain.

12. What associated physical symptoms may exacerbate the pain component?

1. **Neurologic symptoms:** Headache, confusion, hiccups
2. **Gastrointestinal (GI) symptoms:** Dry or sore mouth, dysphagia, nausea, vomiting, constipation
3. **Genitourinary symptoms:** urinary burning, penile spasm, gladder spasm, urinary retention
4. **Respiratory symptoms:** cough, shortness of breath
5. **Other:** Muscle spasms, pruritus, lymphedema, fatigue, insomnia

These factors are enumerated to emphasize pain as a physical symptom that cannot be treated in isolation. Comprehensive evaluation of patients on a daily basis is paramount.

13. What is the generally applied classification of cancer pain?

Cancer pain is conveniently classified into four major categories:

1. **Somatic pain** is caused by tumor involvement of bone, muscle, or other integuments. Patients describe this pain as constant, aching, gnawing, and often well-localized.
2. **Visceral pain** is caused by tumor involvement of solid or hollow viscera. Patients describe it as constant, aching, colicky. Often associated with GI symptoms. Pain may be referred away from the organ of involvement.
3. **Neuropathic pain** is caused by tumor infiltration of peripheral or central neural pathways. Patients describe it as paroxysmal pains, electric shock–like burning, or a constricting sensation.
4. **Central or psychogenic pain** cannot be explained organically and is unrelieved by standard treatments. Pain of this type may result from unmet spiritual needs or associated emotional problems.

Classification of Cancer Pain

CANCER PAIN	PATHOPHYSIOLOGY	PATIENT'S DESCRIPTION	EXAMPLES
Somatic	Tumor involvement of bone/muscles	Constant, aching, gnawing	Bone metastasis, chest wall, muscle involvement
Visceral	Tumor involvement of hollow or solid viscera	Constant, aching (colicky); associated nausea, referred pains away from organ	Pancreatic cancer, liver metastasis, malignant bowel obstruction
Neuropathic	Deafferentation or involvement of afferent pathways of pain. Tumor infiltration of nerves. Nerve damage due to surgical intervention	(Paroxysmal) stabbing or electric shock–like burning ("lancinating"), vice-like	Brachial or lumbar plexopathy. Post herpetic neuralgia cord compression
Psychogenic/ Central	Unrelieved pain with emotional symptoms. Associated with any of the above pains	Never admits relief from standard treatments	Anxiety or depression, unmet spiritual needs

14. What are the common groups of pain descriptors that may help to diagnose the type of cancer pain?

PAIN DESCRIPTOR	CANCER PAIN
Tender, deep, aching, gnawing "all over"	Bone and soft tissue pain
Burning, shooting, stabbing, scalding	Neuropathic
Posterior head pain, intracranial pressure, nausea, headaches	CNS
Spasms, cramping, colicky	Visceral
Patients having more than one type of pain and mixed symptoms	Mixed

15. What are the features of pain due to hepatic involvement with cancer?

Hepatic pain due to cancer may be related to hepatomegaly and the stretching of liver capsule. The traction on hepatic ligaments when standing or walking, intrahepatic hemorrhage, and outward pressure on the rib cage or lumbar spinal strain (as in pregnancy) may cause pain. Hepatic pain is an important visceral pain because most common cancers (lung, colon, and breast) tend to metastasize to the liver.

16. How can lymphedema cause pain?

Lymphedema of the upper or lower limbs can cause considerable pain. Edema increases tissue pressure and muscle tension. Occasionally, lymphedema can cause neuropathic pain as a result of associated lymphatic invasion close to nerves or plexus. Patients with lymphedema are prone to inflammation and infection, which in turn can cause pain.

17. What are the features of pain resulting from bladder spasm?

Pain resulting from bladder spasm may occur because of intravesical, intramural, or extravesical invasion of bladder, prostate, or intrapelvic tumors. Bladder spasm may occur with or without urinary retention. Treatment-related bladder spasm, resulting from indwelling catheters with inflated balloons and fibrosis due to pelvic radiation, for example, also is a common occurrence in cancer patients. Urinary tract infections may occur easily in cancer patients and can cause bladder spasm. Bladder spasm is an important visceral pain and may be difficult to treat.

18. Why is neuropathic pain important?

Neuropathic pain belongs to an enormous spectrum of painful conditions. Description of all neuropathic syndromes is beyond the scope of this chapter. Because of close links with nervous tissue to the musculoskeletal system and locomotion, neuropathic pain can cause severe disabilities and poor quality of life. Control of neuropathic pain is difficult because patients are less responsive to strong opioids given by standard routes. Hence, neuropathic pain can be demoralizing and overwhelming to the cancer patient. When opioids with standard routes and addition of adjuncts fail, patients may need high-tech pain management methods such as epidural or intrathecal analgesia, resulting in considerable cost and burden to the patient and caregiver. Diagnosis and management of neuropathic pain require a multidisciplinary approach toward pain control. Accurate knowledge of neuroanatomy, dermatomal distributions of pain, and neuropharmacology are critical for choosing the best treatment options. Physical rehabilitation of the patient also is important.

19. How is neuropathic pain caused by cancer?

Neuropathic pain is caused by compression or invasion of peripheral nerves, nerve roots, or nerve plexuses by a growing tumor.

20. How do patients describe the pain when it is neuropathic?

"Extremely unpleasant," "burning," or "constricting." "Sharp," "constant," and "severe." It is referred to affected dermatomes and may be accompanied by allodynia (pain provoked by stimuli that normally do not cause pain (e.g., touch). Sometimes the patient may be unable to describe the pain accurately.

21. What is the role of corticosteroids in the management of neuropathic pain?

The theory of corticosteroid action is to shrink tumor-related edema, which may be causing nerve compression. It is more useful on rapidly growing tumors. Dexamethasone is the most commonly used steroid. High-dose intravenous dexamethasone is recommended in the management of acute or impending cord compression.

22. Do antidepressants have analgesic effects on neuropathic conditions?

Antidepressants play a major role in palliative care in the management of neuropathic pain. Amitriptyline (10–20 mg twice a day) is an effective adjunct to pain control with opioids. It takes less time to achieve analgesia than it does to control depression.

23. How do antidepressants help to control neuropathic pain?

Antidepressants have the ability to block the re-uptake of monoamines and modulate pain. Amitriptyline may also increase plasma concentration of morphine in cancer patients on stable doses.

24. How do anticonvulsants help to control neuropathic pain?

Anticonvulsants stabilize nerve membrane firing, consequently reducing pain perception and transmission.

25. Which anticonvulsant drugs are useful in controlling neuropathic pain?

Carbamazepine, phenytoin, and clonazepam have been used as adjuncts with opioids.

26. What are some examples of difficult to treat neuropathic pain?

1. **Plexopathies:**	Brachial
	Lumbar
2. **Epidural:**	Spinal cord compression
3. **Post surgical:**	Radical neck
	Mastectomy
	Thoracotomy
	Amputation
4. **Post chemotherapy:**	Neuropathies
5. **Post radiotherapy:**	Myelopathy
6. **Post herpetic:**	Neuralgia

BIBLIOGRAPHY

1. Ashby MA, et al: Description of mechanistic approach to pain management in advanced cancer. Preliminary Report. Pain 51:153–161, 1992.
2. Fields HL (ed): Core Curriculum for Professional Education in Pain: A Report of the Task Force on Professional Association for the Study of Pain. Seattle, IASP Press, 1997.
3. Galer BS: Neuropathic pain of peripheral origin: Advances in pharmacologic treatment. Neurology 45(suppl 9):17–25, 1995.
4. Grond S, et al: Assessment of cancer pain. A prospective evaluation in 2266 cancer patients referred to pain service. Pain 64:107–114, 1996.
5. Kenner DJ: Pain forum part-2. Neuropathic pain review. Australian Family Physician 23:1279–1283, 1994.
6. Portenoy RK: Cancer pain. Epidemiology and syndromes. Cancer 63:2298–2307, 1989.
7. Shannon MCM, et al: Assessment of pain in advanced cancer patients. J Pain Symptom Manage 41:141–145, 1995.
8. Sykes J, Johnson R, Hanks GW: ABC of palliative care. Difficult pain problems. BMJ 315:867–869, 1997.
9. Twycross R: Cancer pain classification. Acta Anasthesiol Scand 41:141–145, 1997.

12. PAIN ASSESSMENT IN PALLIATIVE CARE

Suresh K. Joishy, M.D., F.A.C.P.

1. With a background knowledge of cancer pain, how will you approach a patient for evaluation?

No two patients will describe pain in the same words. The dialogue on pain between the patient and physician is not finished until the pain is relieved. The following items must be included in the dialogue for a rational approach to pain management:
- The patient must identify the site of pain. The site may indicate the organ of involvement, a referred pain from a distant organ, or dermatomal pain away from the site of the nerve root.
- Duration of pain may indicate acute, subacute, or chronic pain.
- Intensity of pain may be mild, moderate, or severe.
- Exacerbating or relieving factors may be important to be able to assess incidental pain or breakthrough pains.
- Quality of pain, whether constant or lancinating, may help differentiate somatic and neuropathic pain.
- Accompanying symptoms of diaphoresis, nausea, vomiting, or palpitation may indicate visceral pains.
- How the pain interferes with activities of daily living may indicate the need for physical therapy and rehabilitation.
- Impact on the patient's psychological status may show unmet spiritual and emotional needs.
- Response to previous and current analgesic therapies may help to modify, change, or choose a new regimen for pain control.

2. What are the World Health Organization guidelines for evaluating pain?
- Believe the patient's report of pain.
- Initiate discussions of pain.
- Evaluate the severity of the patient's pain.
- Take a detailed history of the pain.
- Evaluate the psychological state of the patient.
- Perform a careful physical examination.
- Order and personally review any necessary investigations.
- Consider alternative methods of pain relief.
- Monitor the results of the treatment.

3. What are the PQRST characteristics of pain?

P   Palliative factors: What makes pain less intense?
Provocative factors: What makes it worse?
Q   Quality: What is it like?
R   Radiation: Does it spread anywhere else?
S   Severity: How severe is it?
T   Temporal factors: Is it constant or sporadic?

4. How do you assess pain on a daily basis in palliative care?

Several measurement tools are available to assess intensity of pain alone (unidimensional) or combinations of factors such as pain intensity, mood, and pain relief (multidimensional). However, multidimensional measurement tools are not suitable in the palliative care setting because patients are too weak to understand and answer numerous questions objectively. This author prefers unidimensional pain measurement scales focusing on pain intensity or relief.

Examples include visual analog, numeric, and categorical scales. Good history taking combined with a numeric pain scale is best suited for palliative care patients.

5. How do you assess pain intensity in a cognitively impaired patient?

Listen to the patient's vocalization, including moaning and groaning. Ask for observations by family members or caregivers. Observe the patient's facial expressions such as furrowed brows. Changes in physiologic responses, such as an increase in pulse rate or decrease in blood pressure, may help but are not consistently useful. Finally, give a trial dose of analgesic and observe the response.

6. When is cancer pain overwhelming?

When severe pain is compounded by insomnia, fatigue, mental exhaustion, loss of morale, and emerging distrust of the caregiver, the pain is considered overwhelming. At times it is overwhelming not only to patients, but to caregivers. Overwhelming pain may be associated with physical reluctance, depression, and dependence on unsatisfactory medications. When a patient is afraid to move, markedly anxious, and agitated, and has no faith in any medication, consider the pain a medical emergency, and hospitalize the patient.

BIBLIOGRAPHY

1. Dudgeon D, Raubertas RF, Rosenthal SN: The short-form McGill pain questionnaire in chronic cancer pain. J Pain Symptom Manage 8:191–195, 1993.
2. Fields HL (ed): Pain measurement in humans. In Core Curriculum for Professional Education in Pain. Seattle, WA, IASP Press, 1995, pp 9–12.
3. Jensen MP, Karloy P, Braver S: The measurement of pain intensity: A comparison of six methods. Pain 27:117–126, 1986.

13. MORPHINE

Suresh K. Joishy, M.D., F.A.C.P.

1. Why is morphine so important in palliative care?

Morphine is the oldest analgesic known to mankind. In these days of drug synthesis using molecular biology, it is humbling to note that the high-tech pharmaceutical industry has not succeeded in manufacturing a better painkiller. We are indebted to the wisdom and observational power of ancient physicians for discovering morphine.

Morphine is an integral part of palliative care because pain is the most important symptom suffered by patients with life-limiting illnesses. The effectiveness of a palliative care physician is very limited unless he or she knows how to use morphine and control pain with confidence.

2. Is morphine a dangerous drug?

Physicians still treat morphine as a dangerous drug when, in fact, it is a "wonder drug." The physician treating a patient with congestive heart failure, pulmonary edema, or cardiac arrhythmia will use digoxin by intravenous titration, without hesitation. Digoxin is a more dangerous drug causing significant mortality because of the sudden and unpredictable development of digitalis toxicity and cardiac arrhythmia. That same physician will invariably hesitate to treat a patient with intravenous morphine to control severe pain. Why?

The very nomenclature used to describe morphine evokes fear of addiction in both medical professionals and the lay public. Morphine is described as a narcotic. This author strongly recommends discarding the word "narcotic" and replacing it with "opioid" or "opiate."

3. What are some of the additional properties of morphine?

Morphine is one of the most versatile drugs available in clinical therapeutics. It can be used by a myriad of routes: oral, sublingual, rectal, intramuscular, subcutaneous, intravenous, epidural, intrathecal, intranasal, and pulmonary. The dosing schedules that can be adopted for patients appear infinite. Most common drugs used today have a therapeutic range for dose beyond which they are ineffective. This is called the "ceiling effect." Morphine is probably the only drug that has *no* ceiling effect for dosing.

Morphine cannot be used indiscriminately, but the toxicity of morphine is patient related and not dose dependent. Patients appear to handle morphine metabolites differently in different pain situations. Thus, the morphine dose can be a fraction of a milligram per hour to hundreds of milligrams per hour.

Lack of education about morphine and pain management principles are the major stumbling blocks when using morphine. Palliative care, and consequently pain and the use of morphine, are not generally part of medical school curricula or physician training. Until this lack of education is rectified, morphine will be underused, much to the unnecessary suffering of palliative care patients.

Although morphine can be used for pain control, it is equally beneficial for treating other distressing symptoms. It is a drug par-excellence in controlling dyspnea in any patient with life-limiting illness. When patients are at the end of their life, there is nothing like morphine to achieve sedation and total comfort.

4. What are the five essential ingredients for successful pain control with morphine?

1. **Determination.** Before contemplating whether to use morphine, make a determination that the pain will be controlled. This confidence should come from the fact that morphine does, in fact, control most types of pain.

2. **Imagination and innovation.** As previously mentioned, morphine is one of the most versatile drugs. Choose from the numerous possibilities arising from the different formulations of morphine, different dose schedules, and numerous routes of administration.

3. **Professional education.** Pain control is a team effort. Explain to palliative care team members, particularly the nurse taking the orders, the rationale behind the use of morphine and the observations that must be made. There is absolutely no room for errors in morphine orders.

4. **Patient education.** The patient needs to know when they are on morphine. They need to be educated about any anticipated side effects. Above all, they should be able to express their own opinion about pain response to morphine. They should be educated about the pain assessment scales used, breakthrough pain, and rescue dosing with morphine.

5. **Family education.** Allaying fears of patient addiction to morphine is paramount. They should be told clearly what to expect and what not to expect. If not well-educated, when the side effects set in, a family member may demand morphine be stopped. Patients and family tend to equate side effects with "allergy."

5. What are the five essentials of the World Health Organization (WHO) recommendations for administration of analgesics?

- By the clock: Schedule doses over 24 hours.
- By the ladder: Use pain medicines "stepwise," according to pain intensity.
- By the patient: Accurately diagnose the type of pain in the individual patient.
- Use morphine for severe pain.
- Continually reassess patient response to analgesics.

6. What is the "WHO ladder" for pain control?

The WHO ladder is a three-step ladder used to illustrate standard guidelines for pain control drug therapy (see Chapter 24). The first step is to use non-opioid, mild analgesics such as acetaminophen for mild pain. For pain of moderate intensity, weaker opioids such as oxycodone are used. If pain is still not relieved, or if it is severe, a stronger opioid such as morphine is used.

7. What are the general principles of pain management?

- Believe the patient's complaint of pain, regardless of your opinion.
- Aim to achieve control at a level acceptable to the patient. It may not be necessary or possible to make the patient completely pain-free.
- Most patients with advanced cancer are polysymptomatic. All symptoms must be addressed with equal concern.
- Psychosocial factors such as anxiety, fear, and depression aggravate the pain experience and should be treated appropriately.
- Always consult palliative care team members to manage "total pain."

8. What guidelines must be followed when starting opioid analgesics in pain management?

1. Use a specific opioid for a specific type of pain. Consult the WHO ladder.
2. Know the pharmacology of the opioids thoroughly.
3. Apply routes of administration to the patient's needs.
4. Administer the drug on a regular basis after initial titration.
5. Use adjuncts judiciously to provide the additive analgesia and minimize side effects.
6. Avoid drug combinations that increase sedation without enhancing analgesia.

9. Which treatments are avoided as first line in cancer pain therapy?

Treatments to be avoided and the reasons that they should be avoided are listed in the table at the top of the facing page.

TREATMENT	REASONS TO AVOID
Meperidine	Low potency. Toxic metabolite accumulation, convulsions
Pentazocin	Increased hallucinations, agitation
Methadone*	Long half-life (48–72 hr), short duration of action. Accumulation of toxic metabolites. Difficult to titrate
IM injections	Painful, not practical in emaciated patients
Suppository forms†	Q 4 hr insertion not practical for titration. Caregiver burden
Pain cocktails	Active ingredient is morphine, which is better given in original form

* May be used when other opioids have failed.
† May be used for stable pain requiring less frequent administration.

10. Is the WHO ladder suitable in a palliative care setting?

It is suitable in principle but not entirely in practice. Palliative care patients with life-limiting illness rarely have the mild pain that can be relieved by acetaminophen or an NSAID. Invariably, these patients have already used numerous analgesics before coming to palliative care. More often, the first step of the ladder is skipped by jumping directly to the second step. All steps of the WHO ladder refer to oral analgesics. In a palliative care setting, parenteral morphine is frequently used. It is understandable that WHO guidelines have taken into account economic factors that are not ideal for parenteral use of opioids. In practice, and even in developing countries if the economic situation allows, indications for parenteral opioids expand for better pain control.

The author has designed an opioid staircase most suitable for palliative care (see below). The three steps represent the opioids used as pain intensity increases. As they become ineffective, the opioid preparations in the higher steps are used. The stairway rails represent the principles of opioid administration: around the clock (ATC), rescue dosing, and adjuncts.

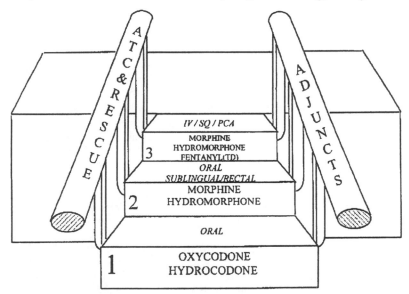

Opioid staircase for pain control in palliative care.

11. When is morphine the drug of choice in cancer pain control?
- Morphine should be used when weaker opioids have failed.
- Morphine can be used as a first-line drug in clinical situations of severe pain.

- Morphine is the drug of choice when the cycle of pain in combination with other symptoms must be broken immediately.
- Morphine should be used as a "portmanteau" drug when a patient has pain associated with dyspnea or cough.
- Morphine is the drug of choice if sedation is required along with pain control.

12. What is the ideal analgesic for cancer pain?

The analgesic chosen for cancer pain should have a rapid onset of action with a short, measurable half-life. It should have strong analgesic potency and should achieve excellent analgesia. The drug should have a high safety profile with few side effects. The patient should be able to maintain clear sensorium. The patient should not develop tolerance to the drug on prolonged administration. Morphine fulfills most of the requirements of an ideal analgesic for cancer pain control.

13. Why is morphine classified as an agonist?

Morphine, hydromorphone, codeine, oxycodone, hydrocodone, oxymorphone, and levorphanol are agonist opioids. These are called "agonist" because they bind to the receptors for their analgesic actions (*mu* receptor agonists).

14. Why are some opioids called partial agonists?

Buprenorphine is an opioid that binds to receptors to produce analgesia. However, unlike morphine, it has a ceiling effect—increasing the drug dose does not produce an increase in analgesia. Hence, it is called a partial agonist.

15. Are there antagonists to opioids?

Naloxone binds to the opioid receptors but does not have the ability to produce analgesia. As a matter of fact, it can block the action of an agonist such as morphine and is used as an antagonist to treat overdose.

16. What are agonists/antagonists?

Pentazocin and butorphanol bind to a specific opioid receptor (kappa) to produce analgesia but also can bind to the *mu* receptor and block the action of the agonist opioids. Hence, these opioids are call agonists/antagonists.

17. Why is morphine preferred over meperidine in cancer pain control?

Meperidine is not to be used for chronic cancer pain, although it is a popular drug in the United States for treating acute and non-malignant chronic pain. The side effects of meperidine outweigh the benefits in treating severe pain in cancer patients. Meperidine has a shorter duration of action than morphine. Toxic metabolites of meperidine may accumulate over time and cause myoclonus, agitation, and convulsions. Besides being analgesic, morphine also has antitussive properties and can aid in respiratory comfort. Meperidine has no such added benefits. Occasionally, a patient in stable pain may refuse to switch to morphine or another opioid. As long as pain remains stable and can be monitored, patient autonomy should prevail.

18. What are the general guidelines used in palliative care in the administration of morphine?

- Start with a specific preparation for a specific patient with a specific clinical situation. For example, if a patient has difficulty swallowing tablets, start with liquid morphine.
- Know the basic pharmacology of morphine, such as its half-life and duration of action, and toxic metabolite accumulation in renal/hepatic impairment.
- Understand the methods of administration such as titration, around-the-clock dosing, and rescue dosing.
- Change the route of administration according to the patient's need, and change the doses according to the route of administration.

- Know how to use the equianalgesic table for morphine when switching preparations and routes.
- Do not stop morphine suddenly. Use titration to prevent precipitation of acute withdrawal symptoms and rebound of severe pain.
- Pre-empt common side effects. To prevent constipation, write orders for a good bowel regimen as soon as orders are written for morphine. Prevent nausea in the initial stages of starting morphine.
- Anticipate uncommon side effects and know how to treat them. These include myoclonus and itching.
- Do not give naloxone in haste just because of reduced respiratory rate. Monitor the patient's respiratory rate and level of sedation. The dose of naloxone in palliative care must be modified (see question 40).
- Do not use morphine as a placebo. A good physician is a good placebo!

19. What are the routes of morphine administration?

Morphine is a versatile drug that can be administered by any route. Strive to administer morphine by the least invasive and most convenient route for the patient, while still achieving effective analgesia.

The oral route is always preferred. If the patient has impaired swallowing, use the noninvasive rectal and sublingual routes. The potency of rectal suppositories is equal to that of oral dosing. Controlled release morphine tablets can be used rectally with good results. The bioavailability of the sublingual route is poor for morphine and the effect is probably related to part of the drug being swallowed. Sublingual administration of injectable morphine may be tried. Parenteral routes are considered for titration in acute severe pain, or for patients with impaired swallowing. Painful intramuscular injections should be avoided in palliative care patients who require frequent dosing. Continuous infusions of morphine can be administered by intravenous or subcutaneous routes.

20. What is meant by an "opioid naive" patient?

One of the most critical pieces of information needed for cancer pain assessment is previous analgesic history. When starting a patient on morphine for severe pain, it is important to 'titrate' the dose of morphine (see question 25). Before writing the orders for morphine, determine the starting dose, the around-the-clock dose, and the rescue dose. The dose calculation depends on principles of equianalgesic dosing (see Chapter 14). It is critical to know if the patient has been on opioids before. If the patient has not, he or she is called "opioid naive." In this case, the starting dose of morphine should be the lowest possible and titrated upward carefully.

21. What are the major side effects of morphine?

Gastrointestinal: Nausea, constipation, opioid bowel syndrome (pseudo bowel obstruction)
Genitourinary: Urinary retention
CNS: Sedation, confusion, hallucinations, dysphoria, depression
Neuromuscular: Myoclonic jerks
Respiratory: Rare, dose limiting

22. What is opioid bowel syndrome?

Morphine and other opioids are known to reduce bowel motility and encourage constipation. Every patient on morphine should be on a good, prophylactic bowel regimen.

When the patient is being titrated upward with morphine over a period of time, symptoms of constipation, nausea, and recurrent vomiting may ensue. These symptoms mimic bowel obstruction. A plain x-ray of the abdomen, flat and upright, may show distended loops of bowel and possible air fluid levels. This condition is reversible, unlike complete bowel obstruction caused by cancer. If pain remains a major problem, morphine can still be used. However, a morphine-sparing drug should be added to bring down the dose of morphine, which may indirectly resolve the bowel obstruction.

23. Why is respiratory depression caused by morphine uncommon?

- Respiratory depression is still the most misunderstood side effect of morphine. Respiratory depression is confused with respiratory failure. Palliative care physicians may rarely have a chance to use the opioid antidote naloxone.
- The principle and practice of titration with morphine are outlined below. If followed diligently, they will provide graded escalation of doses of morphine, thus avoiding respiratory depression.
- Tolerance to morphine leads to tolerance of respiratory depression.
- Morphine is actually regularly used in palliative care to control dyspnea (see question 39).

24. What is meant by titration with morphine?

Starting a patient on morphine by any preparation and route, and trying to determine the optimum dose to control pain with minimal side effects is called "titration." Morphine can be titrated by upward dosing and by downward dosing. Upward dosing is called escalation, which is a common event in severe pain.

This author calls the duration of dosing adjustments until pain is stabilized the "titration period." Several dosing and frequency principles will be observed during the titration period, and these are explained in the questions that follow.

Once pain is controlled after titration, the patient enters the "stable baseline pain" period. Again, dosing and frequency principles are different in the baseline pain period.

25. What are the principles of morphine titration?

- Determine whether the patient is opioid naive or on chronic opioid therapy. The starting dose of morphine in opioid naive patients should be the lowest possible except in cases of extremely severe pain. If the patient has been on opioids other than morphine, or known to be opioid tolerant, equianalgesic dosing principles are followed for starting doses and titration.
- If the patient has been on more than one opioid and more than one route, e.g., fentanyl transdermal patch and rescue doses of oral oxycodone or liquid morphine, all of these opioids are first converted to equianalgesic doses calculated for morphine.
- Apply the principles of around-the-clock and rescue dosing.
- Understand the nature of breakthrough pain to order appropriate rescue doses.
- The oral route is preferable whenever possible in opioid naive patients if pain is not overwhelming and if patient compliance is assured at home or in the hospital.
- If oral titration is indicated, begin with liquid morphine.
- In a hospital setting, if parenteral titration is indicated, the intravenous route is preferred.
- If titration via patient-controlled analgesia (PCA) is indicated, wait for a few hours after beginning IV or SQ morphine titration. Observe the patient to get a sense of the pain. The waiting period can also be used to educate the patient about PCA.
- The orders for titration should be absolutely clear to the attending physician and nurse(s).

26. What is the ATC dose of morphine?

It is that dose of morphine given continuously on a scheduled plan "around the clock" (ATC). The interval between ATC doses can range from a few minutes during the titration period, to many hours during stable pain, or even to continuous release (also called slow release) morphine given every 12 hours. The ATC dose applies to any route of administration. Morphine can be given ATC by the oral, sublingual, rectal, IV, subcutaneous, epidural, and intrathecal routes.

27. What is breakthrough pain?

Breakthrough pain is the transitory increase in pain to a greater intensity than baseline. Baseline pain is pain reported by the patient as the average pain intensity experienced for 12 or more hours during the 24 hours prior to interview. To define breakthrough pain, baseline pain should have been of moderate or less intensity, and the breakthrough pain is severe or excruciating by comparison. If baseline pain is severe or worse, it is considered uncontrolled pain and there is no breakthrough pain. Breakthrough pain is a transitory increase in pain greater than moderate intensity (severe or excruciating) occurring on a baseline pain of moderate intensity or less. In practice, patients are evaluated if there is a relationship between the morphine analgesic regimen and pain occurrence or worsening during dosing intervals.

28. How is breakthrough pain assessed?

Breakthrough pain must be assessed in the same manner as any other pain is assessed, noting location, severity, temporal characteristics, precipitating and relieving factors, pathophysiology (somatic, visceral, neuropathic, and mixed), and etiology.

29. What is the differential diagnosis for breakthrough pain?

When breakthrough pain is precipitated by volitional movements, such as movement in bed, ambulation, and touch, it is called "incidental pain." Non-volitional movements such as cough, hiccups, and bowel and utereric distention may precipitate breakthrough pain. Breakthrough pain may occur because of analgesic failure resulting from inadequate dosing or end of dose failure. Often, breakthrough pain occurs with no identifiable precipitant.

30. What is the rescue dose of morphine?

The rescue dose of morphine is that dose of morphine that is
- given in addition to the ATC dose of morphine
- given on an as-needed basis
- given in defined, pre-ordered intervals PRN
- given to control breakthrough pain (see question 27)
- always given as an immediate-release preparation, oral or parenteral. Never give long-acting (slow-release or continuous-release) morphine for rescue dosing.
- generally identical to ATC preparation with exceptions. When ATC morphine is a slow-release preparation, the rescue dose morphine is an immediate-release preparation, tablet, or liquid. When transdermal fentanyl or methadone are ATC opioids, an oral morphine immediate-release preparation is the rescue opioid.
- sometimes given as a bolus dose on an unscheduled interval to treat incidental pain (see question 29) any time prior to anticipated activity or movement known to cause pain.

31. What is a bolus dose?

Unfortunately, "bolus" is a loosely used word that often refers to a rescue dose. I prefer to reserve the word "bolus" for any single dose or extra dose of morphine given on unscheduled intervals. A good example is a dose of morphine given prior to anticipated incidental pain—such as a pain aggravated by moving a patient out of bed or sending the patient for tests known to cause pain. Another example is when intense pain during the titration period requires an extra dose in addition to the already ordered rescue dose. In this sense, the bolus is actually a supplemental dose to the rescue dose of morphine. Some use the word bolus for the first dose of morphine given in the titration (also referred to by some as the "loading dose").

All bolus doses should be treated similarly to ATC and rescue doses of morphine, and should be included in the calculated total dose of morphine for the 24-hour period.

Generally, the amount of a single bolus ordered is the same as that for the rescue dose. However, if bolus doses are found to be ineffective, morphine should be titrated upward on ATC rescue principles.

32. What understanding is required for calculating rescue doses of morphine?
- Rescue doses are calculated as a percentage of the ATC dose.
- The percentage of rescue doses varies when applied during the titration period or during the stable pain period, based on the pain control required.

- Rescue doses are given PRN at defined, ordered intervals.
- Intervals ordered for rescue doses vary between the titration period and the stable baseline period.
- The PRN interval between rescue doses depends on the time required for peak morphine effect, which varies among different preparations and routes of administration. The rationale is simple. Pain control should be best at the time of peak effect. If not, the patient will need rescue doses at that time.

33. What are the formulas used for calculating rescue doses during the titration period?
- Titration by mouth: Immediate-release morphine, tablet or liquid, is used for ATC dosing. The rescue dose for PO titration is 50% of the ATC dose given every hour PRN until pain is stabilized. Never use slow-release morphine as a rescue drug. The rescue interval in the baseline period is every 2 hours.
- Titration by parenteral route IV or SQ. The parenteral rescue dose is 50% of the ATC dose every 15–30 minutes until pain is stabilized. When pain is overwhelming, the rescue dose can be 100% of the ATC dose for a short time only.
- It is always better to increase the ATC dose rather than to increase the frequency and amount of the rescue doses.
- Rescue doses are concomitantly increased or decreased according to ATC doses.

Rescue Doses During Titration Period

TITRATION MORPHINE PREPARATION	RESCUE DOSE	PRN INTERVAL
PO MS IR tablet or liquid	50% of 4 hourly ATC dose	Q 1 hour
IV/SQ MS IR injectable	50% of hourly ATC dose	Q 15–30 minutes PRN

34. What formulas are used for calculating rescue doses during the stable baseline period of pain?
- When immediate-release morphine is used, such as in tablet or liquid form, 50% of the ATC dose is given as a rescue dose every 2 hours PRN.
- When slow-release PO morphine preparation is used every 12 hours, the MS IR (morphine immediate-release) rescue dose is 10–17% of the total 24 hour dose of slow-release morphine. For convenience's sake, 1/6 of the total 24-hour slow-release morphine is given as immediate-release morphine every 2–4 hours PRN.
- For baseline pain by parenteral route (IV, SQ), the rescue dose is 50% of the hourly ATC dose, given every 2 hours PRN.

Rescue Doses During Stable Baseline Period

BASELINE MORPHINE PREPARATION	RESCUE DOSE	PRN INTERVAL
PO MS IR tablet or liquid	50% of ATC dose	Q 2 hours
PO MS slow-release tablet	1/6 (10–17%) of total 24 ATC dose	Q 2–4 hours
IV/SQ MS IR injectable	50% of hourly ATC dose	Q 2 hours

35. When are ATC doses and, consequently, rescue doses to be increased or decreased?
  1. **Titration period**
     Assess pain every 4 hours while titrating PO or IV. If the patient receives more than 2 rescue doses in a 4-hour period, increase the ATC dose by 50% and calculate the appropriate new rescue dose for each route with appropriate intervals PRN (see question 32).

2. **Baseline period**
   - Assess the patient every 24 hours for the necessity to increase or decrease the ATC dose and, consequently, the rescue dose. If the patient has received more than 5 rescue doses, increase the ATC dose by 25% and increase the rescue doses as previously described.
   - If the patient required no rescue doses in a 24-hour period, maintain the same orders. Decrease the ATC dose and rescue doses only if side effects become troublesome.
   - Know the formulas for the relationships between ATC and rescue dosing during the titration period.
   - The oral route is preferred whenever possible in opioid naive patients, and if pain is not overwhelming.

36. When is morphine ATC IV to be reduced or stopped?
It is rare to do both in severe acute pain during titration in a palliative care setting.
   - If side effects are troublesome, reduce the ATC dose by 25% with an appropriate reduction in the rescue dose.
   - If excessive sedation or severe bradypnea occurs, stop the ATC dosing and rescue infusion until the patient recovers.
   - Restart morphine at 75% of the previous ATC dose.
   - Restart morphine when the next dose of the previously scheduled ATC dose is due.
   - Check IV lines and pumps to ensure that they are functioning accurately.

37. What are the acceptable side effects of morphine continuous infusion (CI)?
Continuous infusion of morphine IV/SQ over a period of time may show acceptable physical signs. There is no direct relationship between plasma concentration of morphine and therapeutic effects.
   - Respiratory rate may be reduced from normal without causing symptoms.
   - PO_2 may drop without new symptoms.
   - Even with high doses, the patient may still remain alert and experience only slight drowsiness.
   - Morphine has no significant effects on PCO_2, blood pressure, or heart rate.
   Note: When patients show both somnolence and bradypnea, consider morphine overdose.

38. What steps should be taken to manage morphine-induced sedation?
   - Polypharmacy is common in palliative care patients. Depression or confusion caused by other drugs such as antiemetics or anxiolytics will be blamed on morphine. The first step is to review all of the medications and discontinue those that are suspected.
   - If pain control is good in the face of sedation, reduce the ATC dose by 25%. Don't forget to reduce the rescue doses too.
   - If morphine cannot be reduced because of persistent pain, try methylphenidate, 5 mg PO BID. This dose may be doubled. An alternate drug is dexamethasone, 4 mg PO BID.
   - Consider a morphine sparing drug to reduce the dose of morphine without compromising pain control (e.g., NSAID PO or ketorolac IV).
   - If sedation is still a problem, consider opioid rotation. Choose an alternative opioid to morphine in an equianalgesic dose.

39. What are the principles of morphine therapy to control dyspnea in palliative care?
   - When general measures have been ineffective, morphine becomes a first choice drug.
   - Morphine can be used safely even in COPD patients by using individual titration and beginning with lower doses.
   - Follow the same principles as for pain management.
   - Increase doses 30–50% q 4–12 hours until the patient becomes comfortable.
   - As part of terminal sedation in patients with intractable dyspnea, use morphine with other drug combinations (e.g., chlorpromazine, atropine, etc.).

40. How might a patient (rarely) go into respiratory failure/depression while on morphine, and how can this be treated?

Sensitivity to PCO_2 is reduced by morphine. Respiratory depression may manifest itself by slow, irregular breathing. Patients may be comfortable without somnolence at a rate of up to 10/mt. Generally, the respiratory depression is detected 7–30 minutes after IV morphine, and 90 minutes after subcutaneous morphine.

If the patient's respiratory rate drops below 10/mt, the morphine must be stopped and the patient must be observed closely for any further drop in respiratory rate. Do not hastily administer naloxone, but be prepared. If the respiratory rate drops below 8/mt, naloxone treatment should start immediately.

Guidelines for using naloxone in non-cancer patients and the acute opioid toxicity of addiction are not applicable in palliative care. Generally, lower doses of naloxone are indicated so that the patient will not rebound with acute, severe pain. Dilute 1 amp of naloxone 0.4 mg in 10 cc of NaCl. Give 1 cc of this diluted naloxone, i.e., 0.04 mg every five minutes IV, until partial arousal has occurred.

41. What are the reasons for incomplete pain relief with morphine?
- The dosage needs to be increased.
- An adjunct pharmaceutical, such as an NSAID for bone pain or amitriptyline for neuropathic pain, may need to be prescribed.
- Breakthrough pains have not been well addressed.
- Vomiting occurred after taking oral morphine.
- Unresolved issues such as anger, fear, or anxiety may be exacerbating pain.
- The pain is truly morphine resistant.

42. What are the patient-related factors for unrelieved pain?

Non-compliance is a major issue. Patients fail to seek medical attention until pain becomes severe. They think they need morphine only "when absolutely necessary." Fear of addiction is also common. Some patients may have less confidence in morphine tablets taken orally, believing that strong pain needs parenteral morphine. Some patients stop taking morphine because side effects such as nausea or vomiting are mistaken for an allergic reaction.

43. What are the physician-related causes for undertreatment with morphine and, consequently, unrelieved pain?

The reasons for unrelieved pain while on morphine are numerous and many of them rest with medical professionals. Failure to fully assess pain intensity at regular or specified intervals leads to underdosing. Physicians may increase the frequency of the ATC dose rather than increase the dose itself. Rescue doses tend to be miscalculated in relation to the ATC dose. A lack of knowledge about the equianalgesic potency of morphine with other opioids, and negligence in referring to equianalgesic tables, may cause undertreatment. There is also the unwarranted fear of respiratory depression, which causes the physician to withhold higher doses of morphine. Unfortunately, higher doses of morphine are withheld until the patient is very close to death. Failure to use appropriate adjuncts with morphine leads to refractory pain syndromes. Physician failure to properly educate patient and family may lead to non-compliance.

44. What are the causes for delays in getting the PRN dose of morphine to a patient in the hospital setting?

There may be 15 minutes to 2 hours of delay in getting morphine, particularly parenteral morphine PRN, to a patient in the hospital setting. The delays may be longer in getting the first dose to the patient after a new order is written by a physician. (See figure on facing page.)

45. How is pain relief from morphine assessed?

Pain relief should be assessed in relation to comfort achieved:

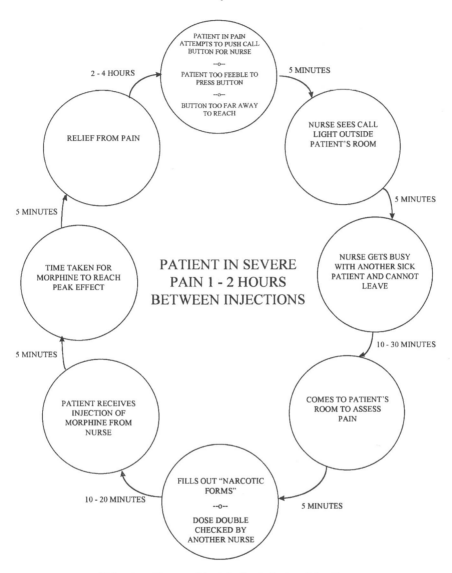

PATIENT IN SEVERE
PAIN 1 - 2 HOURS
BETWEEN INJECTIONS

PATIENT IN PAIN
ATTEMPTS TO PUSH CALL
BUTTON FOR NURSE
--o--
PATIENT TOO FEEBLE TO
PRESS BUTTON
--o--
BUTTON TOO FAR AWAY
TO REACH

2 - 4 HOURS

5 MINUTES

NURSE SEES CALL
LIGHT OUTSIDE
PATIENT'S ROOM

RELIEF FROM PAIN

5 MINUTES

5 MINUTES

NURSE GETS BUSY
WITH ANOTHER SICK
PATIENT AND CANNOT
LEAVE

TIME TAKEN FOR
MORPHINE TO REACH
PEAK EFFECT

5 MINUTES

10 - 30 MINUTES

PATIENT RECEIVES
INJECTION OF
MORPHINE FROM
NURSE

COMES TO PATIENT'S
ROOM TO ASSESS
PAIN

FILLS OUT "NARCOTIC
FORMS"
--o--
DOSE DOUBLE
CHECKED BY
ANOTHER NURSE

10 - 20 MINUTES

5 MINUTES

Delays in getting morphine injection in the hospital setting.

- During the night
- During the day
- During movement

Reassessment remains a continuing necessity; old pains may get worse and new pains may develop. **ALWAYS REVIEW!**

46. Is this information about morphine applicable to other opioids?

Yes. Morphine is the "gold standard" opioid. All of the principles of administration of morphine for pain control are applicable to other opioids. A glossary on morphine in Chapter 34 addresses the principles of administration of other opioids in relationship to morphine. Morphine is also the most versatile drug regarding preparations, dose, schedule, route, and safety profile.

BIBLIOGRAPHY

1. Bruera E, Lawlor P: Cancer pain management. Acta Anaesthesiol Scand 41:146–153, 1997.
2. Cherny NJ, et al: Opioid pharmacotherapy in the management of cancer pain: A survey of strategies used by pain physicians for the selection of analgesic drugs and routes of administration. Cancer 76:1288–1293, 1995.
3. Cleary JF: Pharmacokinetic and pharmacodynamic issues in the treatement of breakthrough pain. Semin Oncol 24(suppl 16):13–19, 1997.
4. Foley KM: Controversies in cancer pain: Medical perspectives. Cancer 63:2257–2265, 1989.
5. Haviley C, et al: Pharmacological management of cancer pain: A guide for health care professionals. Cancer Nurs 15:331–346, 1992.
6. Jadad AR, Browman GP: The WHO analgesic ladder for cancer pain management. JAMA 274:1870–1873, 1995.
7. McQuay HJ: Opioid use in cancer pain. Acta Anaesthesiol Scand 41:146–153, 1997.
8. Portenoy RK: Treatment of temporal variations in chronic cancer pain. Semin Oncol 24(suppl 16):7–12, 1997.
9. Simmond MA: Pharmacotherapeutic management of cancer pain/current practice. Semin Oncol 24(suppl 16):1–16, 1997.
10. Twycross RG: Pain Relief in Advanced Cancer. Edinburgh, Churchill Livingstone, 1994.

14. EQUIANALGESIA DEMYSTIFIED

Suresh K. Joishy, M.D., F.A.C.P.

1. What is equianalgesia?

If the name *morphine* is tainted by myths, *equianalgesia* is shrouded in mystery. Equianalgesia refers to comparison of analgesic potency of one opioid with another, or it refers to the same opioid administered in different routes expressed as a calculated dose in milligrams. The major stumbling block in the understanding and application of equianalgesia is that physicians shun the mathematics required for the calculations.

If one decides to use morphine to control cancer pain, knowledge of equianalgesia is mandatory. The equianalgesic potencies of some opioids have been examined in pharmacokinetic studies. A standardized but not always accurate equianalgesic scale, chart, or table is always readily available for reference. Equianalgesic tables are available in several sizes and shapes, and pocket-sized tables are handy for instant reference.

There are numerous situations in which a palliative care physician needs to apply equianalgesic principles. When morphine is used from the oral to parenteral route, or vice versa, and when morphine is chosen over other opioids, it is best to refer to the equianalgesic table for the appropriate dose of morphine rather than depend on memory. Because dose ranging is wide, opioids are many, and routes are numerous, each opioid has received a numeric conversion factor. By referring to the equianalgesic table, one can find the conversion factor for morphine and determine the equianalgesic dose for a given route.

2. Why do health care professionals not readily refer to equianalgesic tables?

The problem lies with both the tables and the physicians. Equianalgesic tables show lack of clarity and standardization. Health care professionals are not trained how to use equianalgesic tables and feel overwhelmed seeing a dozen opioids listed haphazardly with equally confusing conversion factors. Conversion factors for various routes of administration are often given in different tables or on different pages. It is not clear whether to multiply or divide with the conversion factor.

Some opioids listed in the equianalgesic tables are not even used in the U.S. Conversion factors are not easily available for commonly used weak opioids. Some opioids are listed for single route only. Simply put, equianalgesic tables are not user-friendly. However, when physicians rely on their memory and do not refer to the table, mistakes are bound to happen.

3. Propose a design for a standardized equianalgesic table for palliative care.

1. One side of the table should show all conversions to morphine only.

2. Opioids should be classified according to whether they are weaker than or stronger than morphine. If an opioid is stronger than morphine, obviously the dose of morphine will be higher than the dose of the other opioid. Common sense dictates that the conversion factor should be greater than 1, to multiply the dose of the other opioid. If an opioid is weaker than morphine, the dose of morphine should be smaller and the conversion factor should be less than 1.

3. The same principle should apply for different routes, considering that the parenteral route is always stronger.

4. The table should refer to opioids in day-to-day use.

5. There appears to be no simple way to determine equianalgesia for other opioids in relation to transdermal fentanyl. Fentanyl doses are expressed in micrograms per hour, but all other opioids are expressed in milligrams.

4. In what situations of morphine therapy does one need to refer to an equianalgesic table?

1. To calculate the starting dose of morphine for titration in a patient who previously was taking a different opioid.

2. To switch from oral morphine to parenteral morphine or vice versa.

3. To convert doses of multiple other opioids into morphine only.

4. To switch from morphine to some other opioid when opioid rotation is necessary for troublesome toxicity of morphine.

5. To check the physician's orders so that the nurse can ensure accuracy and safety.

5. Cite some examples using conversion factors in arriving at the equianalgesic dose of oral morphine for other opioids.

The milligram potency ratio of morphine is that ratio indicating its potency in milligrams in relation to other opioids. Most equianalgesic tables give these equivalent doses of opioids in a vertical column and conversion factors in another vertical column.

- Conversion from meperidine to morphine: Meperidine is a weaker opioid than morphine. Equianalgesic potency ratio of PO meperidine to PO morphine = 10:1, which means that morphine is 10 times more potent. Therefore, the dose of meperidine should be multiplied by 0.1., e.g., meperidine 100 mg PO × 0.1 = morphine 10 mg PO.
- Milligram potency ratio of PO oxycodone to PO morphine = 1:1. The conversion factor is 1. Morphine is equipotent with oxycodone PO. Oxycodone 10 mg × 1 = morphine 10 mg PO.
- Milligram potency rate of PO hydromorphone to PO morphine is 1:4, which means that morphine is less potent. The conversion factor is 4: hydromorphone 2 mg PO × 4 = morphine 8 mg PO.

6. How do you arrive at equianalgesic doses of morphine for different routes?

- Morphine PO to morphine IV = 3:1.
- Therefore, IV route is more potent. The conversion factor is ⅓.
- Morphine 60 mg PO × ⅓ = morphine 20 mg IV.
- To arrive at the oral dose from the IV dose, multiply the IV dose by a conversion factor of 3.

7. What are the other opioids for which the equianalgesic dose for morphine should be known in a palliative care setting?

TABLE 1. *Equianalgesic Conversion Table for Morphine*

	CONVERSION FACTORS FOR MORPHINE	
OTHER OPIOID	OTHER PO → MORPHINE PO	OTHER IV/SQ → MORPHINE IV/SQ
Hydromorphone	4	6.7
Meperidine	0.1	0.13
Oxycodone	1 (approx)	IV not available
Hydrocordone	1 (approx)	IV not available
Codeine	0.15	Not recommended
Methadone	1.5	1
Levorphanol	7.5	5

PO = oral; IV = intravenous; SQ = subcutaneous.

To arrive at the equianalgesic dose of morphine with other opioids PO → PO or IV → IV, simply multiply them by the conversion factors.

8. What are the conversion factors for equianalgesia between the same opioids (intraopioids) for different routes?

TABLE 2. *Intraopioid Equianalgesia*

	CONVERSION FACTORS	
OPIOID	PO → IV/SQ	IV/SQ → PO
Morphine	$\frac{1}{3}$	3
Hydromorphone	$\frac{1}{5}$	5
Meperidine	$\frac{1}{4}$	4
Oxycodone	IV not available	IV not available
Codeine	Not recommended	Not recommended
Methadone	$\frac{1}{2}$	2
Levorphanol	$\frac{1}{2}$	2

PO = oral; IV = intravenous; SQ = subcutaneous.

Multiply by conversion factor for desired routes for the same opioid.

9. How can you switch from an oral opioid to intravenous morphine?
1. Refer to Table 2 for different routes for equianalgesic doses between the same opioids.
2. Refer to Table 1 for equianalgesic dosing of morphine (see next question).

10. How do you convert oral hydromorphone to intravenous morphine?
1. Convert the other opioid to the route of your choice.
2. Multiply by the conversion factor in Table 2.
3. Refer to Table 1.

Equianalgesic potency of PO:IV   Hydromorphone = 5:1
                                        Conversion factor = 1/5

Therefore, hydromorphone 7.5 mg PO × 1/5 = 1.5 mg IV.

The conversion factor for intravenous hydromorphone to intravenous morphine in Table 1 is 6.7:

$$1.5 \text{ mg IV hydromorphone} \times 6.7 = 10 \text{ mg IV morphine}$$

11. Under what circumstances and with what drugs can morphine be switched to control cancer pain?
- Oral morphine to parenteral morphine: when there is dysphagia, vomiting, or acute pain or pain that is poorly controlled by oral morphine,
- Parenteral to oral morphine: after stabilization of patient on intravenous/subcutaneous morphine and the patient has not required rescue doses for 24–48 hours.
- Intravenous/subcutaneous morphine to another intravenous/subcutaneous opioid: when troublesome side effects of morphine preclude continuation but the patient still needs pain control.
- Oral morphine to transdermal fentanyl: when the patient has been stabilized on morphine and prefers the transdermal route for convenience and compliance.
- Immediate-release morphine formulation: oral changed to slow-release oral morphine.

12. How do you convert other opioids to morphine for different routes?
Equianalgesic tables give conversion factors for morphine for the same routes. Use the two tables in this chapter as follows:

TABLE 3. *Conversion of Other Opioids to Morphine for Different Routes*

ROUTE OTHER OPIOID → MORPHINE	CONVERSION
PO → PO	Refer to Table 1.
IV/SQ → IV/SQ	Refer to Table 1.
PO → IV/SQ	Convert other opioid PO to IV using Table 2. Refer to Table 1 to convert other opioid IV to morphine IV.
IV/SQ → PO	Not usual practice. Refer to Table 2 to convert other opioid to oral and Table 1 for morphine PO.
Oral → Intrathecal or Epidural	Let pain management specialist do it.
Transdermal fentanyl to PO/IV/SQ	Refer to manufacturer's table.

PO = oral; IV = intravenous; SQ = subcutaneous.

13. What is the role of epidural or intrathecal morphine in palliative care?

If one follows the principles of morphine administration accurately and uses adjunct drugs judiciously, the need for epidural or intrathecal routes is minimized. However, some pains related to cancer may become refractory to parenteral morphine, including neuropathic pain, pelvic pain, cord compression, and plexopathies. Morphine still may be useful if applied directly at central nervous system sites via epidural or intrathecal catheters. Management of the dose of morphine and schedule by these routes is best left to the pain management experts who install these devices. However, the palliative care physician will be attending these patients, and it is worthwhile to have some basic knowledge about morphine administered at central nervous system sites.

The conversion factor for the epidural or intrathecal route is 1/10 dose of the intravenous route. The titration is carried out much more gradually than with intravenous administration. Rescue dose principles are the same but the intervals are much more prolonged. Dose escalations are carried out once in 24 hours only. The maximum volume of morphine solution instilled in cerebrospinal fluid is no more than 2–3 ml every 24 hours. The maximum concentration of morphine in saline is 50 mg/ml. Side effects of morphine are the same and possibly less than intravenously. However, systemic absorption of morphine may occur through nearby blood vessels. Despite the high-tech nature of administration, problems administering morphine by these routes are not uncommon and include catheter breakage, displacement, kinks, and infection. Constant vigil is required. Ambulation may be limited and postural hypotension is common.

In summary, epidural and intrathecal morphine is useful only in select cases and at great expense.

14. What are the possible indications for starting transdermal fentanyl?

1. Stable chronic cancer pain while the patient is taking other opioids.
2. Inability to take opioids by standard routes.
3. Infrequent episodes of breakthrough pain.
4. Noncompliance, or inconvenience of other opioids.
5. Opioid abuse by other routes.

15. What is meant by opioid rotation?

The switching of one opioid to another to achieve a therapeutic benefit. A patient's cancer pain may well be controlled on morphine, but side effects may be troublesome. It may be necessary to find another opioid with a different side effect profile that can give equally good pain control. Morphine may be replaced by hydromorphone. Opioid rotation is not an irreversible decision. For instance, if a patient's creatinine level was transiently high and morphine was switched to hydromorphone, reverse rotation can be achieved when renal function returns to normal.

16. What should you do with all the equianalgesic tables you already have in your collection?

The tables in this chapter are to be used for selected opioids only. You may still need to refer to your large collection of tables for other, less commonly used opioids. The tables here are designed to be user-friendly and to help readers learn to decipher more complicated, larger tables. The practical use of these tables is illustrated by actual cases in the next chapter.

BIBLIOGRAPHY

1. De Stoutz ND, Bruera E, Suarez-Alomar M: Opioid rotation for toxicity reduction in terminal cancer patients. J Pain Symptom Manage 10:378–384, 1995.
2. Dupen SL, Williams AR: The dilemma of conversion for systematic to epidural morphine. A proposed conversion tool for treatment of cancer pain. 56:113–118, 1994.
3. Ferrell BR, McCaffrey M: Nurses knowledge about equianalgesia and opioid dosing. Cancer Nursing 20:201–212, 1997.
4. McQuay HJ: Opioid clinical pharmacology and routes of administration. BR Med Bull 47:703–717, 1991.
5. Sheidler R: Equianalgesia dosing: Oral to IV conversions. Nursing 23:12, 1993.

15. DAY-TO-DAY USE OF MORPHINE

Suresh K. Joishy, M.D., F.A.C.P.

1. What are the palliative care challenges in controlling cancer pain with morphine?

No two cancer patients have the same pain nor suffer from the same intensity of illness, even with identical diagnoses and staging. Therefore, it is a wonder how medicine achieves a success rate approaching 90% in controlling cancer pain with morphine. Of course, the physician alone cannot take credit for this success: it is the result of a team effort including nurses, social workers, physical therapists, and clergy.

Success aside, the challenges are numerous. Textbook guidelines on morphine are useful, but practical knowledge and innovations are required to tailor therapy for each patient. The response to morphine is not a predictable event. The appropriate dose to control pain and duration of treatment to maintain a stable baseline are totally unpredictable. Side effects vary from patient to patient, as well. The physician needs to be proactive and vigilant, constantly assessing and reassessing the patient's response.

The clinical course of pain in *any* patient is not a static process. In some patients, pain may change hour by hour. It is not known why some patients experience "breakthrough" pain. Old pains may disappear and new pains may arise at any time. Incidental pain may immobilize a patient despite absence of fracture or neurologic sequelae. The challenge lies in prescribing the most appropriate around-the-clock (ATC) dose and proper intervals for rescue doses without causing side effects. Incidental pain also must be preempted. There are patients who receive pharmacologic doses of morphine—hundreds of milligrams per hour—and do not show side effects mentioned in textbooks, but still have pain.

The palliative care physician should know how to use morphine in all possible doses, formulations, and routes. This knowledge should be matched with intuition, imagination, and innovation. Finally, in the interest of the patient, the palliative care physician can set aside his or her ego and consult a colleague in the interventional pain management service for advice on high-technology pain control. Fortunately, such ego displacement is not often necessary.

2. How should continuous infusion morphine be started in a 65-year-old patient with severe cancer pain?

Find out from the patient or caregiver if the patient is "opioid naive" or on chronic opioid therapy. Refer to old medical records.

- If the patient is **opioid naive**, start with lowest dose of morphine infusion: 0.5 mg/hr CI.
- If the patient is **opioid tolerant** but does not know the drug and dosage, start with 2–5 mg IV every 10 minutes until pain is relieved, and then start ATC and rescue doses accordingly.
- If uncertainty exists about whether or not the patient has been on opioids, treat as opioid naive.
- If other opioid is known to be other than morphine, convert to an equianalgesic dose and start equianalgesic IV morphine. Some authors recommend 75% of the dose to other corresponding opioids because there is no cross-resistance among opioids. Reducing the ATC starting dose unnecessarily compromises calculations and risks under-treatment in the palliative care setting.
- If it is known that the patient was receiving oral morphine, convert to equianalgesic IV morphine as a starting dose, and titrate up to an ATC dose as described previously.
- If the patient has been on more than one opioid, convert all of them to equianalgesic morphine to calculate the starting dose.

Some authors recommend a starting dose for all patients equal to 75% of the usual recommended dose for the elderly population. This is unnecessary in a palliative care setting.

Do not forget directions for rescue doses and bowel regimen.

3. What are the five essentials to remember before prescribing morphine to control cancer pain?

- Pain type: visceral, somatic, neuropathic, mixed, central
- Pain assessment: numeric verbal scale, 0 = no pain and 10 = worst pain; or visual analogue scale 1–10
- Knowledge of morphine dosing and equianalgesia
- Knowledge of adjuncts to use with opioids: NSAIDs, corticoids, antidepressants, anticonvulsants, radiotherapy, other nonpharmacologic treatments
- How to prevent and manage side effects of opioids: nausea, sedation, constipation, cognitive impairment

4. What is the formula for calculating a rescue dose of morphine in a patient currently maintained on continuous-release morphine 60 mg PO every 12 hours?

This patient's physician forgot to write a prescription for a rescue dose. The formula is:

$$(15–17\%) \times \text{24-hour total dose, or } \frac{1}{6} \text{ of the total daily dose.}$$

In this case, 24-hour total dose = (60 mg × 2) = 120; rescue dose = 120 × (15–17%) = 20 mg. When prescribing liquid morphine, choose a solution in higher concentrations that can be given in lower volumes for the patient's convenience. If the patient finds liquid morphine distasteful, offer tablets.

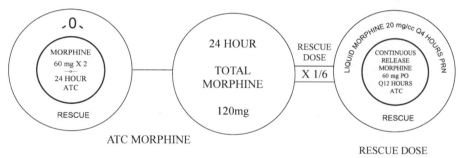

Calculation of oral rescue dose for morphine (from ATC morphine P.O.) in baseline period.

5. How is a cancer patient taking Tylenol #4 (codeine plus paracetamol) switched to oral morphine?

Tylenol #4 contains 40 mg of codeine and 325 mg of paracetamol. In this case, the patient is self-medicating with 4 tablets every 4 hours because of unrelieved pain. Note that this dosage exceeds the safe daily limit of paracetamol.

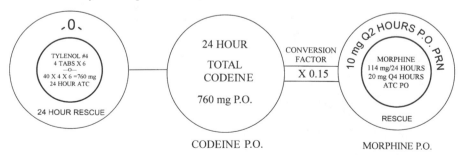

Conversion of codeine P.O. to morphine P.O. in titration period.

Remember: Codeine can cause severe constipation. Therefore, question the patient about bowel history and regimen.

6. What is the formula for switching from oral to IV morphine in a patient receiving MS Contin (slow release) 60 mg PO every 12 hours and MS-IR (immediate release) 20 mg PO every 4 hours as required (three doses in the previous 24 hours)?

This patient is NPO for surgery.

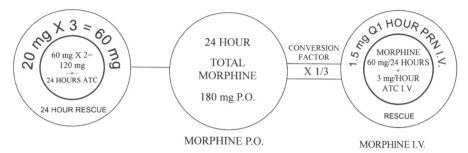

Conversion of oral morphine to parenteral morphine in titration period.

Remember: The patient may need a postoperative dose escalation for surgical pain. Institute a bowel regimen once the patient begins oral intake of food. Switch back to oral morphine when the pain has been controlled for 24–48 hours on IV.

7. What is the equianalgesic dose for oral morphine in a patient taking Percocet (5 mg oxycodone plus 325 mg paracetamol) 2 tablets PO every 4 hours ATC?

This patient also ingested 1 Percocet every 4 hours four times in the previous 24 hours. The safe daily dose for paracetamol has been exceeded.

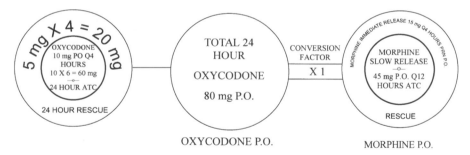

Conversion of oxycodone P.O. to morphine P.O.

- Use MS-IR tablets or liquid morphine for rescue.
- If the patient refuses morphine, consider giving oxycodone in liquid form and add paracetamol in safe doses as an adjunct.
- If the patient finds the liquid distasteful, consider slow release oxycodone, which can be given in tablet form every 12 hours. The patient may still need rescue oxycodone and an adjunct.
- Morphine is the best choice for patients requiring large doses of oxycodone.

8. What is the equianalgesic dose for oral morphine in a cancer patient receiving 6 mg/hr IV morphine ATC?

In the previous 24 hours, this patient received 3 mg every 2 hours four times. She is being discharged home tomorrow on oral morphine.

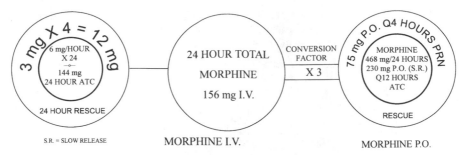

Conversion of parenteral morphine to oral morphine in baseline period

9. How is a cancer patient on IV morphine 4 mg/hr ATC and 2 mg every 2 hours as required for rescue switched to equianalgesic IV hydromorphone?

The patient had received six rescue doses, and her blood urea nitrogen and creatinine were rising due to renal impairment. Morphine metabolite accumulation in the presence of renal impairment can produce troublesome side effects. Therefore, a replacement opioid is necessary. Hydromorphone was selected because it does not depend on renal clearance. Hydromorphone also is a good choice in patients with hepatic failure.

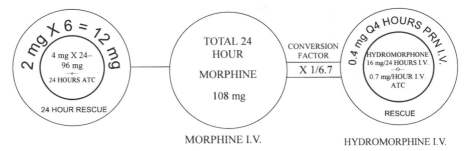

Conversion of parenteral morphine to parenteral hydromorphone in baseline period.

Remember: Continue IV morphine for at least 2–4 hours after starting slow-release morphine to compensate for delayed absorption. Choose liquid morphine in higher concentrations (20 mg/ml) for rescue, because it is easy to administer in smaller volumes.

10. What is the calculation for switching a patient from self-controlled hydromorphone 2 mg/hr subcutaneous to subcutaneous morphine?

For some reason, the physician started this hospice patient on hydromorphone without first trying morphine. The hospice reports the high cost of using hydromorphone compared to morphine, and the patient agrees to switch to morphine but refuses oral preparations.

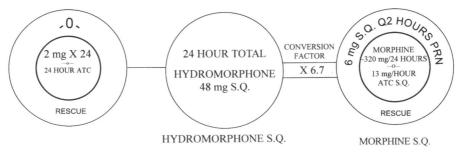

Conversion of parenteral hydromorphone to parenteral morphine in baseline period

Remember: Check the patient's renal and hepatic function before starting morphine: he might have been started on hydromorphone due to hepatic or renal compromise. Watch carefully for side effects and treat preemptively.

11. How is a cancer patient taking slow-release morphine 150 mg PO every 12 hours switched to transdermal fentanyl?

This patient's cancer pain is well controlled; he is on rescue doses of liquid morphine, but has not needed any recently. However, he is tired of taking pills and has heard about transdermal fentanyl.

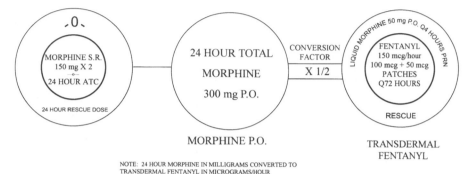

NOTE: 24 HOUR MORPHINE IN MILLIGRAMS CONVERTED TO
TRANSDERMAL FENTANYL IN MICROGRAMS/HOUR

Conversion of PO morphine to transdermal fentanyl in baseline period.

Remember: The conversion factor does not imply milligram potency ratio in this case. The fentanyl dose is calculated in micrograms per hour. Prescribe rescue doses of morphine to any patient on transdermal fentanyl. Calculating ⅙ of total 24-hour morphine, the rescue dose is 50 mg PO.

BIBLIOGRAPHY

1. Cherney NI, Portenoy RK: Cancer pain management: Current strategy. Cancer 72:3393–3415, 1993.
2. Donner B, Zenz M, Tryba M, Strumph M: Direct conversion of oral morphine to transdermal fentanyl. Pain 64:527–534, 1996.
3. Dunbar PJ, Chapman CR, Buckley FP, Gavrin JR: Clinical analgesic equivalent of morphine and hydromorphone with prolonged PCA. Pain 68:265–270, 1996.
4. Portenoy RK: Treatment of temporal variations in cancer pain. Seminar Oncol 24(Suppl 16):516–512, 1997.

16. PALLIATIVE PHARMACOLOGY

James B. Ray, Pharm.D.

1. Is there a need for a pharmacist in palliative medicine?

With the evolution of palliative medicine in the United States, and especially the development of hospital inpatient units, the involvement of a pharmacist is a logical extension of their expertise in pharmaceutical care. For the past 20 years, pharmacists have been involved in hospice care in multiple capacities. Their expertise in drug therapy and dosage form compounding, as well as in the provision of drug information and patient counseling, can be valuable assets to a palliative care team. Pharmacists can assist the team by diagnosing patient symptoms; choosing the most cost-efficacious drug(s); determining the proper dose, schedule, and route of administration; providing ongoing monitoring for efficacy, side effects, adverse reactions, and drug interactions; assessing patient/caregiver compliance; and developing methods to measure patient outcomes.

2. How would a pharmacist diagnose patient symptoms?

Pharmacists who have recently completed their education are trained in physical assessment. Those pharmacists who have ongoing experience in hospice and palliative care settings have acquired the necessary physical assessment skills to aid team members as new symptoms evolve. The symptoms of advancing disease can sometimes be difficult to distinguish from the side effects of some drugs used to control other symptoms. The pharmacist can help the team determine the cause of the symptoms.

Assume, for example, that there is a new onset of confusion in a patient. Does the patient assessment demonstrate deficits in cognition? Are agitation and combativeness present? Are hallucinations present? Are there other physical symptoms, such as intractable constipation or urinary retention? Confusion may be related to altered metabolism and clearance of one or more drugs or may be related to another symptom that has not been treated. A pharmacist can compare the current regimen of medications to the patient's current status of disease progression. Their findings may point to drug delirium as the cause of the patient's confusion.

3. How can a pharmacist assist with pain management?

Many pharmacists are called on to provide pain management suggestions in palliative care. Team members may ask for dose escalation suggestions when patient pain worsens. In these situations, the pharmacist's ongoing bedside assessment of the patient's pain is invaluable. Sudden increases in pain or diminishing pain relief from the current pharmaceutical regimen may require more than a simple increase in the dose of the current analgesic. In a patient with metastatic cancer, sudden increases in back pain might be an early sign of spinal cord compression. The inability to bear weight while standing or walking may suggest an impending pathologic fracture. Changes in the description and intensity of the pain may indicate the need to add other agents to the current regimen rather than a need to increase the dose of the current agents. Ongoing patient evaluation by a pharmacist can provide input to the team regarding both symptoms and management. A model for this care has been termed "collaborative drug therapy management." Treatment algorithms developed by the interdisciplinary team detail the types of symptoms and treatments to be used for the most common problems. These algorithms can then be used by pharmacists and nurses to manage patients.

4. How does the pharmacist provide cost-effective therapy?

By knowing the patient's medical history and current symptoms. By being actively involved with the team and at the patient's bedside, the pharmacist can provide meaningful input. Review of the current pharmaceutical regimen will focus on duplicative therapies and therapies that have been used to treat comorbid conditions that may no longer be important or active. The pharmacist may then be able to substitute less expensive yet equally efficacious agents for current symptoms.

The Medicare Hospice benefit provides for a daily capitated fee that must provide for all of a patient's care, including medications. Medications are often the most expensive provisions in a hospice program. The pharmacist can help the team "balance" these economic pressures by suggesting appropriate choices for ongoing therapy to control costs while simultaneously providing highly effective therapy.

Palliative care can be viewed as a "cheaper" alternative to the aggressive supportive care provided in an institution. However, any aggressive symptom control can be costly. The pharmacist can educate hospital administrators, insurance providers, and others about the futile aggressive curative/supportive care so often used in patients with incurable illness.

5. Can a pharmacist assess patient or caregiver compliance?

An ongoing relationship between the patient and caregivers must exist to achieve successful compliance. Thus, the pharmacist must be an active bedside member of the palliative care team. It is often difficult to achieve patient compliance when administering pain medications. This is because patients and caregivers may have fears regarding addiction, respiratory depression, and side effects. The use of patient diaries coupled with the frequent reassessment of medication usage can help determine if compliance is a problem. Additional education may be warranted to ensure that the patient and caregivers understand medication use and the goals of care. It is always important to ensure that the team goals of care match those of the patient and caregivers. Differences in goals can lead to the perception of noncompliance by the team members. Ongoing communication is essential!

6. How are methods to measure patient outcomes developed?

This is an area of palliative medicine that requires much work. Many of the common symptoms at the end-of-life have not been systematically studied to fully understand their rates of occurrence or their response to treatment. Treatment algorithms, as previously mentioned, use a standardized approach to symptom treatment. The algorithm must include a standardized method of assessment (e.g., a visual analog scale for pain) to allow measurement of the problem. The outcome measured (e.g., pain relief) may need to be combined with secondary measures of quality of life, functional improvement, and patient and caregiver satisfaction in order to rank outcome measures. Application and monitoring of the algorithm will allow for continuous quality improvement in the care of future patients.

Outcome measures will most likely be responsible for the future advancement of palliative medicine within the United States. With the establishment of ICD-9 codes for palliative medicine, reimbursement (especially increased reimbursement) will be linked to demonstrated outcome measures. There are many validated tools for assessment and outcome measures (see Field and Cassel, 1997). The team, with the assistance of the pharmacist, should begin to use these tools to scientifically answer questions about end-of-life care. This can be done without sacrificing the "caring" we want to provide to our patients and their families.

7. Pain is a common symptom in palliative care. Are there any analgesics to avoid?

Meperidine (Demerol), one of the most commonly prescribed opiates in the United States, is a poor choice for use in chronic dosing situations. Meperidine is biotransformed by the liver via hydrolysis and N-demethylation to various by-products, one of which is normeperidine. Normeperidine possesses half of the analgesic effect of meperidine but **twice** the central nervous system toxicity potential. Elimination of normeperidine occurs via the kidneys, and the half-life of normeperidine is 24–48 hours as compared to meperidine's half-life of 3–6 hours. The repeated dosing of meperidine allows for accumulation of the active metabolite. Accumulation may occur more quickly in patients with renal dysfunction because of the impaired clearance of normeperidine. Normeperidine can produce the objective signs of CNS excitation, including tremors, twitches, multifocal myoclonus, and grand mal seizures. Myoclonus may precede a convulsion, but seizures can occur without the warning signs of CNS excitation.

The development of normeperidine-induced neurotoxicity in patients with renal impairment is unpredictable and other factors may contribute to this toxicity. These include prolonged duration of meperidine therapy, a high daily dosage, an elevated normeperidine-to-meperidine serum ratio, an alteration in urinary pH, a previous history of seizures, and the co-administration of other potentially neurotoxic agents (e.g., phenothiazines).

Propoxyphene (as a single agent or in combination—Darvon, Darvocet, Wygesic) is a synthetic derivative of methadone possessing weak analgesic activity. At low doses it is equal in potency to 325 mg of aspirin. It has roughly one-half to two-thirds the potency of codeine. As with meperidine, propoxyphene is biotransformed by the liver to norpropoxyphene, which carries the same potential of CNS toxicity as normeperidine.

Mixed agonist-antagonists include pentazocine (Talwin), butorphanol (Stadol), nalbuphine (Nubain), buprenorphine (Buprenex), and dezocine (Dalgan). With the exception of pentazocine, these agents lack oral formulations. In addition, they demonstrate a ceiling to their analgesic properties, making dose escalation useless. Dose escalation often leads to a high incidence of psychotomimetic effects. All of these agents have the potential to precipitate withdrawal in opiate-dependent patients; thus they are unsatisfactory options for use in palliative care patients.

8. Which opiates are used to control pain in the palliative care setting?

Healthcare professionals should be familiar with the following opiates for palliative care use. The chart below provides "starting points" for dose manipulation and titration. These figures are not "written in stone," but serve as guidelines for dose conversions and adjustments. It is important to note that many of these ratios were determined from single dose crossover studies done many years ago. There is ongoing re-evaluation of the potencies of many of the agents listed and practitioners should understand that current recommendations may change in the near future.

Opiate Analgesics: Equianalgesic Doses, Half-Life, and Duration of Action

DRUG	IM*	PO	IM:PO RATIO	HALF-LIFE (HOURS)	DURATION OF ACTION (HOURS)
Morphine	10	30	1:3	2–3.5	3–6
Codeine	130	200	1:1.5	2–3	2–4
Oxycodone	15	30	1:2	3–4	2–4
Hydromorphone	1.5	7.5	1:5	2–3	2–4
Methadone	10	20	1:2	15–120	4–8
Levorphanol	2	4	1:2	12–16	4–8
Oxymorphone	1	10	1:10	2–3	3–4
Fentanyl	0.1[†]	—	—	1–2[‡]	1–3[‡]

* Dose (mg) equianalgesic to 10 mg IM morphine.
[†] Empirically, transdermal fentanyl 100 mcg mcg/hour approximately equals 2–4 mg/hour IV morphine.
[‡] Single dose data. Continual infusion produces lipid accumulation and prolonged terminal excretion.
(Adapted from Cherny NI: Opioid analgesics. Comparative features and prescribing guidelines. Drugs 51:713–737, 1996.)

Discussions about which opiate to use and at what dosage are common for most pharmacists involved in palliative care. This is especially true when patients are continuing to experience pain and side effects. The pharmacist must be prepared to discuss the possibilities of metabolite accumulation (e.g., morphine-6 MG metabolite) as a possibility for side effects, and to recommend alternatives, particularly in patients with renal insufficiency. In this situation, oxycodone would be a good alternative.

Discussions about switching from one opiate to another often focus on the incomplete cross tolerance between opiates and the need to reduce the dose rather than to use the "equianalgesic" dose found in the previous chart. However, the pharmacist must evaluate this fact against whether the patient continues to have pain on the current dose of opiate and whether the patient has developed any side effects. If so, changing opiates and using the full equianalgesic dose would be appropriate. The pharmacist can help ensure the success of the team by regular reassessment of the change in opiate to allow for faster and smoother dose titration.

9. How can the pharmacist help eliminate barriers to opiate use for pain relief?

The pharmacist is commonly in a position to educate the nursing, house, and attending staff in issues associated with opiate dosing. The points must be made that there is no maximum dose of opiate and that the dose that works is the dose that works, as long as it does not produce intolerable or untreatable side effects. Many health care professionals continue to be confused about physical dependency, addiction, and tolerance, and continue to be overly concerned about the risk of respiratory depression. The pharmacist can play a vital role in clarifying these issues while ensuring that this lack of knowledge or these misbeliefs are not barriers to effective pain relief.

10. What is the role of the palliative care pharmacist after the patient goes home?

Patients preparing to leave the hospital or inpatient setting need "behind the scenes" action to ensure a smooth transition to the home. This is especially true for patients returning to rural settings. The palliative care pharmacist contacts the community pharmacy to ensure that the opiate and its correct dosage are available. Thus, the family is not left to search for the needed medication. This also assures the community pharmacist that the prescription is valid, particularly if the pharmacist is not familiar with the physician. All of this requires anticipation and early planning on the part of the palliative care pharmacist. If a patient is returning across state lines to a state that has triplicate prescription forms, the pharmacist will need to work with the palliative care team to locate a physician in that state to write further prescriptions.

11. What route should be used when administering opiates?

As long as the patient can swallow, the oral route is always preferred. In patients with chronic sustained levels of pain, sustained release delivery systems of oral morphine and oxycodone are available, as is fentanyl in transdermal form.

12. What about dosing for "breakthrough" pain?

Patients must **always** have an immediate release preparation of an opiate available for "breakthrough" pain to be used as a "rescue" dose. A common dose of breakthrough opiate has been described to be 12–15% of the total daily dose administered every 2–3 hours as needed for breakthrough pain. The consistent use of more than two breakthrough doses per 24 hours signals the need for an upward adjustment of the maintenance dose. Again, the pharmacist can play an active role in dose titration. Increases in sustained release opiates are commonly made without thought to adjusting the breakthrough doses. Each time the total daily dose is increased, the breakthrough dose must be proportionately increased. By being involved on an ongoing basis the pharmacist can prevent problems such as transdermal fentanyl being used with Percocet (oxycodone with acetaminophen) for breakthrough pain, which is common. As the doses of fentanyl are increased for analgesia, the Percocet may also be increased to keep pace with the sustained release product. The pharmacist must intervene because of the dose limiting, potential toxicity carried by the acetaminophen. To avoid potential liver toxicity, patients should not be receiving more than 4 g of acetaminophen per day. It is not uncommon for patients to be taking acetaminophen alone for other reasons without realizing that it is also in their fixed combination opiate. This is why many pharmacists advocate the use of single entity rather than the use of fixed combination opiates.

13. What routes of administration are available for patients who cannot swallow?

The **sublingual route** is a simple route and morphine has often been described as administered this way when patients are no longer able to swallow. However, sublingual absorption is very poor with drugs that are not highly lipophilic, such as morphine. Both fentanyl and methadone are relatively well-absorbed by the sublingual route and an injectable formulation of fentanyl or methadone administered sublingually may be a useful alternative in patients who lose their ability to swallow.

Rectal suppositories containing morphine, hydromorphone, and oxymorphone are commercially available in the United States, and controlled-release morphine tablets can also be administered rectally. The rectal dosage is often equivalent to the oral dosage. Pharmacists can extemporaneously compound suppositories of morphine or hydromorphone in higher dosage units or with opiates that are not commercially available in suppository form (e.g., methadone). The clinical pharmacist involved in the palliative care setting is not usually the pharmacist who will compound the suppository for the patient. However, this individual can provide a vital link to the palliative care team and provide additional information to the compounding pharmacist to ensure that the product is made correctly for the patient.

Parenteral routes, either by the continuous intravenous route or by subcutaneous infusions can also be used. In patients with indwelling venous access devices such as mediports or PICC lines, stable access for continued therapy is often assured. But in patients without these devices, the subcutaneous route (an under-utilized route) can be used successfully. Use a 25–27 gauge "butterfly" or "soft-set," needle placed subcutaneously. This needle can remain in place for up to one week. The site is rotated as needed for skin irritation. Morphine or hydromorphone are commonly used by this route; fentanyl and oxymorphone would also be alternatives. A pharmacist can help determine the optimal concentration of drug, flow rate, and method of delivery for these routes. The pharmacist is often the "interface" between the physician or the palliative care team and the nurses caring for the patients. The pharmacist speaks both "languages," translating the meaning of orders into practice by facilitating the proper delivery of medications, especially when it is by the parenteral route. The palliative care pharmacist often possesses knowledge about the infusion devices in the institution and understands the necessary components of drug delivery to know if what is desired by the team is practical and achievable. The pharmacist must also "interface" with home healthcare agencies, home hospice, insurance case managers, and other providers when patients are discharged to their homes. It is not uncommon that different infusion technologies will exist in the home setting because of the different providers involved. This will require anticipation and ongoing communication by the palliative care pharmacist with out-of-hospital caregivers.

Other routes of administration may also be utilized. One example would be the evolving practice of using inhaled morphine for the control of dyspnea. Again, interacting between respiratory therapy, nursing, and the patient must occur, with the pharmacist being the common link. The type of opiate preparation to be used, dosing questions, compatibility of the opiate with other inhaled agents, the potential side effects, and the monitoring for effectiveness and titration of dose are issues that the pharmacist is prepared to address. This information must be shared with all parties involved.

14. How do I get a drug dosage formulation made when a commercial product does not exist?

The rapid growth of hospice and palliative care over the past 20 years has increased the need for extemporaneously compounded medication dosage forms. Good pain and symptom control sometimes necessitates the preparation of medication dosage forms not commercially available. Compounded prescriptions, like all other prescriptions, must be initiated by a licensed prescriber and must be based on a prescriber-patient-pharmacist relationship.

Before any drug is compounded in a unique dosage form, the pharmacist must determine that no commercially available alternative exists, that it can be formulated as a reasonably stable product, and that the ordered medication has a chance of producing the desired clinical endpoint. Many pharmacists do not perform extemporaneous compounding because of a lack of expertise or equipment, or because the policies of the institutional or community pharmacy discourage the practice. It is therefore important that the prescriber satisfies him/herself that the pharmacist indeed has the expertise and resources needed to produce an acceptable dosage form for their specific patient. This process can be facilitated by the palliative care pharmacy team member interfacing with the physician and the compounding pharmacist. An ongoing relationship and active communication regarding each individual patient will help ensure that this aspect of palliative care can be successful.

15. How are extemporaneously compounded medications formulated?

Medications can be formulated into capsules, troches, suspensions, rectal suppositories, and topical dosage forms, as well as into sterile products with the pharmacist considering the physical-chemical properties of the drug as well as the intended use and desired outcome. An example would be the prescribing of suppositories. The physician should state whether a local or systemic action is needed. As a general rule the pharmacist will use a suppository base that has the opposite physical characteristics of the drug when systemic action is desired. When using a drug for local effects, the base and the drug should be of the same type to decrease drug absorption into the systemic circulation. Again, communication between the prescriber and the pharmacist is key along with attention to continued re-assessment of the patient about therapeutic effect.

16. What other agents are used for controlling pain in palliative medicine?

These agents are often referred to as "adjuvants." This describes a drug that has a primary indication other than pain but has been shown to be useful for certain pain states. The most common adjuvant analgesics include antidepressants, anticonvulsants, and corticosteroids.

Antidepressants have been especially useful for neuropathic pain that responds poorly to opiate therapy. The tricyclic antidepressants (e.g., amitriptyline, desipramine) have demonstrated greater activity than have the newer selective serotonin reuptake inhibitors (SSRIs). While the majority of the literature documents amitriptyline efficacy, agents with lower anticholinergic activity such as desipramine would be preferred, especially in the elderly. The dose should be started low (e.g., 10 mg qd) and slowly increased every 3–5 days until analgesia or side effects occur. Analgesia often occurs with doses lower than needed for antidepressant effect, and their pain relief is independent of mood elevation. The pharmacist can assist the team in understanding failure or intolerance to amitriptyline or desipramine; such failure does not mean these agents do not work. There are many tricyclic antidepressants available and sequential drug trials may need to occur with the pharmacist tracking progress and ensuring that patients are not given agents that have failed or have been poorly tolerated in the past.

Anticonvulsants such as carbamazepine (Tegretol), phenytoin (Dilantin), divalproex (Depakote), and clonazepam (Klonopin) have all been shown to be analgesic for neuropathic pain, especially pain with lancinating or paroxysmal qualities. Dosing of these agents is similar to the clinical rules used in treating seizures. Considerable variation exists in analgesic response to these agents and rotation to an alternative compound may be necessary to find the most useful agent. Plasma concentration monitoring of carbamazepine, phenytoin, and valproate may be warranted to ensure that therapeutic concentrations are achieved while avoiding toxicity.

These agents are highly protein bound. In patients with advanced disease and lowered albumin, a higher free fraction of the drug may occur, increasing the risk of toxicity, especially in frail patients. Pharmacists have been involved for many years in the monitoring of these agents for seizure control. If a team member recognizes a new central nervous system effect in a patient, the palliative care pharmacist may clarify it not as a sign of advancing disease but as a potentially toxic effect of increasing drug concentrations that may require dosage adjustment or the choosing of an alternative agent.

Anecdotal reports indicate that the newer anticonvulsants gabapentin (Neurontin), lamotrigine (Lamictal), and topiramate (Topomax) have analgesic activity in neuropathic pain. Controlled trials of gabapentin have just begun but, based on the large amount of positive anecdotal reports as well as its low toxicity profile, it may become the preferred anticonvulsant agent, especially for patients with advanced disease. The usual starting dose of gabapentin is 300 mg at bedtime (lower in the elderly or frail). That dosage is increased as needed for analgesia. Doses > 3,600 mg/day are probably not useful because of gabapentin's ability to limit its own absorption.

The "landscape" for anticonvulsant use in neuropathic pain has changed considerably in the last couple of years with the three new agents listed previously. Many questions remain unanswered about their use for this indication. The pharmacist serves as a source of drug information to the team about these compounds but also as a careful observer, evaluating efficacy and being vigilant for new or unusual side effects arising from these agents in palliative care patients.

Corticosteroids. There is a great deal of favorable anecdotal experience to promote the use of corticosteroids for analgesia. These agents have been shown to be useful in alleviating bone pain, refractory neuropathic pain, pain from bowel obstruction, pain caused by capsular swelling or duct obstruction, pain from spinal cord compression, and in headaches caused by increased intracranial pressure. Prednisone, 5–10 mg, or dexamethasone, 1–2 mg, is given orally once or twice a day.

Treatment is continued based on patient response and side effect development. If the patient's disease worsens and corticosteroid response wanes, dose increases are acceptable as long as side effects are tolerable. When a pain crisis fails to respond to escalating doses of opiates, high-dose steroids (e.g., dexamethasone 100 mg IV, followed by 96 mg in four divided doses per day) may be useful. This dose can then be gradually tapered to the lowest effective dose over the next several weeks. Much of palliative care medicine involves the administration of medications for uses other than their original indications. These medications are often administered by routes and dosing not typical for that medication. Pharmacists by both nature and their training tend to be very "black and white" professionals. The palliative care pharmacist must be open to "shades of gray," understanding that because exact information about a particular medication may not exist, it may not mean that it is contraindicated for that use. The pharmacist must remain close to the case and provide ongoing monitoring for effectiveness, side effects, and titration.

17. Constipation is a common problem in the palliative setting. What laxative(s) are preferred?

Constipation is a symptom frequently encountered in hospice and palliative care patients. More than 50% of patients will require the regular use of laxatives. In addition to opiates, many agents used in palliative medicine can contribute to constipation (especially those with anticholinergic activity). The pharmacist can aid in determining the causes of the patient's constipation by reviewing their current list of medications and then reducing or removing any unnecessary drugs.

Patients who are bed bound and have reduced fluid intake are at an increased risk for constipation. Regular laxative use should only be initiated *after* ensuring that the patient is not obstructed.

Oral Laxatives Available for Use

AGENT	DOSE	COMMENTS
Bulk-forming agents	10 g/qd	Can cause flatulence or worsen obstructive symptoms. Avoid in severely debilitated patients unable to take in adequate fluids (200–300 ml). Makes colonic cement!
Osmotic Laxatives Lactulose or sorbitol	15 ml bid	Flatulence, abdominal cramping. Lactulose tastes sickeningly sweet to some patients. Sorbitol is cheaper and may be less nauseating
Saline Cathartics Magnesium hydroxide or Magnesium citrate Na phosphate	15–30 ml bid	Severe diarrhea and dehydration may occur with overuse. Electrolyte abnormalities of fluid overload may occur from the absorption of sodium, magnesium, or phosphorus; avoid in renal insufficiency or heart failure.
Lubricants Mineral oil	15–30 ml qd	Can be used for acute management of severe constipation or impaction. Long-term use can cause perianal irritation, impaired absorption of fat-soluble vitamins, and lipoid pneumonia with aspiration.

(Table continued on following page.)

Oral Laxatives Available for Use (Continued)

AGENT	DOSE	COMMENTS
Surfactants		
Docusate Na (Colace)	200–400 mg/dl	Combined with a contact cathartic such as casanthranol-(Peri-Colace), this is a good starting point for patients in whom constipation has not been an ongoing problem.
Contact Cathartics	1 tablet bid,	Useful for long-term management of opiate-induced
Senna (Senokot)	inc q 2–3 d	constipation. May result in laxative bowel with prolonged
Bisacodyl (Dulcolax)		use. Consider alternative in patients with a long life expectancy.
Prokinetic Drugs		
Metaclopramide (Reglan)	10 mg qid	Try when patients have responded poorly to other measures
Cisapride (Propulsid)	20 mg qid	
Colonic Lavage Agents		
Polyethylene glycol (GoLYTELY)	250–500 ml	Expensive, poor palatability, and useful in the most refractory of cases.
Oral Naloxone	0.8 mg bid, inc as needed	Cramping and possible opioid withdrawal caused by the absorption of naloxone. Costly! May be useful when all other conventional measures fail.

18. Are there any special considerations regarding laxative use?

Patients may require ongoing titration of laxative(s) just as they would with analgesics for pain. A combination of the previously mentioned agents in addition to rectal interventions (suppositories or enemas) may be required. The goal of laxative therapy is *comfortable* bowel movement and *not* a particular number of bowel movements. Remember, the need for disimpaction is no more enjoyable for the disimpactee as it is for the disimpactor!

To guard against problems related to constipation, many pharmacists have worked with team members to develop bowel programs for use in the inpatient setting. These are stepwise, progressive protocols to help guide the nursing staff to titrate laxatives to bowel movement frequency. While this may seem on the surface as a "cookbook" approach to the problem, it tends to provide focus and attention to a detail that is too often neglected until it is too late.

The pharmacist can aid the team by obtaining a bowel history from the patient and educating the patient and family members about the goals of laxative therapy. Patients need to understand that the regularity that they enjoyed prior to their illness and prior to receiving medications is not a realistic goal. The team will work toward the goal of consistent regularity, without the discomfort of constipation.

19. What if intestinal obstruction is present?

In the setting of intestinal obstruction with nausea and vomiting, a trial of dexamethasone, 4 mg twice a day, for five days, may help symptoms by reducing tumor edema. In addition, octreotide (Sandostatin) 300 mcg given as a continuous infusion, may help reduce the nausea and vomiting associated with intestinal obstruction. It reduces the volume of gastrointestinal secretions and inhibits gut peristalsis from the stomach to the large bowel.

The palliative care pharmacist may be challenged to be creative when requested to provide an antiemetic "cocktail" for patients with refractory nausea and vomiting. This will involve assessing for drug interactions as well as compatibility information if drugs must be given intravenously or subcutaneously. It will also mean interfacing with a community pharmacist if preparations of multi-agent suppositories (e.g., metoclopramide, dexamethasone, diphenhydramine) are needed for patients at home who cannot take oral medication and the intravenous or subcutaneous routes are not practical.

20. What drugs can be recommended for treating nausea and vomiting?

The pharmacist would begin by reviewing the patient's medical history and current medication list to identify a possible cause of the nausea and/or vomiting. A useful pharmaceutical agent is then selected to address the nausea and/or vomiting.

Possible Drug Choices for the Treatment of Nausea and Vomiting

DRUG	TYPES OF NAUSEA AND VOMITING	ORAL	SUBCUTANEOUS (CONTINUOUS INFUSION)	COMMENTS
Haloperidol (Haldol)	Opiate drug induced chemical metabolic	1.5–5 mg/d, inc to 20 mg/d	1.5–5 mg/d	Can cause dystonias. Side effects uncommon at low doses. Compatible with morphine or Dilaudid for subcutaneous use. Can be formulated as a suppository.
Metoclopramide (Reglan)	Gastric stasis, ileus	10–20 mg qid	30–120 mg/d	Metaclopramide can be formulated as a suppository.
Cisapride (Propulsid)		20 mg qid	Not used	
Prochlorperazine (Compazine)	General use anti-emetics	10–20 mg q 4–6 hours	Not used	Rectal 10–25 mg every 6–8 hours. Less potent than Haldol
Chlorpromazine (Thorazine)		10–25 mg q 4–6 hours	100–200 mg per 24 hours	Rectal 50–100 mg q 6–8 hours Very sedating, less potent than Haldol
Scopolamine	Intestinal obstruction	Not used	1.2 mg/24 hours	Available as a transdermal patch. 1–3 patches/72 hours. Can cause agitation.

The newer 5-HT$_3$ receptor antagonists, granisetron (Kytril) and ondansetron (Zofran), while effective for chemotherapy induced nausea and vomiting, have not been tested for nausea and vomiting in patients with advanced cancer or AIDS. Because of their high cost, their use should be restricted to patients who have failed all conventional therapy.

21. What other suggestions can the pharmacist provide in the palliative care setting?

Drug interactions can be a significant issue. Palliative care often utilizes "polypharmacy"— multiple drugs are often used to treat pain and other symptoms. This is especially difficult in patients who may still be in the "transition" from treatment with active curative intent (cancer patients) and patients with active palliative intent (HIV infected patients or patients with early AIDS). These patients are often taking multiple agents that may already cause concern about drug interactions (e.g., protease inhibitors, antineoplastics).

Induction or inhibition of biotransformation of drugs via the P450 hepatic enzyme system requires close review of not only possible drug-drug interactions but also drug-food, drug-disease, and drug-lab interactions. The pharmacist can be called upon to assist in this ongoing review as medications are added or deleted from therapy.

The pharmacist should be much more than the person in the basement or at the other end of a telephone. He or she should be sought out to be an active member of the palliative care team, to be available to do bedside rounds for inpatients, and to assist in patient and family discussions involving care of the patient. The palliative care pharmacist must be prepared to talk about non–drug-related issues such as advanced directives, avoidance or withdrawal of life support, and physician-assisted suicide. These are all areas that may require the use or avoidance of medications.

The pharmacist must be careful to not allow his/her own feelings to influence the patient or family members in these discussions while remaining open to patient and family issues and team communication.

If possible, the pharmacist should be available to make home visits with the nursing staff or with the physician to identify problems and suggest solutions to symptom control issues. Involvement of the pharmacist at team meetings may help identify unrecognized side effects from medications that had previously been viewed as advancing disease. With the pharmacist's help, a chance to medicate is a chance to palliate.

BIBLIOGRAPHY

1. Anderson RP, Forman WB: Alternate routes of opioid administration in palliative care: Pharmacologic and clinical concerns. J Pharm Care Pain Sympt Control 6:5–21, 1998.
2. Barry CP, Fuller TS: Home and hospice care. Hosp Pharm 33:797–799, 818, 1998.
3. Cherny NI: Opioid analgesics. Comparative features and prescribing guidelines. Drugs 51:713–737, 1996.
4. Dube JE: Hospice care and the pharmacist. US Pharm 6:25, 1981.
5. Field MA, Cassel C: Approaching death: Improving care at the end of life. Institute of Medicine, Washington, DC, National Academy Press, 1997. Chapter 5—Accountability and quality in end-of-life care, pp 122–153.
6. Kaiko RF, Foley KM, Grabinski PY, et al: Central nervous system excitatory effects of meperidine in cancer patients. Ann Neurol 13:180–185, 1983.
7. Lichter I: Nausea and vomiting in patients with cancer. In Cherny NI, Foley KM (eds): Pain and Palliative Care. Hematol Oncol Clin North Am 10:207–220, 1996.
8. Lipman AG, Berry JI: Pharmaceutical care of terminally ill patients. J Pharm Care Pain Sympt Control 3:31–56, 1995.
9. Portenoy RK: Nonopioid and adjuvant analgesics. In Pain in Oncologic and AIDS Patients. Newtown, Pennsylvania, Handbooks in Health Care Co., 1997, pp 126–155.
10. Storey P: Primer of Palliative Care, 2nd ed. Gainesville, Florida, American Academy of Hospice and Palliative Medicine, 1996.
11. Virani A, Mailis A, Shapiro LE, Shear NH: Drug interactions in human neuropathic pain pharmacotherapy. Pain 73:3–13, 1997.
12. World Health Organization: Cancer pain relief and palliative care. Report of a WHO Expert Committee. WHO Technical Report Series 804. Geneva, WHO, 1990.

17. SUBCUTANEOUS INFUSION OF MORPHINE

Suresh K. Joishy, M.D., F.A.C.P.

1. What are the indications for administration of morphine subcutaneously?

- When the patient is unable to take oral medications due to intractable vomiting or nausea, dysphagia, cognitive dysfunction, altered consciousness, or when the patient is in his or her last days or hours of life.
- When the rectal route is not feasible because (1) the drug is not available in the suppository form, (2) frequency of administration makes it difficult to administer suppositories, and (3) caregivers have difficulty administering suppositories.
- When sublingual morphine is impractical for some of the same reasons oral administration is impractical.

2. What are the advantages of giving morphine by patient controlled analgesia (PCA) subcutaneously?

Morphine by PCA should be considered when oral or transdermal routes for opioids are not possible. It eliminates communication barriers, and patients can monitor their own analgesic requirements. It eliminates delays in getting morphine to the patient. The physician can set around-the-clock and rescue doses, and patients can treat themselves for breakthrough pain. Patients cannot administer excessive doses. PCA allows dosing to the maximum effect due to 100% availability of morphine by the subcutaneous route. Titration of PCA considers individual variability, sensitivity, response, and susceptibility to adverse effects.

PCA is practical in the home setting as much as in the hospital setting. Frequent injections are not needed because continuous infusion is possible. Patients have freedom and control. As opposed to intravenous infusions, there is less danger of inadvertent overinfusion or overdosing.

3. Are there disadvantages to subcutaneous infusion of morphine?

Yes. It is difficult to adjust doses rapidly because the drug effect can be assessed for 24 hours only. Expensive equipment such as infusion pumps may be required. When used at home, nursing and pharmacy back-up is needed. One needs to be aware of problems at the infusion site.

Subcutaneous PCA may be inappropriate in patients with confusion or cognitive deficits or in very young patients. Some patients may be physically unable to operate the PCA device.

Subcutaneous PCA morphine does not eliminate the need for adjuvant drugs. There are technical and logistic problems when PCA is being used over the long term. Catheters and pump devices tend to malfunction. Technical expertise is needed to calibrate and set up the dosage of morphine. Even though morphine is inexpensive, the operation of PCA could be costly.

4. What are some useful drugs in palliative care that are compatible with morphine and can be given in solution together by the parenteral subcutaneous route?

Metoclopramide:	To control nausea and gastroparesis
Haloperidol:	To control confusion, delirium, and nausea
Dexamethasone:	To help patients facing multiple symptoms, fatigue, nausea, bowel obstruction
Octreotide:	To reduce secretions in the fistulas, control secretions in bowel obstruction, and prevent vomiting
Atropine:	To reduce oropharyngeal secretions and to control death rattle

5. Are there any contraindications for subcutaneous infusion of morphine?

Severe thrombocytopenia may lead to subcutaneous hematoma and preclude absorption of morphine. Patients with anasacra may have little subcutaneous tissue to hold the needle.

6. What are the essentials for a successful subcutaneous infusion of morphine?

1. Daily inspection of the infusion site to check for signs of local inflammation and the need for change of site.

2. Prevention of kinking of tubes and battery failure in battery-operated pumps.

3. Availability of oral or sublingual morphine, if morphine infusion requires discontinuation for any reason, until the subcutaneous line is reinstated.

4. Frequent checks of rate, calculations, and settings.

5. Education of the patient and family and provision of the on-call nurse's telephone number for any problems.

BIBLIOGRAPHY

1. Mouline DE, et al: Subcutaneous narcotic infusions for cancer pain: Treatment outcomes and guidelines for use. Can Med Assoc J 146:891–897, 1992.
2. Pasero CL: PCA: For patients only. AJN 96:22, 1996.
3. Shaw HL: Treatment of intractable cancer pain by electronically controlled parenteral infusion of analgesic drugs. Cancer 72:3416–3425, 1993.
4. Storey P, et al: Subcutaneous infusions for control of cancer symptoms. J Pain Symptom Manage 5:33–41, 1990.

18. THE ROLE OF RADIOTHERAPY

Bharati D. Bhate, M.D.

1. What is radiation therapy?

The delivery of ionizing radiation into a defined volume of the body to eradicate or substantially depopulate the tumor cells within that volume, without exceeding the tolerance of normal tissues. Radiation therapy is curative or palliative. In curative radiation therapy, many small fractions will be delivered to a small or medium-sized volume. A standard treatment regimen might be 650 Gy in 30 fractions over 6 weeks to 70 Gy in 35 fractions over 7 weeks. In palliative radiation therapy, a few larger fractions often can be given, such as 30 Gy in 10 fractions over 2 weeks, 37.5 Gy in 15 fractions over 3 weeks, 20 Gy in 5 fractions over 1 week, or a single dose of 6–8 Gy.

2. Describe some of the terminology used in radiotherapy.

1. Dosing terminologies: rads; external beam radiation therapy consists of photon beams and electron beams; gamma knife for stereotactic radio surgery.

2. Conformal radiation: radiation is delivered to a cancerous spot with margin.

3. Treatment planning: the process in which a patient's CT (computed tomography) scan, radiographs, and bone scans are reviewed. Treatment is planned on a treatment planning computer. In the past, only two-dimensional treatment planning was done. However, with the recent advancement of computers and spiral CT scanning, three-dimensional computer planning is now common, which makes it easy to see where the radiation dose is being delivered so the clinician can avoid delivering radiation to normal tissue.

4. Fraction: the number of treatments.

5. Tissue tolerance: dose that the tissue can tolerate, and dose at which only 5% of patients at 5 years can develop serious side effects to that tissue as a result of radiation. For example, the lens of the eye has tissue tolerance of at least 120 Gy in 1 week; otherwise a cataract will develop. For the whole lung, tolerance is 17.5 Gy in 9 fractions in 2 weeks; otherwise pneumonitis can occur. For the whole kidney, tolerance is 23 Gy in 12 fractions in 2½ weeks; otherwise clinical nephritis can occur.

3. What is palliative radiation therapy?

Radiation treatments that are given to relieve symptoms in advanced cancer such as pain, bleeding, and blockage of hollow viscera. It is a short course of radiation treatments given 5 days a week for 3–5 weeks. This noninvasive form of treatment relieves pain in 80–85% of patients. It is used in advanced cancer patients and treatment relapses.

4. What is advanced cancer?

A cancer is localized if it exists only in the organ in which it started. When it metastasizes to bones, the brain, the liver, or any other organ, it is called advanced cancer. Cancers of the lung and breast commonly metastasize to bone, the liver, and brain. Colorectal cancers metastasize to the liver and lungs. Prostate cancer commonly metastasizes to bones.

5. What is the significance of bone metastasis, and what are the symptoms?

About half of the most common tumor types (cancer of the lung, breast, and prostate) have bone metastasis. Vertebral bodies, hips, and the long bones of the upper and lower extremities are commonly involved sites. Pain is the most common symptom. Weightbearing bones may fracture because cancer softens the bones. Radiotherapy is indicated, preferably after orthopedic consult and surgical correction. Typical radiation involves 30 Gy given in 10 treatments and 37.50 Gy given in 15 treatments.

6. How does radiation help in cases involving bone metastasis?

Radiation kills the cancerous cells, provides pain relief, and strengthens the bones to prevent them from fracturing. Fractures sometimes occur during the course of radiation because radiation takes a few weeks to work. Pathologic fracture and spinal cord compression have been reported in 36% of breast cancer patients with skeletal metastases. Lytic lesions that are 2.5 cm or larger in weightbearing bones or that cause more than 50% loss of cortical bone place patients at high risk for pathologic fracture. Patients with such lesions may benefit from prophylactic surgical fixation before starting irradiation.

Spinal cord compression associated with vertebral collapse due to bony or epidural metastases requires emergent radiation therapy, sometimes in coordination with surgical intervention to preserve neurologic integrity.

7. What are the symptoms of metastasis to the vertebral bodies?

Pain is the first symptom. When vertebral bodies soften, a compression fracture occurs, which may cause spinal cord compression. This situation is an emergency. The patient could develop paralysis of upper or lower extremities and may lose control of the bowel and bladder depending on the location of metastasis to the vertebral bodies. Radiation is indicated on an emergency basis in about 80% of patients if there is spinal cord compression. If there is no diagnosis of cancer, if the cancer is resistant to radiation, or if previous radiation has been given to the same level, a neurosurgical consult is obtained on an emergency basis to relieve cord compression.

8. Should bone metastasis be treated if a patient is asymptomatic?

Radiation is usually not recommended in asymptomatic patients, even in the case of a positive bone scan, except for suspected metastasis in weightbearing bones such as the femoral neck, trochanteric region, and femurs. Signs of impending fracture also are indications for radiotherapy.

9. How do you treat symptomatic bone metastasis at multiple sites?

Radiopharmaceuticals are used in situations in which multiple metastases are present throughout the skeleton, making external beam treatment not feasible.

10. What is the role of radiopharmaceuticals in controlling bone metastases?

Strontium 89, a radiopharmaceutical that acts biologically as a calcium analog, has a role in the treatment of selected patients with metastatic cancer. Strontium 89 is appropriate for patients with hormone-refractory prostate cancer and painful osseous metastasis, either as the sole form or as therapy for patients who are also receiving palliative external radiation therapy. Patients with other primary sites of involvement, with symptomatic metastases with an osteoblastic component, also may be candidates for strontium 89.

11. What are the symptoms of brain metastasis?

Headache, nausea, and vomiting are the most common symptoms. They occur as a result of increased intracranial pressure. Depending on the location of the metastasis in the brain, other symptoms include confusion, seizures, and inability to write, walk, or easily talk.

12. Should brain metastases be treated if the patient is asymptomatic?

Yes, to prevent increased intracranial pressure and seizures.

13. What is the treatment for brain metastasis?

All patients are started on steroids to lower increased intracranial pressure. If there is only one brain metastasis, no metastasis anywhere else in the body, and the patient's general condition is good, surgery is indicated to remove the single brain metastasis. Radiation therapy follows. Patients typically receive 30 Gy in 10 treatments or 37.50 Gy in 15 treatments. With multiple brain metastasis, radiation therapy usually is the treatment of choice.

14. What is the impact of radiation therapy on brain metastasis?

Radiation improves quality of life by decreasing the symptoms caused by brain metastasis. If radiation treatments are started as soon as diagnosis is made, the patient can start to walk, talk, write, and have an improved quality of life. Radiation therapy prevents relapse in 80–90% of patients.

15. Describe superior vena cava syndrome.

The superior vena cava may become obstructed, most commonly by lung cancer and lymphoma, causing engorgement of the veins of the neck and over the chest, a swollen face, and difficulty breathing.

16. What is the treatment for superior vena cava syndrome?

Elevation of the head of the bed and administration of diuretics and steroids is the early treatment. Once the diagnosis of lung cancer is made, external radiation therapy is the treatment of choice to help relieve symptoms by shrinking the cancerous spot in the lung. With localized lung cancer 45 Gy in 5 weeks is given to the primary lung cancer and regional lymph nodes, which is followed by a boost dose of 15–20 Gy in 1½ weeks to the primary lung cancer and cancerous nodes that are seen on the CT scan of the chest. If superior vena cava syndrome is due to lymphoma, chemotherapy is also needed.

17. What is the treatment for blockage of bronchi?

Lung cancer arising in bronchi may cause blockage of it and sometimes leads to atelectasis of the lung. The patient experiences shortness of breath, which is the main symptom. Oxygen is required. If radiation therapy, the treatment of choice, is started within 2 weeks of the onset of atelectasis, there is higher probability of expansion.

18. What is the role of radiation therapy in malignant bleeding?

When surgery is not feasible, radiation therapy is very effective in stopping cancer-related bleeding anywhere in the body: bleeding from the esophagus (hematemesis), the rectum (hematochezia), the bladder (hematuria), the lung (hemoptysis), and fungating or ulcerating skin lesions.

19. What is hemoptysis, and how is it treated?

Coughing up blood is called hemoptysis. Lung cancer is the most common cause of hemoptysis. Symptoms of lung cancer are cough, shortness of breath, pain in the chest, and hemoptysis. Radiation can effectively stop hemoptysis by shrinking the cancerous spot in the lung. A course of 45 Gy in 5 weeks is given to the primary lung cancer and regional lymph nodes, which is followed by a boost dose of 15–20 Gy in 1½–2 weeks to primary lung cancer and lymph nodes that are seen on the CT scan of the chest.

20. How is gynecologic bleeding treated?

Bleeding from the vulva, vagina, or cervix is usually the result of venous ooze from the tumor. Pressure dressings or vaginal packing and bedrest coincident with the beginning of irradiation are successful in most clinically emergent conditions. In a typical patient, 45 Gy in 5 weeks is given to the whole pelvis. If possible an intracavitary implant is performed to give the tumor a total dose equivalent to 65 Gy in 6½ weeks. Intravascular replacement is recommended when the hemoglobin level is 7 g/dl or less and hypotension exists. Hypogastric arterial ligation is done for intractable bleeding.

21. What are the causes and treatment of urinary bleeding?

Invasion of the urinary tract by recurrence of carcinoma of the rectum, bladder, prostate, or cervix are the most common causes for urinary bleeding. Urology consultation is obtained if there is obstruction of the urinary tract with bleeding. Bladder irrigation and indwelling catheters may be needed.

Irradiation may be recommended for bleeding, which can be palliated in more than half of patients. Typically 45–50 Gy to the whole pelvis in 5–5½ weeks is given to stop bleeding. With localized cancer, this course is followed by a boost dose of 15–20 Gy in 1½–2 weeks for cancer of the rectum, bladder, or prostate; for cervical cancer, an intracavity implant is done if possible.

22. What is the role of radiation therapy for relieving obstruction of visceral conduits?

Radiation therapy is a nonsurgical way to relieve obstruction of visceral conduits, e.g., biliary tract obstruction due to cancer of the head of pancreas, obstruction of portahepatis due to lymph nodes, retroperitoneal tumors occluding the renal pelvis or ureters, and pelvic tumors blocking ureters. Typically 45 Gy in 5 weeks in 25 fractions is given.

23. Is there a role for radiotherapy in the treatment of lymphedema?

Yes. If axillary lymph nodes, inguinal lymph nodes, and pelvic lymph nodes are causing lymphedema, radiation therapy can help relieve lymphedema.

24. What is the role of radiotherapy in the management of pain other than osseous metastasis?

The five major situations in which tumors produce pain are infection, obstruction, pressure, nerve involvement, and tissue destruction. Infections results from anatomic changes caused by the tumor, resulting in a nidus for microorganisms to grow. The most common situation resulting in infection is obstruction of an organ by a tumor. Pain secondary to pressure occurs when tumors involve closed spaces, such as the central nervous system. Nerve involvement is commonly associated with head and neck cancer. Tissue destruction is a cardinal feature of bony metastasis. In pain due to soft tissue metastasis, visceral pain due to liver metastasis, splenomegaly, neuropathic pain, brachial plexopathy, Pancoast tumors, nerve root compression, pelvic pain, cord compression, and lumbar and sacral plexopathy, radiation therapy helps 70–80% of the time.

25. What are the cancerous causes of pelvic pain?

Recurrence of cancer of the rectum after abdominal perineal resection; neuritic pain after cystectomy or prostatovesiculectomy for cancer of the bladder; recurrence of cancer of the cervix causing sciatica or obturator pain, back pain, hydronephrosis, and leg edema; metastatic involvement of the pelvic bones, lumbosacral neuroplexus, or cauda equina.

26. What is the treatment for pelvic pain?

Pelvic pain can be effectively relieved by irradiation if the lesion causing the pain is in a well-defined area. Marked pain relief may be achieved with only minor shrinkage of the pelvic mass. Substantial relief of pain from osteolytic defects in the pelvic bones or vertebrae occurs despite absence of recalcification.

27. What are the advantages of treating cancer pain with radiotherapy?

1. Radiotherapy directly treats the tumor and is especially useful for bone metastasis.
2. Radiotherapy can provide fast onset of pain relief.
3. Radiotherapy is widely available.
4. Radiopharmaceuticals can often treat multiple disease sites.
5. Radiotherapy is associated with limited toxicity with standard fractionation.

28. What are the disadvantages of treating cancer pain with radiotherapy?

1. Giving multiple fractions may lead to prolonged inconvenience and discomfort for patients.
2. Myelosuppression may occur, especially with prior chemotherapy, when large external beam fields or radiopharmaceuticals are used.

29. Are any side effects associated with radiotherapy?

Yes. Examples include xerostomia, mucositis, and skin reactions.

30. What is radiation-induced xerostomia, and how is it managed?

Xerostomia is a dryness of the mouth. When radiation is used to treat head and neck cancers, the salivary glands are in the treatment field, which causes radiation-induced xerostomia. Temporary symptomatic relief can be provided by moistening agents and saliva substitutes and is the only option for patients without residual salivary function. In patients with residual salivary function, oral administration of pilocarpine, 5–10 mg three times a day, is effective in increasing salivary flow and improving the symptoms of xerostomia and should be considered as the treatment of choice.

31. How do you manage mucositis due to radiation?

For mucositis in the mouth, patients are advised to avoid commercial mouthwash. Instead, patients should rinse with 1 teaspoon of salt and 1 teaspoon of baking soda that is dissolved in 1 quart of tap water and then rinse again with a large glass of warm water. Patients should rinse and cleanse their mouth every 2 hours, especially before and after eating.

For candidiasis, clotrimazole is used 3 times a day.

For esophagitis, patients should eat soft, moist foods. Sauces and gravies can improve the taste of food and aid in swallowing. Patients also should eat many small meals, avoid alcoholic beverages, and use 1 tablespoon of liquid Mylanta before each meal and at bedtime, which helps in 80–90% of patients. Patients can be given a "GI cocktail" consisting of 1 tablespoon of benalyn, 1 tablespoon of cherry Maalox, and half a teaspoon of xylocaine liquid; ingredients are mixed thoroughly, and the patient swishes, gargles, and swallows for 1 minute immediately prior to a meal.

For cystitis, patients should drink 2–3 quarts of fluid each day. If that does not help, the physician can prescribe Pyridium, 200 mg three times a day, and Bactrim DS two times a day for 10 days.

32. How do you treat skin reactions due to radiation?

1. Always cover treated skin with a scarf, hat, or cotton clothing.
2. Always use a sunscreen with a number 15 protective factor on treated skin for at least 1 year after treatment.
3. In the shower, let lukewarm water run over the skin and gently pat the skin dry.
4. If you must shave treated skin, dry shave with an electric razor.
5. Prescription creams or ointments can be used, including Aquaphor, Damor, Silvadene, and Carafate suspension. Clean skin with a solution of 50% hydrogen peroxide and 50% water.
6. Wear comfortable, loose-fitting clothes, preferably cotton, over treated areas.
7. To air dry, leave treated skin exposed as much as possible.
8. Do not expose treated skin to direct sunlight, heating pads, or ice packs.
9. Do not scrub with a washcloth or brush.
10. Do not massage the treated area.
11. Do not use deodorant, cologne, or perfume on treated skin.
12. Do not apply creams to the skin prior to daily radiation treatments.
13. Do not take baths.

33. Is old age a barrier to radiation therapy in palliative care patients?

Cancer is largely a disease of aging. Radiation therapy appears suitable for older patients because it is effective both for curative and palliative purposes and has limited symptomatic toxicities. Old age by itself is never a contraindication to radiation therapy.

Radiotherapy has negligible acute mortality, can be used to treat patients whose general condition and concurrent diseases contraindicate surgery or aggressive chemotherapy, preserves organs and function, and protects normal tissues. A clear disadvantage of radiotherapy is that patients may require treatment 5 days a week for as long as 4–7 weeks.

34. When should patients be hospitalized for radiation therapy?

About 90–95% of patients take radiation therapy as outpatients. Patients need short-term hospitalization when they are dehydrated and require intravenous fluids, have severe bleeding that requires changes in packing, need pain control, or are short of breath and require oxygen.

35. What kind of palliative care patients should be treated as outpatients?

Most palliative care patients are treated as outpatients once acute problems are regulated and patients know how to take care of themselves or family members know how to help them.

BIBLIOGRAPHY

1. Guchelaar HJ, Vermes A, Meerwaldt JH: Radiation induced xerostomia: Pathophysiology, clinical course, and supportive treatment. Support Care Cancer 5:281–288, 1997.
2. Hoegler D: Radiotherapy for palliation of symptoms in incurable cancer. Curr Probl Cancer 21:129–183, 1997.
3. Kerkbride P: The role of radiotherapy in palliative care. J Palliat Care 11:19–26, 1995.
4. Olmi P, Cafaro GA, Balzi M, et al: Radiotherapy in the aged. Geriatr Med 13:143–168, 1997.
5. Tong D, Gillik L, Hendrickson FR: Palliation of symptomatic osseous metastasis: Final results of the study by the Radiation Therapy Oncology Group. Cancer 50:893–899, 1982.

19. COMPLEMENTARY MEDICINE AND PALLIATIVE CARE

Suresh K. Joishy, M.D., F.A.C.P.

1. Why should we discuss ancient medical systems in palliative care?

Palliative medicine evolved because of deficiencies of modern medicine—in its preoccupation to cure disease, modern medicine has ignored the symptoms and suffering of terminally ill patients and has not found adequate means to relieve patients from the discomfort and side effects of tests and treatments. Hence, iatrogenic illnesses are common, particularly in teaching hospitals. When symptoms remain unresolved, disgruntled patients and family members often seek ancient medical therapies that are believed to be noninvasive, less toxic, and noninjurious. Above all, patients need not fear painful needle sticks, endoscopies, radiographs, and surgeries.

Patients with cancer and other terminal illnesses spend billions of dollars each year seeking ancient medical systems. Most are also receiving modern medical treatments but do not reveal this use of other approaches to their physicians. It is important to understand why palliative care patients seek ancient medical systems and whether they are beneficial or harmful. This chapter provides insight into common ideologies of ancient medicine and palliative care—for this is essential to understanding the strengths and weaknesses of ancient medicine in relation to palliative care.

2. How widespread is the use of ancient medical systems?

Most people alive today continue to depend on ancient medical systems: ayurveda in India, Srilanka, and Indonesia; Chinese medicine in most of China and Southeast Asia; unani in India, Pakistan, and the Middle East; and homeopathy in some European countries.

Various ramifications of these ancient medical systems are practiced officially and unofficially in the United States under the name "alternative medicine" or "complementary medicine." Medical schools in the United States have opened subspecialty departments to teach alternative or complementary medicine. Conferences in palliative care offer workshops on complementary medicine regularly.

3. What principles form the basis for the practice of ancient medical systems?

Chinese medicine, ayurveda, and unani resemble each other in their organization of practice, formulated from physiologic and cosmologic concepts. They all adopt humoral theories in some form, believing that the equilibrium of these qualities maintains health and that disequilibrium causes disease.

Equilibrium, or health, is considered to be regulated by each individual's age, sex, temperament, and constitutional type, and by his or her relationship with the climate, season, food consumption, and other activities. Diagnosis requires skill in correlating physical symptoms with the environment. Therapy uses physical manipulation, modification of the patient's surroundings, and numerous medications.

Ancient medicine did not limit anatomy and physiology to the human body but considered them to be bound to physical surroundings and the universe itself. This concept is extremely important for palliative care physicians to remember. It rationalizes the relationship of humans to the environment to maintain or restore "cosmic equilibrium." Patients who were terminally ill in ancient medical systems traveled to the end of life's journey with tranquility.

4. What are some common characteristics of ancient medical systems?

Characteristics of Ancient Medical Systems

Disease causation	Humours, yin yang (opposing forces), ancestral spirits and cosmic forces
Diagnostics	Sphygmology (examination of the pulse), astrology, planetary influences, astute patient observation
Medical ingredients	Herbs, fruits, precious metals, animal products
Dietary manipulations	Specific diets by inclusions or exclusions
External applications	Hot baths with medicated oils, massage, acupuncture, medicated pastes, balms
Spiritual and religious influences	Important
Proven effective	Symptom control in chronic diseases, neurologic diseases, and psychosomatic illnesses

5. Is there any scientific basis for ancient medical systems?

Ancient medicine lacks scientific research, instrumentation, standardization of technologies, and refinement of experimental methods. Nevertheless, ancient medical systems are capable of furnishing detailed and rational diagnoses. They apply naturalistic ideas to organize and treat diseases systematically. Explicit and orderly ways of recording and teaching are available. Elements of modern medicine such as health education, diagnosis, prognosis, treatment, and prevention are integral parts of ancient medical systems. In addition, ancient systems practice medicine on both body and soul, enshrined in rituals that govern every aspect of life. The ceremonies are designed to have therapeutic values—to reduce stressful situations and their ill effects on physical and mental health.

6. Describe some scientific dogmas of modern medicine that are counterproductive in palliative care.

- *Modern medicine is perfect science, and no alternatives are accepted accordingly.*
  Ayurveda or Chinese and other alternative or complementary medicine systems are rejected.
- *Every disease or condition recognized by a physician is best treated by introducing drugs or other agents into the body.*
  Dietary manipulation and external applications are rejected.
- *Every disease has a physical basis, such as bacteria, viruses, or chemical changes.*
  Psychomatic conditions or a patient's spiritual needs are not readily accepted.
- *Documentation of every disease should be supported by instrumentation or laboratory tests.*
  Ancient medical systems have no instrumentation.

7. What terminologies are used to describe ancient medical systems in the U.S.?

Any medical system other than modern medicine that does not employ biochemical substances and instrumentation is considered *alternative medicine*. Other terms, which are often used interchangeably and tend to confuse the public and medical professionals, include *unconventional medicine, unorthodox medicine, traditional medicine, unproven methods,* and *complementary medicine*.

8. What is the attitude and knowledge of modern physicians about the use of ancient medical systems in palliative care?

Modern physicians have little knowledge of ancient medical systems for several reasons. The study of ancient medical systems is not included in the curriculum of medical schools. Physicians take the Hippocratic oath to practice medicine without reading how Hippocrates practiced ancient medicine. Most physicians view alternative cancer therapies as quackery because they are scientifically unproven. Such a viewpoint is understandable when the condition is one for which modern medicine has already achieved a curative therapy. Some physicians have become generally tolerant and even encourage a patient's use of alternative therapies unless they are invasive or considered harmful to the patient physiologically, psychologically, or financially. Physician reactions also are influenced by the efficacy or inefficacy of standard treatments against cancers. Some physicians support ancient medical systems such as imagery, positive thinking, and biofeedback comcomitantly with modern medical treatments, feeling that they are useful complements to standard therapy.

9. Is quackery limited to ancient medical systems?

There is a general perception that any medical system other than standard therapies of modern medicine is quackery. Ancient medical systems lack standardization, which makes one question the authority of some practitioners. However, not all modern therapies are standardized, and modern medicine is not devoid of quackery. Among other practices, this author considers as quackery the use of futile therapies simply to appease a patient. The important question to ask in palliative care is if any therapy becomes an additional burden to the patient and causes more suffering. Giving any such treatment should be considered quackery.

10. What are the merits of modern medical systems in helping palliative care patients?

The advancement of modern medicine in the treatment of cancer has been dazzling. Scientific advances in surgery, radiotherapy, and chemotherapy have led to breakthroughs in the cure of childhood and adolescent cancers and some early-stage cancers in adults. Unless the patient is actively dying, palliative surgical methods can be applied for symptom control, such as placement of stents, bypasses, and ostomies. These approaches help to improve the quality of life in some patients. Modern radiotherapeutic principles are increasingly applied to control somatic pain and other selective symptoms.

Although morphine is developed from ancient herbal medical systems, new synthetic analogues of morphine and modern methods of administration by nonoral routes have greatly helped control pain in palliative care.

11. What are the major modalities of complementary therapies that are practiced to help palliative care patients?

The common ground on which complementary therapies stand is the belief that the body has the power to heal itself. The mind and emotions play a part in causing disease or maintaining health. The complementary therapies give attention and listening, which themselves can be therapeutic. Common complementary therapies include touch, massage, aromatherapy, reflexology, relaxation, guided imagery, visualization, meditation, biofeedback, and therapeutic touch.

12. Describe touch.

The theory behind touch is that a chronically ill patient with an altered body image may have an unmet need for touch. Nurses know well that touch is an effective way of communicating warmth and acceptance to patients with terminal illnesses. Touch is used only when the patient accepts it. It can be as simple as a handshake or hugging the patient when the patient is emotionally upset.

13. Describe massage.

Massage is touch given in a systematic fashion. A little oil, cream, or powder is used on the area to be massaged. Massage invariably relaxes patients and helps them to feel invigorated to face the rest of the day.

14. Describe aromatherapy.

Aromatherapy, which has grown in use in recent years, entails the smelling of aromatic essential oils extracted from herbs, flowers, trees, and fruits. Several devices are available to dispense the aroma of these oils. Some oils can be used as bath oils. As a treatment, aromatherapy should be dispensed by experienced professionals. Aromatherapy has a place in palliative care in the management of stress and insomnia.

15. Describe reflexology.

Reflexology, also called reflex zone therapy, is a form of massage concentrating on the feet or hands. It induces relaxation and helps the patient to sleep, provides a feeling of well being, and conveys warmth and caring from the therapist.

16. Describe relaxation.

This does not mean socializing or not working. Relaxation involves focusing on tension or contracting and relaxing each muscle group. Sometimes guided imagery or meditation is included in relaxation teaching.

17. Describe guided imagery.

Guided imagery makes use of imagination to focus the mind and induce relaxation through pleasant thoughts; it is a form of planned daydreaming. Techniques include using words to create a pleasant picture for the mind and visualizing travel to a place that is special to the patient. One also may listen to audiotapes of cool breezes, ocean waves, or bird sounds. This is an excellent way to divert the mind from stressful situations in palliative care, provided that the patient does not have too many complex undifferentiated symptoms.

18. Describe visualization.

The underlying hypothesis of visualization is that the physical processes in the body are affected by what the imagination creates and that, with training, patients can learn to use their own powers of imagination to control the disease process and physical symptoms. The main picture to be visualized is that of strong, powerful force that is battling a weak, feeble opponent, such as the cancer or physical symptom. An important end to this visualization is patients seeing themselves becoming healthy. This also may be helpful to palliative care patients who do not have too many complex undifferentiated symptoms.

19. Describe meditation.

Meditation is not necessarily a religious experience. The aim is to quiet the mind and the body. Books about meditation teach how to concentrate on an object, a special word, or a mantra and how to learn to let go of unnecessary chatter of the mind—letting thoughts come and go until they reach a state of inner quiet, a silent space. Although it takes a long time to master the technique of meditation, it is certainly suitable for ambulatory palliative care patients.

20. Describe biofeedback.

Biofeedback is a technique of learning to govern body states that are not normally under control of the conscious mind. For example, stress-monitoring machines issue a high-pitched beeping noise when a person is tense; the aim of biofeedback is to learn how to relax until the machine held by the patient emits a low-pitched hum. Relaxation techniques, meditation, or guided imagery may be used as biofeedback to the stress monitor.

21. Describe therapeutic touch.

Therapeutic touch is not to be confused with massage. It is believed that an energy field surrounds each of us and that it is constantly changing according to our emotions. When we are healthy, the field is expanding and we feel open to others. When we feel ill, the energy field contracts and we feel closed in. The therapeutic touch practitioner, usually a nurse, places her hands a few centimeters from the body and passes them over the patient so she has felt all the energy fields. With practice the nurse can detect subtle differences in sensation and can smooth them out by hand motions, thereby helping to balance the energy field and enhance the feeling of relaxation to the patient. Therapeutic touch is a widely practiced therapy.

22. What is known about music therapy?

In palliative care, music therapy offers nonintrusive opportunities for patients to express their feelings at their own pace. It fosters supportive interaction between the patient and their loved ones and enables patients to maintain some degree of physical well being. Music therapy also offers increased opportunities to communicate with brain-impaired palliative care patients. In music therapy patients may listen to music, sing to the music of their choice, and may sing or play an instrument by themselves. Music therapists usually accommodate the patient's choice of music.

Numerous reports support the role of music in the alleviation of pain in palliative care patients. Music probably reduces the intensity of pain by distraction. Reducing anxiety aids in relaxation and acts as a vehicle for supportive psychotherapy. Music therapy is an aesthetic and creative option offered to palliative care patients to reduce their pain.

23. Is it possible to integrate ancient medical systems with modern medicine?

Palliative care appears to be an ideal place for ancient medical systems and modern medicine to come together. Ancient medical systems can help modern medicine put its goals in proper biologic and spiritual prospective. The ancient concepts of constitutional pathology need to be learned and integrated into modern medicine.

"Unproven" remedies can be tested in clinical trials alongside modern medicine. Ancient medical systems need not lose their identity but, rather, may find enhanced utility by adopting scientific teachings.

It may prove to be extremely difficult to integrate diverse disciplines that culturally and philosophically have so little in common. However, much might be achieved if a start is made by modern medicine's adopting some of the simple remedies of ancient medical systems.

24. How do modern physicians compare with ancient physicians?

We have several major weaknesses today. We often fail to recognize a patient as a psycho-spiritual as well as biologic entity. There is a dogmatic commitment to scientifically proven physical and chemical treatments. Specialization, which has fragmented medicine into increasingly narrow and specific elements, is undermining the physician's role. At the very moment the patient is admitted to the hospital, when the patient is most in need of reassurance about his illness, he may only catch a glimpse of the doctor. He may feel without an ally.

Modern palliative care still lacks patient-physician interaction, which is so vital for recovery. Many doctors and patients perceive this lack, but few have any clear idea of how to change things.

The physicians of ancient medicine were expected to perceive every circumstance that caused a patient's illness and forecast its exact course by examining the patient without diagnostic instruments. Ancient medical texts reveal that there was no room for probability or for acknowledging uncertainty. The physician was expected to do his utmost in whatever condition he was called upon to treat, and he was considered competent to work miracles. Above all, his moral assistance was of prime value to the patient.

The ancient physician must have been an impressive sight (as described in an ancient text) as he made his rounds to the patients, with a "calm mind, speaking pleasantly, a friend of all beings" and, in the house of patients, he would be treated courteously. The ancient physician was able to instill such confidence in his patients that they trusted him as fully as they trusted their parents. He cared for them as he would care for his sons and daughters.

BIBLIOGRAPHY

1. Bourgeault IL: Physicians' attitudes toward patients' use of alternative cancer therapies. Can Med Assoc J 155:1679–1685, 1996.
2. Joishy SK: Towards Ideal Medicine: What Traditional Medicine Can Teach Us [monograph]. Basel, Switzerland, Documenta Geigy, 1981.
3. O'Collaghan CC: Complementary therapies in terminal care: Pain, music, creativity, and music therapy in palliative care. Am J Hospice Palliative Care March/April:43–49, 1996.
4. Penson J, Fisher R (eds): Complementary Therapies in Palliative Care for People with Cancer. London, Arnold, 1995, pp 233–245.

20. THE ROLE OF PHYSICAL MEDICINE

Kathleen Ellis, P.T.

1. What is physical medicine?

A branch of medicine that provides patient care using agents such as light, heat, cold, water, electricity, therapeutic exercise, and mechanical equipment.

2. Who are the members of an interdisciplinary team that provides physical medicine?

The physical therapist, occupational therapist, speech therapist, rehabilitative nurse, recreational therapist, and massage therapist are the main members of a physical medicine program.

3. What are the goals of "traditional" physical medicine?

To help the patient return to the preillness level of physical function.

4. What are the goals of the physical medicine professional in working with the palliative care patient?

To improve quality of life, provide for the highest level of function, assist in pain control, and provide teaching and support to caregivers. With assistance, much anxiety and fear can be alleviated as patients learn there are methods to cope with daily activities and that they can be independent with the use of an adaptive device or minimal assistance of another. In addition, the common problems in the home environment can be assessed and plans can be made for any anticipated declining mobility.

5. What are the differences in services offered by an occupational therapist and physical therapist?

The occupational therapist deals mostly with adaptive equipment and what is needed for the patient to perform activities of daily living (ADLs) such as bathing, grooming, dressing, transferring from bed to commode, and light housekeeping. The physical therapist deals mostly with strength, balance, coordination, range of motion of the lower extremities including gait training, and the need for assistive devices for ambulation. Both professionals may address upper extremity weakness, lack of coordination, and mobility. For patients who have many deficits in movement, both professionals have a role in helping the patient and family achieve the highest quality of life.

6. In what areas can a physical medicine specialist help a palliative care physician control symptoms?

Pain, immobility, muscle weakness, balance and coordination problems, lymphedema, loss of sensation, loss of bowel and bladder control, difficulty in performing ADLs, and speech or swallowing difficulties.

7. Is physical therapy useful for hospice patients at home?

Yes. The homebound hospice patient can benefit from symptom control described above.

8. Who can initiate a referral for a patient who needs palliative care rehabilitation services?

A physician. The referral also can be initiated by a nurse but needs to be authorized by the physician under most licensure regulations and third-party payor rules.

9. When is the best time to refer a patient to physical medicine?
As soon as possible. Early referral allows for planning and coordination, with the result being discharge of the patient with the appropriate equipment and training by the therapist in its use. Early referral allows for repetition of exercises and establishment of a home exercise program and continuity of care. If the patient is seen in the hospital setting, recommendations can be made for follow-up in the home or other placement.

10. What are the most common rehabilitative needs of the palliative care patient?
Most patients who have been quite ill have been deconditioned and have considerable loss of mobility. They need exercises, gait training with an assistive device, and careful planning for equipment that facilitates transfer to the commode, tub, and wheelchair at home.

11. Define "deconditioned."
When muscles, nerves, and bones are not used in regular upright ambulation, they become weakened and function poorly. Without the gravitational pull of earth, even astronauts become deconditioned to walking with gravity. Patients with prolonged bedrest or inactivity may experience a similar lack of function related to not using their skeletal structure in the usual manner.

12. What is the role of the rehabilitation nurse?
To see the big picture of the patient's physical medicine needs. The nurse can assess the patient's mobility and function and can assist in the referral process for physical therapy, occupational therapy, speech therapy, recreational therapy, discharge planning, home health referral, and for medical equipment. The nurse is particularly trained to recognize the need for maintaining mobility and knows how to use therapy for pain control in palliative care patients. The nurse acts as liaison with the nursing staff to ensure that the level of activity achieved by the patient is maintained in day-to-day care. The nurse's ability to function as a coordinator is invaluable to the team effort.

13. How can the physical therapist help provide pain control for a cancer patient?
The application of a transcutaneous nerve stimulator by a physical therapist can reduce pain in a localized area without the side effects of medication and can help plan medications to be more effective. Other local modalities also may be helpful, including hot packs, cold packs, and neuromuscular massage.

14. What is lymphedema, and why is it important in palliative care?
Lymphedema is swelling of an extremity. It usually is caused by obstruction to the normal lymph drainage by surgical removal of lymph glands or by radiation to the main lymph nodes in the groin or axilla. To reduce swelling, manual lymph drainage and comprehensive decongestive physiotherapy can be applied by a specially trained occupational therapist or physical therapist.

15. Is lymphedema a cause of pain in the cancer patient?
Some patients with lymphatic swelling complain of an aching pain that is similar to that experienced by a person who has swollen glands in the tonsils. Usually, this pain and discomfort is greatly reduced with treatment by the occupational or physical therapist, who performs manual lymph drainage and teaches the patient self-management techniques.

16. What is comprehensive decongestive physiotherapy?
A type of massage that encourages lymph drainage and incorporates multilayer bandaging, skin care, and compression garments when the limb size is reduced to its lowest level. It may include some vasopneumatic pumping but not as an initial modality. A vasopneumatic pump is an air-filled sleeve that rhythmically applies pressure to the limb gradually from the distal to the proximal part of the limb.

17. What is the average duration of lymphedema treatment?

It depends on the severity and duration of the swelling, the initial cause of the swelling, and the patient's general mobility status. Most patients are seen initially five times weekly for 2–3 weeks; a home program is then established and the frequency can be reduced. Duration of treatment also depends on the patient's compliance with the home program. Therapy usually averages about 20 visits.

18. Are diuretics useful in controlling lymphedema?

Not usually. Lymph swelling is caused by a large protein molecule that is trapped in the small lymph vessels. Diuretics simply call the water back to the same area and the swelling rapidly returns. Only manual lymph drainage massage and multilayer bandaging can remove the protein molecule.

19. How is recurrence of lymphedema prevented?

Usually, patients will need to wear a compression garment and perform self-management techniques the rest of their life. The damage in the lymph system remains and patients cannot drain the limb with daily activity alone. Keeping the limb elevated is only a small portion of the treatment and is not practical for everyday activity.

Measurements for special compression garments are made by a professional usually after the limb has been reduced by other measures to its smallest size. The garments are then made to order specifically for that patient. Compression garments do wear out and need to be replaced periodically; remeasurement is necessary if the limb has changed significantly in size. A well-fitting compression garment that is donned upon arising can keep additional swelling from pooling in the limb during the day.

20. What types of exercise can help palliative care patients achieve the goals of ADLs?

Flexibility exercises help maintain or regain range of motion. A certain amount of mobility is always required to be able to transfer, walk, and perform ADLs. Without this basic mobility, function is compromised. A flexibility exercise program can be included in a basic therapy regimen.

21. What is the role of strength training in palliative care?

When the patients are very ill, they become deconditioned. When they try to walk, they feel weak and demonstrate imbalance and weakness in their mobility. They can regain some of their strength with an individually designed exercise program constructed by the physical therapist or occupational therapist, depending on which extremities are involved. When the upper extremities are involved and the weakness interferes with activities such as eating and grooming, an occupational therapist could be requested for consult. Together, the therapists can design a comprehensive exercise program that the patient can work at independently or with family assistance. The patient can learn to do "little bits often" so as not to tire and overextend but to gradually regain function.

22. What is endurance training?

Training that counteracts the reduced level of fitness associated with severe illness and its accompanying prolonged immobility. Endurance exercises usually require the use of large muscles to increase heart rate and breathing. The heart rate and the breathing function usually are monitored by a professional during endurance exercises, and the return to resting levels is also noted. Walking, calisthenics, and bike riding are considered forms of endurance training. Just sitting up sometimes can be the beginning of fitness training for a severely deconditioned patient.

23. Is massage therapy a part of physical medicine?

Massage therapy is becoming a recognized profession that is sometimes provided by the physical medicine team. Massage therapists can add a manual approach to pain control and relaxation that can be helpful in achieving the therapeutic goals.

24. Is relaxation training helpful to patients with advanced cancer?
Yes. Relaxation training helps to decrease pain, helps patients handle the daily stresses their illness causes, and helps to lessen anxiety over the unknown. Relaxation techniques are also helpful for caregivers because they are in a new and stressful role. These techniques can help them be more effective in their roles and more supportive to the patient.

25. How can a speech therapist help to manage swallowing difficulties?
Surgery or radiation can affect a patient's speech or ability to swallow. Swallowing incorrectly can lead to aspirating food or fluid into the lungs and developing pneumonia. The speech therapist can perform a modified barium swallow study to identify dysphagia and subsequently recommend a diet with a specific consistency. For instance, a diet that does not include liquids could make it safe for the patient to eat. A speech therapist also can provide special exercises to improve swallowing, including oral-motor exercises, sensory stimulation, postural adjustments, and swallowing techniques.

26. What are the signs and symptoms of dysphagia?
Coughing or choking during or after meals, residual food left in the oral cavity after meals, chronic weight loss, painful swallowing, sensation of liquid boluses stuck in the throat, and elevated temperature with no other known cause.

27. Can a speech therapist help a patient who has had surgery or radiation regain the voice?
Yes. Depending on the type of problem, the speech therapist determines the voice quality that is desired and works with the patient to attain the therapeutic goals. Techniques can include strengthening exercises, breath control, desensitization, tongue strengthening, and working with an artificial voicebox.

28. Does the physical medicine professional have a role in bowel and bladder retraining or continence?
Specially trained physical therapists or nurses can be of great assistance with retraining of normal function of the bowel and bladder, especially after surgery or injury secondary to radiation scarring. Both professionals may use bladder drills and pelvic muscle exercises to help the individual to gain control of this area. They also may use surface electromyography to help the patient gain awareness of the pelvic floor muscles and to strengthen them so that continence can be attained. They can address constipation, which is caused by many medications and immobility.

29. Is the use of braces, splints, and slings appropriate for the palliative care patient?
The use of a brace can sometimes reduce pain; a splint can reduce metastatic bone pain; and a sling can be used to support a painful arm or to assist a weakened leg into bed.

30. For what types of adaptive equipment might patients and caregivers need special instructions by a therapist?
1. Sliding boards—a device used to transfer the patient from bed to chair without needing the patient to stand. The patient slides across a smooth board from bed to chair and back.
2. Hydraulic lifts, which are used to transfer the patient safely from bed to chair in a sling type of apparatus.
3. Adaptive equipment ordered by the physical therapist or occupational therapist.

31. What is the role of the recreational therapist?
To help the patient engage in activities that are meaningful and challenging and that can prevent disuse atrophy. Recreational therapists can design activities that can build function and do not appear to be exercises. They can use humor, art, music, or creative adaptation of the patient's own hobbies to help the patient continue the highest possible quality of life. Sometimes, they can

assist with the creation of a memory book so a person can organize his pictures and have a sense of regrouping his life. They can create a gardening program with elevated beds so that the patient can have a chance to take care of something at a time when he or she is being taken care of by so many others. These often overlooked professionals can make a big difference in a patient's satisfaction and quality of life.

32. What other types of noncancer patients might benefit from palliative physical medicine services?

Patients with endstage diseases such as congestive heart failure, kidney failure, endstage neurologic diseases, and breathing disorders. Whenever a person has prolonged bedrest, deconditioning starts within a few days, mobility becomes a problem, and performing ADLs becomes difficult.

33. What is the difference between rehabilitation provided at home and at a health care facility?

Homecare rehabilitation is usually established because there is difficulty taking the patient to a rehabilitation facility for outpatient care. The homebound status can be determined by the inability of the patient to walk without assistance or by a patient's need for oxygen and frequent rests. Therapists providing homebound services are required to document homebound status and to work closely with the other team members. They usually set a routine time to visit and work with the patient on the therapeutic goals. They sometimes work with family members on transfers and the use of adaptive equipment to facilitate their taking care of the patient. The great advantage of the homecare setting is being able to use the patient's own railings, steps, ramps, and bathroom. The furniture in the patient's room can be rearranged for optimal placement and patient function.

34. How are therapy services paid for in the United States?

Most therapy services are paid by the health insurance carrier. It always is a good idea to check with the insurance company ahead of time to determine coverage and limitations. Health maintenance organizations may require preapproval for therapy services.

35. Are there restrictions on payment for durable medical equipment for use by palliative care patients in the home?

Again, it is best to check with the insurance company before delivery. Some medical equipment companies know which insurance companies will pay for what items and are thus a good source of information. Their job is to assist in the determination of the payment before delivery. In some cases, a patient will need a specially designed item such as a roller walker with wheels and glide brakes and the insurance company will only pay for the wheels and not the brakes. Some insurance companies will not authorize the payment for a walker if a wheelchair is also ordered. It is good to know these kinds of restrictions in advance so the patient, therapist, and family can make informed decisions. Helping the patient to obtain the appropriate devices for home use can be a team effort involving therapists, the medical supply company, insurance company, and the physician.

36. When is it appropriate to consider placement in a facility instead of a homecare setting?

If the patient does not have help in the home and cannot safely provide for himself, placement in a facility is appropriate. There, rehabilitation professionals can help the patient attain independence and solve safety issues before the patient returns home. Most homecare professionals do not provide 24-hour care. An individual who requires 24-hour care and does not have family support would need to seek placement in a facility.

37. Should physical medicine professionals be a part of the interdisciplinary team that provides palliative care?

Yes. Physical medicine professionals offer an expertise and services that can enrich, enhance, and restore the quality of life in terminally ill patients. Referrals should be made as soon as possible during the patient's care.

BIBLIOGRAPHY

1. Braddom RL: Physical Medicine and Rehabilitation. Philadelphia, W.B. Saunders, 1995.
2. Brennan MJ, DePompolo RW, Garden FH: Cardiovascular, pulmonary and cancer rehabiliation. III. Cancer rehabilitation. Arch Phys Med Rehabil 77:S52–S58, 1996.
3. Burkhardt A, Joachim L: A Therapist's Guide to Oncology: Medical Issues Affecting Management. San Antonio, Therapy Skill Builders, 1996.
4. Chalker R: Overcoming Bladder Disorders. New York, Harper Collins, 1991.
5. Ebel S, Langer K: The role of the physical therapist in hospice care. Am J Hospice Palliat Care 10:32–35, 1993.
6. Marcant D, Rapin CH: The role of the physical therapist in palliative care. J Pain Symptom Manage 8:68–71, 1993.
7. Swirshy J, Nannery DS: Coping With Lymphedema. New York, Avery Press, 1998.

21. CONSTIPATION

Suresh K. Joishy, M.D., F.A.C.P.

1. Why is constipation important in palliative care?

Constipation is an extremely common symptom in palliative care patients. It affects 50% of patients admitted to hospice, and will afflict almost every patient (95%) on chronic opioid therapy. Like pain, constipation may lead to a variety of associated symptoms, including anorexia, nausea, fecal impaction, and large bowel obstruction. Constipation is often ignored by patients until complications develop. From the physicians' and nurses' points of view, constipation can frequently become a formidable symptom to treat despite a large armamentarium of laxatives. Constipation is as important a symptom as pain, nausea, or vomiting.

2. What epidemiologic factors are important in understanding constipation?

The normal population in Western countries is at risk for constipation because of a high meat, low fiber diet. Constipation is more common in the normal elderly (20%), and a large percentage of palliative care patients are elderly. As many as 2–3 million people in the United States take laxatives on a chronic basis. Constipation is more common in the southern United States, and more common in low income groups. One study showed that congenital constipation correlated with fingerprint patterns. Of patients with congenital constipation, 64% had increased numbers of fingers with arches (this is not a recommendation for palm reading to diagnose constipation in palliative care!). Pre-existing epidemiologic factors should be kept in mind when evaluating and treating constipation in palliative care patients.

3. Is it possible to define constipation?

Obviously constipation involves difficulty in evacuating feces. But, what is considered difficult for one patient may not be so for another. It may be normal for a patient to move the bowels only 3 times per week, even before illness, whereas some patients move their bowels more than once a day. Certain factors should be considered when defining constipation for the sake of treating an individual patient.

• Frequency: Failure to defecate at least 3 times per week.
• Straining at stools: More than 25% of the duration of the act.
• Duration of the bowel movement: Taking longer than 10 minutes.

4. What anatomic and physiologic factors of the colon are important in understanding constipation?

The colon is the organ for fecal evacuation. Flow digesta from the ileum are presented to both the cecum and the right colon. The carbohydrate and plant fiber fermentation is high in the right colon because of the high growth rate of fermenting bacteria. This leads to bulk presentation to the rest of the colon for better motility. There is little bacterial growth in the left colon for fermentation of carbohydrates. However, protein fermentation is increased without forming bulk. These factors should be taken into account in the dietary manipulation of constipation.

Colonic motility is key for evacuation. The colon is endowed with a rich mat of axons and interstitial cells that lies on the submucosal surface of its circular muscle layer. The bulk of the stool, resulting from water content and fiber, stimulates this intricate neuromuscular mechanism to provoke evacuation. Any factor adversely affecting this system may lead to constipation.

5. What are the common causes of constipation in the palliative care setting?

By the time patients present to palliative care, their diet has changed considerably due to lack of taste, anorexia, or nausea. Due to poor intake of food and fluids, the bulk of the stool is reduced drastically, leading to constipation.

Common Causes of Constipation in Palliative Care

FACTORS	CAUSES
Physiologic	Age, inactivity, change in diet
Psychological	Depression, physical/social impediments
Metabolic	Dehydration, hypercalcemia, hypokalemia
Commonly used drugs	Opioids, anticholinergics, oral contrast barium, muscle relaxants, antacids (calcium-containing), anticonvulsants
Neurologic	Visceral neuropathy, compression of neural structures, cord compression, lumbar or sacral plexopathy
Colorectal	Intraluminal tumor, extraluminal tumor, strictures, fissures of the anus, hemorrhoids

6. When taking the patient's history, what information is sought relative to constipation?

Ask first when the last bowel movement took place. This may provide an immediate clue to constipation. It is important to obtain a history of bowel movements when the patient was healthy. The following questions may help to pinpoint the causes of constipation.

QUESTION	USEFUL INFORMATION
What is your bowel movement frequency?	Constipation if fewer than 3 bowel movements per week
Do you ever have urges to have a bowel movement but find you are unable to do so?	Neurological damage
Have you experienced worsening hemorrhoids or blood in your stools?	Pathology above the hemorrhoids
How often do you take laxatives?	Will certainly need good bowel regimen
What medications do you take on a regular basis?	Identify drugs causing constipation
What is the appearance of your stools?	Ribbon like, pencil like, hard pellets indicate constipation
What are your dietary habits?	Fiber content, fluid intake
Have you ever had abdominal surgery?	Mechanical causes

7. What aspects of physical examination are important for determining constipation?

Pay attention to the patient's appearance. Are they weak, frail, or fatigued? A lack of ambulation predisposes the patient to constipation. Examine the abdomen carefully for any visible or palpable masses or distention. Hard stools may feel like masses along the colonic areas in poorly nourished patients. Bowel sounds may be increased on auscultation. Rectal examination is important. Large soft stools or hard stools may indicate constipation. The rectum may be devoid of stools but constipation may still be present in the colon above. Fecal impactions, if present, are readily felt by rectal examination. Intrinsic and extrinsic masses may be palpated rectally.

8. Will the rectal examination cause discomfort to frail patients?

Rectal examination is not comfortable for any patient. If it will help in the diagnosis of constipation, a one-time examination may not cause too much discomfort if performed gently. Digital evacuation may provide considerable comfort to patients suffering from large impactions diagnosed on rectal examination. An empty rectum in a constipated patient may suggest a higher impaction with colonic loading. Suppositories may not help this type of constipation. The presence of rectal ballooning may indicate a fecal mass beyond the examining finger. Thus, rectal examination combined with abdominal examination is very valuable in the initial management of constipation.

9. Is it necessary to order abdominal x-ray films in the diagnosis and management of constipation?

Abdominal films are not necessary for the diagnosis of constipation, which is readily ascertained by good history taking and abdominal and rectal examination. When there are difficulties obtaining accurate information and the patient has symptoms related to complications of constipation (nausea, vomiting, and abdominal pain), plain x-ray films of the abdomen taken upright and flat are useful. Masses of stools become readily visible and their amount and location in the colon may indicate the need for enemas. Distended loops of small bowel, air fluid levels, and bowel gas patterns may help to differentiate the ileus versus obstruction. The presence of a large amount of stool in the abdominal or pelvic colon may reveal constipation as the etiology. Abdominal x-ray films are extremely valuable in the diagnosis of pseudo bowel obstruction or opioid bowel syndrome.

10. What is opioid bowel syndrome?

This syndrome is the product of poorly controlled constipation that resulted from opioid treatment. It may occur with chronic opioid use during the baseline period or with the use of high-dose opioids during the titration period. The symptoms of opioid bowel syndrome are the same as those experienced by a patient with bowel obstruction. These symptoms include nausea, vomiting, abdominal discomfort, abdominal distention, and severe constipation. A flat plate and upright x-ray films of the abdomen may reveal classic signs of bowel obstruction, including air fluid levels. The presence of a large amount of stool, the absence of active abdominal malignancy, and the history of opioid use will help to clinch the diagnosis. Difficulties in diagnosis arise when the patient has active abdominal malignancy and is also taking opioids. In the presence of large amounts of stool, opioid bowel syndrome is suspected before mechanical bowel obstruction due to tumor is considered. Some refer to opioid bowel syndrome as pseudo bowel obstruction. I prefer to call it "opioid bowel syndrome" to specify the etiology. The mechanism of opioid bowel syndrome is not well known. It is postulated that opioids have a direct action on gut motility by acting on the mu and delta receptors of the myenteric plexus and submucus plexus, respectively.

11. Does diarrhea occur in patients having symptoms of constipation and abdominal x-rays showing hard stools in the colon?

A patient with poorly controlled constipation may experience occasional diarrhea. This is a result of bacterial liquefaction of the surface of the impacted feces. Although this diarrhea is not profuse, because it is watery the patient is quick to bring it to the physician's attention. Careful digital examination or x-ray films will reveal impaction. Some call this "spurious diarrhea." This author calls it "paradoxical diarrhea." In the presence of constipation the patient may need enemas and not antidiarrheals.

12. What are the consequences of uncontrolled constipation?

Palliative care patients rarely have one isolated symptom. Any new symptom that appears will compound pre-existing symptoms. Constipation may cause or aggravate anorexia, nausea, and vomiting. Bowel obstructions of various degrees and forms may occur. These include partial, functional, or complete obstructions, and pseudo and opioid bowel syndromes. Distention, abdominal pain, and urinary retention become added sources of discomfort to the patient. A rapidly deteriorating performance status leads to a vicious cycle of constipation that is further aggravated. Elderly patients may develop delirium (acute brain syndrome) with constipation, the mechanism of which is unknown. The drugs used to control the symptoms of delirium may also further aggravate constipation. Thus, uncontrolled constipation is an extremely serious and overwhelming symptom to a patient and may require hospitalization.

13. Can patients with colostomy get constipated?

Depending on the location of the ostomy, they may experience constipation. Colostomies at the proximal colon rarely cause constipation because there is little chance for water reabsorption and the feces remain liquid. Patients with colostomies at more distal sites, particularly left-sided colostomies, may develop constipation as a result of the same factors that affect patients who have an intact colon.

14. What are the strategies used to treat constipation?

The goals of treatment should be to achieve easier passage of stools and to obtain relief within a reasonable period of time. The drugs or procedures to relieve constipation should be practical and acceptable to the patient. The results of treatment must be monitored to avoid overtreatment, which can lead to diarrhea. Once constipation is relieved over a period of time, bowel protocol should be observed to prevent recurrence. Patient education and compliance are as important as the laxatives. Caregiver education is also mandatory in treating dependent patients.

15. What are the major components of medical management of constipation in palliative care patients?

Constipation in palliative care is treated by laxatives in the form of oral medications, rectal suppositories, or enemas. There are no parenteral laxatives.

Laxatives are non-absorbable chemicals designed to increase the bulk of the stool or lubricate stool and indirectly or directly stimulate the motility of the colonic wall.

16. What is the difference between treating constipation in palliative care patients compared to other patient populations?

There is not much room for dietary manipulation and physiologic increase of the bulk of stools. Time is also critical. One must choose laxatives that will give good results in hours, not days. If already constipated at presentation to palliative care, it is likely that the patient will need stronger laxatives or a combination of laxatives even after relief of constipation. The patient will probably need prophylactic laxatives. It may not be possible to eliminate constipation-causing drugs, such as opioids and antidepressants. Just as in treating pain, treatment of constipation is a team approach, coordinated by patient, physician, nurse, and caregiver.

17. If constipation is observed and recorded by the nurse or caregiver, should it be treated even if the patient isn't complaining?

Yes. There are dietary manipulations, exercise programs, and laxatives gentle enough to be practical in severely ill patients. Prophylaxis of constipation may save the patient from medical interventions and hospitalization.

18. What are the mechanisms of action of oral laxatives?

Increasing the bulk of the stools. Dietary fibers absorb water and expand, increasing stool bulk and decreasing transit time in the colon. The plant fibers methylcellulose and psyllium are commonly used.

Emollient action. Laxatives with emollient action act as surfactants. By facilitating the interface between the aqueous (hydrophilic) and fatty acid (hydrophilic) components of the stool, they cause emulsification. These agents may also alter the mucosal secretory activity of the small and large bowels, increasing luminal water and sodium chloride to keep stools soft. Decusate sodium is the most commonly used stool softener in the United States.

Osmosis. Saline laxatives have osmotic properties that cause water retention in the intestinal lumen. Various magnesium salts (magnesium hydroxide, sulfate, or citrate), lactulose, and sorbitol are commonly used in palliative care.

Increasing peristalsis. Some laxatives have a direct action on the walls of the distal ileum and colon. They not only promote water and electrolyte movement into the lumen, but increase peristalsis mediated by cyclic AMP, and prostaglandins. The laxatives in this category most widely used in the United States are bisacodyl, senna, castor oil, and cascara.

19. What are rectal laxatives?

Rectal laxatives are administered as suppositories or enemas. Suppositories act locally by softening and lubricating the fecal mass (e.g., glycerin suppository), or by directly stimulating the bowel mucosa (bisacodyl suppository). Enemas are designed to act immediately by present-ing large volume to the colon and stimulating peristalsis. Tap water, soap suds, and sodium phos-phate are commonly used agents for enema. Innovations in using synthetic and natural substances as enemas are numerous but are not used in day-to-day practice.

20. How long does it take for oral laxatives to cause bowel evacuation?

Bulk-forming
Methyl cellulose   2–4 days
Psyllium
Lubricants   Overnight
Mineral oil
Osmotic diuretics   3–6 hours
Magnesium citrate
Sodium phosphate
Intestinal stimulants   6–12 hours
Senna, cascara
Bisacodyl

21. How does the knowledge of mechanism of action help you to choose the most appropri-ate laxative?

- If the patient is suffering from complications of cancer with nausea and vomiting, abdomi-nal distention, and a large volume of stool in the colon, it is best to give an enema.
- If the patient is simply uncomfortable, and lower abdominal and rectal examination indi-cates bulky or hard stools, consider using a glycerin suppository. Follow up with mainte-nance oral laxatives.
- If the rectum is not loaded but stool is present higher up, insert 1 or 2 bisacodyl supposito-ries into the empty rectum to stimulate peristalsis.
- If the patient is constipated, but in stable condition, oral laxatives are indicated. If the con-stipation is opioid induced, a combination of stool softener, decusate 100 mg PO BID, and stimulant laxative, senna 7.5–15 mg PO, is indicated. If senna causes cramping, a mineral oil at night or a suppository in the morning may be used instead.

22. Do oral laxatives have side effects?

Like any other pharmacologic agents, laxatives have side effects. Fortunately, most of these side effects are predictable, manageable, and easily reversed. There are plenty of safe and alter-native laxatives; thus, good laxative treatment is *not* to be withheld when needed.

LAXATIVE	POSSIBLE SIDE EFFECTS
Bulk-forming laxatives	Flatulence, eructation, occasionally diarrhea, rare allergy (psyllium), hyperglycemia in diabetes
Emollients	Increases systemic absorption of mineral oil
Lubricants	Chronic use impairs absorption of vitamins A, D, and K. Increase in prothrombin time
Osmotic cathartics	Absorption of salts. Sodium and magnesium may aggravate congestive heart failure or renal insufficiency
Stimulant laxatives	Cramping, diarrhea

23. How is opioid-induced constipation treated?

Whenever an order is written for an opioid, a laxative should simultaneously be prescribed, following the principles of ATC and rescue. A stool softener should be prescribed twice a day even if the patient does not complain of constipation. A rescue laxative can be given QOD PRN. Mineral oil or senna may be chosen as a stimulant laxative PRN. Some patients may need a stim-ulant laxative on a daily basis and a suppository as a rescue laxative QOD PRN.

24. Is there a role for prokinetic agents in the treatment of constipation?

Metoclopramide and cisapride are prokinetic agents. Both agents decrease gastric emptying time. There is evidence for the prokinetic action of cisapride on the colonic smooth muscle. It may be worth trying in selected patients, at a rate of 5–10 mg PO TID for 8–12 weeks.

25. What day-to-day nonpharmacologic measures are helpful to combat constipation?

Guidelines for nonpharmacologic measures are difficult to follow in patients with life-limiting illness. If the patient's performance status is good and if the patient is ambulatory, dietary fiber supplementation is advisable. If the patient is resting most of the time, an exercise program to promote abdominal muscle strength, abdominal massage, and appropriate positioning for defecation may be advocated by the physical therapist. Training patients to make use of high colonic motility periods such as upon rising in the morning or post prandial, 10–15 minutes after meals, is also helpful for bowel evacuation.

26. What are some of the difficulties encountered when treating constipation and how are these difficulties managed?

- **Constipation with colicky abdominal pain.** Use higher doses of stool softeners (decusate 200 mg PO TID) or use higher doses of sorbitol (30 cc PO TID)
- **Stimulant cathartics are not working.** Try lactulose 30–60 cc PO BID. Increased doses of sorbitol may also be effective, 30 ml PO TID.
- **Opioid bowel syndrome.** When reduction in opioid dose is not possible, consider opioid rotation with an alternative opioid, in equianalgesic doses. If the patient is hospitalized and is still being titrated with escalating doses of opioid, an opioid sparing drug may be considered to bring down the dose of opioid and indirectly relieve opioid bowel syndrome. Intravenous ketorolac, a strong parenteral NSAID, may help bring down the dose of morphine quickly without losing pain control.
- **Constipation with partial or near complete bowel obstruction.** Stimulant cathartics should be avoided because they may increase abdominal cramping. Low-dose, oral sorbitol is useful. If the patient is experiencing considerable abdominal pain, morphine can still be used subcutaneously with subcutaneous metoclopramide.

27. How is constipation treated in a patient who has lost innervation to the colon?

Spinal cord compression is not an uncommon event in patients having vertebral metastases previously known or unknown. A high index of suspicion should be maintained when the patient develops a new pain in the back and neurological symptoms in the limbs. Fortunately, not all patients lose bowel control or develop neurological sequelae when the cord is just encroached. However, if the patient has associated neurological sequelae, loss of bowel control may occur.

Patients with cord compression may develop constipation because of loss of gastrocolic reflex, altered colonic motility, or loss of sphincter control. The multifactorial nature of constipation requires multimodal therapy to treat these challenging patients.

- **Bowel training.** The goal here is to establish a routine regimen for defecation by establishing a new, conditioned reflex. A dietary consult is obtained to educate the patient to drink sufficient fluids (6–8 glasses of water each day) and to choose high fiber foods.
- **Laxatives.** Emollients or stool softeners are used on an ATC basis. Daily suppositories are also used ATC for a few days and then every other day.
- **Enemas.** Some patients may need enemas. Because there may be loss of voluntary control of the external sphincter, enemas are placed higher up or given by continence catheter devices.
- **Drugs to stimulate colonic motility.** Erythromycin is well known as a prokinetic agent for the upper gastrointestinal tract. Cisapride is another. It may be worthwhile to try these agents, in addition to stimulant suppositories, in patients with cord compression.
- **Colostomy.** If a patient has intractable constipation, they may benefit from colostomy. However, this decision should be left to an experienced colorectal surgeon. Colostomy

improves quality of life for such patients, and they can be taught to irrigate the colostomy for evacuation at regular intervals.

28. How safe are enemas for debilitated palliative care patients?

Enema therapy for constipation has been practiced since ancient civilizations. Each physician or patient seems to have their own preference for enemas. Horrible complications of enema administration have been sporadically reported in the literature, even for the most commonly used soap suds enema. Mucosal abrasions, bleeding, perforation, and gangrene have been reported. However, in an experienced nurse's hands, such events are rare.

Enemas are not convenient for the patient or the caregiver. Tap water, soap suds, and saline enemas are the most commonly used enemas in palliative care when immediate symptom control is desired. Innovative recipes abound when the above simple enemas fail:

Molasses enema:	powdered milk	1 cup
	molasses or corn syrup	1 cup
	warm water	1000 ml
Clezy enema:	paraffin oil	30 ml
	glycerin	30 ml
	enema soap	30 ml
	olive oil	60 ml
	warm water	400 ml

29. When is the manual evacuation of stools indicated?

If large amounts of hard feces are found in the initial evaluation of the patient, and if the patient is symptomatic, digital evacuation may bring immediate relief. The patient may still need an enema for stools higher up.

Digital evacuation is not comfortable for either the patient or the caregiver. It is best to sedate the patient with lorazepam 1 mg IV or midazolam 5 mg SQ.

BIBLIOGRAPHY

1. Burk A: The management of constipation in end-stage disease. Austral Fam Phys 1248–1253, 1994.
2. Cameron JC: Constipation related to narcotic therapy. A protocol for nurses and patients. Cancer Nursing 15:372–377, 1992.
3. Campbell J: The soap bubble bursts!…There is a risk factor associated with giving any enema. World Council Enterost Ther J 15:28–29, 1995.
4. Hall GR, et al: Managing constipation using a research based protocol. Medsurg Nursing 4:11–20, 1995.
5. Jensen JE: Medical management of constipation. In Wexner SD, Bartolo DCC (eds): Constipation. Etiology, Evaluation and Management. Oxford, Butterworth Heinemann, 1995, pp 137–152.
6. Longo WE, Ballantyne GH: Constipation in patients with spinal cord injury. In Wexner SD, Bartolo DCC (eds): Constipation. Etiology, Evaluation and Management. Oxford, Butterworth Heinemann, 1995, pp 243–250.
7. Portenoy RK: Constipation in the cancer patient: Causes and management. Med Clin North Am 303–311, 1987.
8. Sonnenberg A, Koch TR: Epidemiology of constipation in the United States. Dis Colon Rectum 32:1–8, 1989.

22. MALIGNANT BOWEL OBSTRUCTION IN ADVANCED CANCER PATIENTS

Suresh K. Joishy, M.D., F.A.C.P.

1. Why is it important to consider malignant bowel obstruction in the palliative care setting?

Bowel obstruction is a frequent complication of advanced-stage abdominal malignancies. The incidence and cause of bowel obstruction are summarized below.

PRIMARY CANCER	INCIDENCE (%)	MECHANISM
Ovary	14–42	Benign adhesions, extrinsic occlusion of bowel wall, widespread peritoneal metastasis ("caking")
Colorectal	16–24	Anastomotic recurrence, intraluminal occlusion-polypoid/annular metastasis, bowel muscles and nerves
Stomach	6	Linitis plastica of small bowel extending from stomach, abdominal metastasis
Pelvic tumors, bladder, gynecologic, prostate		Pelvic metastasis

2. What is pseudo bowel obstruction?

Metastatic tumors of the abdomen or pelvis may cause intestinal motility disorders by infiltrating the mesentery and nerve supply to the bowel muscle, or by malignant involvement of the celiac plexus. Extra-abdominal tumors such as lung cancer may cause paraneoplastic neuropathy affecting the bowel. Opioids may affect intestinal motility adversely and cause symptoms and signs of bowel obstruction (opioid bowel syndrome). In these conditions the obstruction is "functional" rather than mechanical. Hence, the term "pseudo bowel obstruction" is applicable.

3. What risk factors might predict future development of bowel obstruction in advanced cancer patients?

Bowel obstruction should be strongly suspected in patients with a primary diagnosis of ovarian and colorectal cancers if persistent nausea or vomiting develops. Patients with advanced stages of malignancy upon first diagnosis, or patients presenting with a short interval of relapse after treatment are more prone to develop bowel obstruction. Obviously, patients with known abdominal metastasis are also at high risk. Patients who have had previous abdominal surgeries and radiotherapy are more prone to develop adhesions.

4. How can bowel obstruction be recognized in polysymptomatic palliative care patients?

A strong suspicion of bowel obstruction helps the physician to recognize the symptoms. Unfortunately, there may be delays in diagnosis because bowel obstruction in such patients is rarely an acute event. The symptoms may develop over several days and spontaneously resolve only to recur. Symptoms may gradually worsen and become continuous.

The symptoms of bowel obstruction include vomiting, abdominal pain, and intestinal colic. Vomiting develops early and in large amounts in upper GI obstruction. It develops later in large bowel obstruction. Many patients are already on opioids and may not have acute abdominal pain and colic. The "textbook" triad of abdominal distention, visible peristalsis, and intermittent borborygmi may not be present.

5. What investigations are appropriate for diagnosis of bowel obstruction?

Abdominal x-ray, taken in supine and standing positions, should suffice in patients who are already ill. If a patient is too feeble to travel to the x-ray department, supine and lateral views of the abdomen may be taken at bedside. The films may reveal dilated loops of small bowel, air fluid levels, or both, confirming the diagnosis.

If the films show a large amount of stool in the colon, constipation, rather than bowel obstruction, may be the cause of the vomiting. If the patient has been on escalating doses of opioids, and is constipated, opioid bowel syndrome should be considered rather than malignant bowel obstruction.

Further investigation is unnecessary unless the patient is being considered for surgery and is strong enough. A small bowel series with contrast medium can distinguish an obstruction resulting from metastasis, radiation damage, or adhesions. Motility disorders are revealed by the slow passage of barium. These studies may help the physician ascertain the level of obstruction.

6. What is the difference between complete and partial bowel obstruction?

Clinicians tend to diagnose partial bowel obstruction when not all of the symptoms of bowel obstruction are present. In debilitated patients taking opioids and other drugs who are vomiting persistently, the distinction between partial and complete bowel obstruction is difficult. Sometimes the obstruction may change from one type to the other. If the patient is having bowel movements (albeit very little) or passing gas, it is probably partial bowel obstruction. If the symptoms persist and worsen, the patient should be treated as having malignant bowel obstruction.

7. When is surgical consultation appropriate for a patient suspected of malignant bowel obstruction?

The decision to obtain a surgical consultation rests with the palliative care physician. This decision depends on two factors:

1. **The patient's performance status.** If the patient's pre-morbid condition was good with adequate nutritional status and the patient was ambulatory, the patient is probably operable. A surgeon may be contacted.

2. **Extent of the disease.** If the patient has widespread abdominal carcinomatosis, and obstruction at multiple levels, it may not be feasible to resect the obstruction. It may not be useful to call a surgeon for definitive treatment.

8. Which poor prognostic factors will cause a surgeon to decide against operating on a patient suspected of malignant bowel obstruction?

PROGNOSTIC FACTOR	CONTRAINDICATION
Cachectic patient over 65 years of age	High postoperative mortality
Ascites	Will recur. Leakage, peritonitis
Low serum albumin level	Poor wound healing, anastomotic dehiscence
Previous radiotherapy to the abdomen/pelvis	Poor tissue healing, bleeding
Palpable intra-abdominal masses	Further postoperative obstruction. Unresectable
Multiple levels of obstruction	Unresectable

9. What is the drip and suck method for treating bowel obstruction?

The traditional treatment of intravenous fluid drip and nasogastric suction is called "drip and suck." This method is indicated as an immediate measure to make the patient comfortable in the hospital setting. Intravenous fluids help to hydrate the patient and correct electrolyte imbalance. Nasogastric suction helps the patient by relieving abdominal distention and vomiting.

10. What are the indications for nasogastric suction?

Nasogastric suction is indicated for short periods of time only. It is useful for symptom relief at initial management or in preparation for surgery on a patient who is operable and has a resectable obstruction. Nasogastric suction is most useful for cases of upper bowel obstruction with profuse vomiting. If the bowel obstruction is truly partial, decompression of the bowel and rest by nasogastric suction may temporarily restore bowel function. Recurrent obstruction is common.

11. Why is prolonged nasogastric suction not feasible for relief of malignant bowel obstruction?

If the patient is inoperable, prolonged nasogastric suction for symptomatic treatment is not indicated. The nasogastric tube is very uncomfortable to the patient. It interferes with cough, predisposes to nasal cartilage erosion, and may lead to esophagitis and bleeding. Some patients feel it is more unpleasant than their abdominal condition.

12. If the patient is not operable or the lesion is not resectable, how can the symptoms resulting from bowel obstruction be controlled?

When surgery is not possible, traditional pharmacotherapy is applied to relieve symptoms. Traditional pharmacotherapy consists of antispasmodics, antiemetics, H2 blockers, and analgesics. The goal is to obviate the need for nasogastric suction. The use of corticosteroids and newer drugs such as octreotide to relieve bowel obstruction is discussed later.

13. What is the role of pharmacotherapy in the management of inoperable bowel obstruction?

Currently recommended drugs can be administered in the hospital or at home with equally good results. Obviously, the drugs need to be given parenterally. Fortunately, most of these drugs can be given subcutaneously for patients at home, and continuously infused using any pump device. These recommended drugs are also advantageous in that they are compatible with morphine when mixed in solution and can be subcutaneously administered via the same tubing and needle.

14. How effective is pharmacotherapy for inoperable malignant bowel obstruction?

SYMPTOM	DRUG	RELIEF	ACTION
Colic	Hyoscine butyl bromide 60 mg/24 hr	68% 89%	Reduces gastrointestinal secretions and motility
Abdominal pain	Morphine: titrate dose subcutaneously	13%	Centrally acting

15. What other drugs are useful for controlling the nausea and vomiting that result from malignant bowel obstruction?

If haloperidol is ineffective, cyclizine 100–150 mg/24 hr can be substituted. Watch for crystallization of cyclizine in the infusion device. Sometimes haloperidol and cyclizine may be used in combination. Interestingly, metoclopramide, a prokinetic agent, has been used subcutaneously, 160 mg/24 hr or 10 mg every 4 hours. Metoclopramide can be used when the obstruction is at the distal bowel. It should not be used for proximal bowel obstruction.

Methotrimeprazine is a highly effective antiemetic and sedating agent. It can be administered subcutaneously 12.5–75 mg/24 hr.

16. What is the role of corticosteroids in the management of malignant bowel obstruction?

The mechanism of corticosteroid action is unknown, but it is postulated that corticosteroids reduce peritumoral inflammatory edema and thus improve intestinal passage. Dexamethasone is the steroid of choice and is given at a variable dose range, 8–60 mg/24 hr. It is worthwhile to consider a trial with dexamethasone as early as possible, or as an adjunct with standard treatments.

17. What is the role of octreotide in the pharmacologic management of bowel obstruction?

Octreotide is emerging as a very effective drug for controlling vomiting in malignant bowel obstruction. It inhibits gut hormones and blocks pancreatic secretions, gastric acid, and pepsin. These actions also inhibit gastrointestinal motility. Octreotide can be conveniently administered

100 µg TID IV or subcutaneously, and can be increased up to 600 µg/24 hr. No acute side effects have been noted. It can be combined with other drugs in solution. When standard antiemetics fail or when the total volume of each vomitus is large, octreotide is recommended.

18. How can the patient be kept hydrated while the symptoms of malignant bowel obstruction are treated?

If the patient's performance status is good, or if nausea and vomiting are being controlled well, the patient can resume taking oral liquids. The need for parenteral hydration should be decided on an individual basis, and depends on the performance status. If the patient is not totally bedridden and life expectancy is reasonable, parenteral hydration by IV or hypodermoclysis is recommended. Good mouth care (including keeping the mouth wet to prevent thirst) may suffice in bedridden, obtunded patients.

19. What can be done to relieve symptoms when pharmacotherapy fails?

A small group of patients, usually with high obstruction, may continue to vomit profusely. If a trial of nasogastric suction is ineffective, octreotide may be considered to hopefully wean the patient from the nasogastric tube. If this fails, a venting gastrostomy may be considered.

20. How useful is venting gastrostomy in the management of malignant bowel obstruction?

When either pharmacotherapy fails or a nasogastric tube is necessary but cannot be used over prolonged periods of time, percutaneous gastrostomy as a venting procedure is extremely useful. A tube is percutaneously introduced through the abdominal wall while the patient is under local anesthesia. Venting of the bowel proximal to the inoperable bowel obstruction permits continuous decompression of fluids and gas and thereby relieves the symptoms. Some patients become adept at venting the tube intermittently, with small amount of fluids or food intake in between.

21. Should every patient with bowel obstruction be managed by pharmacotherapy only?

Surgery is either not indicated or not feasible in a large percentage of patients with malignant bowel obstruction and limited life expectancy. Pharmacotherapy is the logical approach to symptom control when the patient is found inoperable and when the obstructing lesion is unresectable. If the patient has partial bowel obstruction, symptoms may be relieved by pharmacotherapy. Pharmacologic control of symptoms is possible with morphine, antiemetics, steroids, and octreotide. Prolonged intravenous hydration and nasogastric tube suction are not indicated. Percutaneous gastrostomy is a safe venting procedure.

BIBLIOGRAPHY

1. Baines M, Oliver DJ, Carter RL: Medical management of intestinal obstruction in patients with advanced medical disease. A clinical and pathological study. Lancet ii:990–993, 1985.
2. Baines MJ: ABC of palliative care. Nausea, vomiting, and intestinal obstruction. BMJ 315:1148–1150, 1997.
3. Mangili G, et al: Octreotide in the management of bowel obstruction in terminal ovarian cancer. Gynecol Oncol 61:345–348, 1996.
4. Ripamonti C: Malignant bowel obstruction in advanced and terminal cancer patients. Eur J Palliat Care 1:15–18, 1994.
5. Steadman K, Franks A: A woman with malignant bowel obstruction who did not want to die with tubes. Lancet 347:944, 1996.

23. SURGERY AND PALLIATIVE CARE

Geoffrey P. Dunn, M.D., F.A.C.S.

1. Is there a need for surgical expertise in palliative care?

Palliative medicine endorses the concept of patient-centered treatment instead of disease-centered treatment and, on this basis, the surgeon has a definite place if he or she has had previous contact with a patient. The technical and other information a surgeon has pertaining to a given individual can be invaluable in planning future palliative strategies. The surgeon can help review a patient's history in light of newer developments, reinforce earlier understandings or, in some cases, help a patient "sign off" a doubtful surgical option that the patient may have been offered or may have wished for. The surgeon's personal credibility to the patient in this instance cannot be overemphasized.

2. Is major surgery ever indicated in palliative care or hospice?

Depending on the wishes of the patient, the scope of the procedure, the skill of the surgeon, and the likelihood of palliative benefit, an operation as major as a craniotomy or abdominal surgery can occasionally be justified, particularly in patients with good functional status and reasonable anesthetic risk. These decisions must be made on an individualized basis, focusing on symptom control.

3. What attributes of the surgeon's experience come to the aid of the palliative practitioner?

Surgeons are trained how to "make wounds that heal." They have knowledge pertinent to natural or iatrogenic wounds. They are familiar with the management of mechanical obstruction, whether it be respiratory, digestive, urinary, or circulatory. They are probably at their best and happiest doing drainage procedures, such as related to pus in an abscess causing opiate-resistant pain, ascites refractory to pharmacologic management, or a distended bladder that may require a skilled catheterization. Surgeons have sophisticated knowledge in nutritional support, which can be helpful in discussions of aggressive nutritional interventions such as enteral or parenteral nutrition. Their more recent role in transplantation and oncology gives them valuable insight into the problems of immunosuppression that are prevalent in patients receiving palliative care. Trauma has been the most ancient of challenges to the surgeon, and what has been learned is certainly applicable to patients with problems such as pathologic fractures or brisk hemorrhage.

4. How can a surgeon participate in the decision-making process on behalf of a patient with advanced cancer?

If the surgeon is already acquainted with the patient and has a well-established, trusting relationship, the surgeon may serve as the primary medical advocate for the patient in an interdisciplinary forum. In this scenario, the surgeon's advice will not be based on mere knowledge of surgery but knowledge of the individual obtained under unique circumstances. This is what appropriately positions the surgeon as the primary medical advocate.

Another duty the surgeon may be asked to perform is restaging the patient's disease by endoscopy and tissue biopsy. Endowed with knowledge of the person and the person's disease, the surgeon is ready to offer the advantages and disadvantages of any surgical procedure to be considered for palliation. Advice would include statistics relating to the chance of a desired outcome, morbidity, complications, and recommendations for the necessary preoperative preparations to maximize the chance of success and minimize morbidity.

5. How does the surgeon weigh the risks and benefits before operating on a patient with advanced cancer?

The more precarious the patient's overall condition, the more careful the weighing of risk versus benefit must be. A careful preoperative assessment of risk must include social, psychological, spiritual, emotional, and even economic issues. The only sensible fulcrum for this weighing is knowledge of the patient in his or her totality. To assist this process, much data is available to surgeons regarding morbidity, such as wound complications and bleeding. However, data is scarce with respect to other parameters, such as the degree of symptomatic improvement and patient satisfaction in general following palliative procedures for advanced cancers. This experience closely parallels the criticism of medical oncologic trials.

6. What are the important preoperative supportive care measures required for safe surgery in advanced cancer patients?

Patients frequently have already received chemotherapy or radiation therapy and, in some cases, surgical therapy. The sequelae and complications of these treatments must be assessed and corrected when possible. This assessment often directs the surgeon's attention to correction of clotting problems, nutritional deficits, and insufficiency of any other system that may have been compromised by previous cancer therapy or noncancer-related disease. In urgent situations, these preparations may need to be abbreviated, but operability is usually quickly determined. The most important supportive preoperative measure is reassurance to the patient by the surgeon that preparation is thorough. If this is the truth, there should be few surprises at surgery. A close, nonadversarial partnership with the anesthesiology team is critical because many of the considerations for operability and degree of risk are related to the anesthetic risk. There must be evidence of capacity to adequately oxygenate tissues and maintain hemostasis to justify anesthesia.

7. Surgical procedures are traditionally described as "minor" and "major." Are these terminologies suitable to describe the surgeries with palliative intent?

These are highly relative terms because what is minor from the point of view of anesthesia or tissue trauma may be a major event for a patient emotionally. It is not uncommon for a patient to forget details of a previous major operation such as cholecystectomy or hysterectomy but to recall vividly details of a minor procedure such as a biopsy. The traditional use of the term often reflected the type of anesthesia. The relative nature of these terms applies to palliative procedures as well as curative ones. Overall, these terms reflect the degree of risk.

8. What happens to the status of "do not resuscitate" (DNR) during and after surgery for a patient undergoing anesthesia?

A general anesthetic is a form of continuous resuscitation because breathing is assisted and circulatory stability is under the anesthetist's control. This makes DNR difficult to interpret during an operation. To minimize confusion, it is best to have a preoperative statement among the surgeon, anesthesiologist, operating room nursing staff, and the patient about goals of treatment and the limits of treatment. The same should apply postoperatively. Different institutions have varying policies regarding this scenario.

9. Are there any psychosocial and emotional emergencies for which a surgeon's help may be needed?

Any cause for patient distress that might be relieved by surgical knowledge or a surgical procedure is worthy of a surgeon's attention. A common psychosocial and emotional emergency is discovery of a mass. A professor of surgery at Harvard once taught that seeing a distraught 18-year-old girl with a newly discovered breast mass (almost certainly a benign lump) was as much a matter of urgency as seeing a patient with suspected appendicitis.

10. What are the unique features of the surgeon-patient relationship as opposed to the physician-patient relationship?

The relationship between a surgeon and a patient is one of the most intimate medical relationships possible. No therapeutic encounter leaves as obvious a mark in its aftermath as that with a surgeon, whether it is the physical scar or the degree of trust. The dramatic change possible following surgery fills the patient with a mixture of awe and fear: this makes abandonment or indifference, even after a brief encounter, extremely destructive. A surgeon can do or undo in an hour what a physician can do or undo in a lifetime.

11. For what gastrointestinal conditions in advanced cancer patients would you call a surgeon rather than a gastroenterologist? Why?

Conditions suspicious for intestinal perforation, obstruction, or infarction or conditions presenting similarly to these due to gynecologic, thoracic, or urologic disease should steer the referring physician toward a surgical opinion. Hemorrhagic problems of the gastrointestinal system can be comfortably managed by a gastroenterologist skilled in endoscopy, but it is prudent to arrange for surgical back-up at the outset of these problems so that a consensus can be reached prospectively about the extent of nonoperative trials of management. Infectious and metabolic problems of the gastrointestinal system are best initially evaluated by a gastroenterologist.

12. What are the surgical options available to alleviate symptoms of dysphagia due to esophageal and nonesophageal malignant conditions?

Depending on the patient's functional status, extent of disease, and preference, there is a spectrum of surgical options, ranging from resection to stenting or ablative procedures, either with radiation or laser photodynamic therapy. Because treatment for carcinoma of the esophagus is rarely curative, all surgical therapies are essentially palliative. In general, resection for palliation is reserved for patients with better functional status and less advanced disease. Surgical resection has the advantage of providing staging of the disease and the rare chance of cure. Stenting avoids both general anesthesia and the risks and morbidity of an open operative procedure and provides immediate palliation for dysphagia.

13. Which candidates are suitable for relief of malignant bowel obstruction by surgical procedures rather than nonsurgical management?

Any patient with a known or suspected malignant condition who can tolerate surgery should be considered for exploration. In several series, the cause of bowel obstruction proved to be benign in about a third of cases. In advanced cancer, the decision to operate for a condition even as compelling as unrelieved obstruction is difficult because so many factors can influence the recommendation for surgery and the acceptance of the recommendation by the patient. There is no longer any excuse to consider surgery only because "obstruction is a terrible way to die," since obstructive symptoms can be effectively relieved by pharmacologic techniques.

Adverse factors for favorable surgical palliation include advanced age, poor medical or nutritional status, previous surgery documenting extensive intraabdominal involvement with tumor, signs of diffuse or advanced disease such as ascites, palpable masses, distant metastases, previous radiation therapy to the abdomen or the pelvis, previous combination chemotherapy, evidence of multiple sites of bowel obstruction, and small bowel obstruction. Most of these are reflections of extremely advanced disease with its related problems: increased chance of infection, poor wound healing, and tissue deficits related to earlier therapies. Open discussion of these general problems may help the patient to recognize their interrelatedness. This type of decision provides an opportunity for discussing the meaning of the symptoms and may require more than what surgical expertise alone can offer.

Because of the unpredictable findings at laparotomy, the patient needs to know a wide range of possible operative solutions before granting consent. These choices include (1) resection of a segment of the bowel followed by reanastomosis and (2) removal of a segment of the bowel and formation of a stoma, which is bringing the opened portion of the bowel to the skin. A stoma made from small intestine is usually called an ileostomy; if made from colon, a colostomy. Other choices include bypassing the obstruction internally without removal of any tissue or cutting obstructing adhesions. Any of these operations may include placement of a gastrostomy tube. The best choice of procedure in a situation with high-grade obstruction in a nutritionally exhausted patient with widespread tumor in an area of previously irradiated bowel, with a history of chemotherapy and possibly receiving steroid therapy, can be challenging to even the most experienced surgeon. In some cases an expeditious and orderly retreat leaving only a venting gastrostomy may be the wisest course of action. Doing nothing is not palliation!

14. What are the indications for ostomy procedures at various sites along the gastrointestinal (GI) tract?

The primary indication for creation of a stoma from any level of the GI tract in advanced disease is a relief of obstruction, but a stoma can be used as an access port for feedings and medications.

At the level of the stomach, the stoma is called a gastrostomy and may be performed as part of a more comprehensive operation or as the sole procedure. It is now possible to perform a gastrostomy under local anesthesia without opening the abdominal cavity, making it much more suitable for palliative situations than the traditional open procedure. A gastrostomy can be considered in decompressing a diffusely obstructed GI tract at the time of laparotomy for conditions such as ovarian carcinomatosis as an alternative or adjunct to pharmacologic management with opiates, anticholinergics, and antiemetics. In rare cases it can be considered for feeding and medication when starvation and acute dehydration are likely to result from mechanical obstruction instead of the consequences of systemic disease.

The indications for creation of a stoma from the jejunum follow similar guidelines. A tube is inserted through the stoma at both sites. An ileostomy or colostomy is formed for relief of obstruction when primary anastomosis is not possible or safe. Depending on the patient's anatomy and disease and the preference of the surgeon, the ileostomy or colostomy can take the form of a loop or end colostomy. In cases when an end colostomy is fashioned, the distal segment of divided bowel can be brought up as a mucous fistula, or it can be stapled or sewed shut and left inside the abdomen. The mucous fistula can be a handy site for administering suppositories. Suppositories also can be given safely through a colostomy. Absorption is less predictable for suppositories given through an ileostomy because of the more continuous drainage.

15. What are some recommendations for solving ostomy problems at various sites of the GI tract?

The most common problem related to gastrostomy or jejunostomy sites is displacement of the tube or leakage around the tube. Significant bleeding is uncommon. Intermittent trivial bleeding from the edges of the stoma with minor trauma or manipulation is common. Prompt attention from a surgeon is necessary in cases of suspected tube displacement because a malpositioned tube can cause obstruction with pain and aspiration; if the tube comes out, the stoma can rapidly close, making reinsertion difficult and traumatic. Gastrostomy and jejunostomy sites usually have a small area of redness (several millimeters) with mucus discharge that can be misinterpreted by the novice as infection. For stomas of the ileum and colon, problems such as mucosal separation, obstruction, variceal bleeding, hernia, and prolapse can occur. Most of these problems will yield to nonoperative measures, but surgery can be considered in patients with good functional status and refractory stoma-related problems.

16. What are debulking procedures, and what are the indications?

Debulking, or cytoreduction, procedures refer to operations in which tumor is removed to the extent possible even if cure is not expected. These operations are usually part of a comprehensive program of management that includes chemotherapy and radiation therapy. In carefully selected cases, debulking can be done as a sole measure, e.g., in a symptomatic patient with a slow-growing sarcoma unresponsive to nonsurgical therapy.

17. Can respiratory distress be surgically relieved by a direct approach that actually removes the cause of distress?

Yes. An example is resection of a tumor obstructing or compressing the tracheobronchial tree, such as an anaplastic thyroid tumor or tracheoesophageal fistula caused by a tumor. With the availability of laser surgery and cryosurgery, an endoscopic approach for removal of tumors is now available even for advanced lesions no longer amenable to radiation or chemotherapy. In advanced cases these operations can be tailored just to the point of providing relief and then repeated as needed. Resection may be indicated in certain abdominal conditions that are causing respiratory distress by compromising diaphragmatic function. Examples include debulking a large ovarian tumor or liver resection in polycystic liver disease associated with polycystic kidney disease.

If resection is not an option, maintaining patency through an obstructing or fistulized area can be achieved endoscopically and maintained by placement of a stent. In some cases a stent can be used to provide brachytherapy even in previously irradiated regions. For obstructing lesions of the upper airway or dyspnea due to the demands of breathing through an anatomically normal airway in neurodegenerative illnesses such as amyotrophic lateral sclerosis, a tracheostomy is an option and can be done in an outpatient setting under local anesthesia. To preserve the ability to speak, a fenestrated tube that allows air to pass through the larynx can be used.

For management of pleural effusions, thoracoscopy drainage and instillation of talc or open pleurodesis remain options but require complete reexpansion of the lung. In situations in which this is not possible, drainage via a pleuroperitoneal shunt is effective; no operative mortality was reported in one series.

18. How can a surgeon be expected to improve quality of life?

A surgeon can use operative means or knowledge related to perioperative care (nutrition, pain management) to relieve distressing symptoms and increase functionality as ways of improving quality of life. A surgeon can improve quality of life simply by bringing hope to the patient. As one patient put it: "If they sent in a surgeon, they must mean business even if they don't want to operate!"

19. How can surgeons contribute to the development of palliative care and hospice for the year 2000?

By becoming engaged in the palliative care community and beginning the exchange of disease-oriented medicine for patient-oriented medicine. The trend of increasing subspecialization by surgeons is making this transition even more difficult. One patient put it bluntly when referred to a women's health center for evaluation of a newly discovered breast lump: "I don't want to go to a place that's focused on my breast, I want to go to a place that's focused on me!"

The first contribution surgeons can make is their endorsement of the concept that palliation alone is a legitimate focus of practice, research, and self-esteem. Following this will be reexamination of surgery's vast experience from the perspective of patient advocacy instead of disease control. It is hoped that this will inspire a recataloging of surgical data and outcomes to make this vast potential more readily available to the immediate concerns of the patient. The rapid acceptance of laparoscopy—a patient-driven development—and increased attention to cosmetic outcomes in breast surgery are examples of this kind of transition.

BIBLIOGRAPHY

1. Ashby MA, Game PA, Devitt P, et al: Percutaneous gastrostomy as a venting procedure in palliative care. Palliat Med 5:47–50, 1991.
2. Baines MJ, Oliver DJ, Carter RL: Medical management of intestinal obstruction in patients with advanced malignant disease: A clinical and pathological study. Lancet 2:990–993, 1985.
3. Butler JA, Cameron BL, Morrow M, Kahng K: Small bowel obstruction in patients with a prior history of cancer. Am J Surg 162:624–628, 1991.
4. Doyle D, Hanks GW, MacDonald N: Oxford Text of Palliative Medicine. 2nd ed. New York, Oxford University Press, 1998.
5. Dunphy JE: Annual discourse—On caring for the patient with cancer. N Engl J Med 295:313–319, 1976.
6. Gallick HL, Weaver DW, Sachs RJ, Bouwman DL: Intestinal obstruction in cancer patients. An assessment of risk factors and outcome. Am Surg 52:434–437, 1986.
7. McCarthy D: Strategy for intestinal obstruction in peritoneal carcinomatosis. Arch Surg 121:1081–1082, 1986.
8. McDermott WV: Lecture. Harvard Surgical Services, New England Deaconess Hospital, Boston, 1979.
9. Milch RA, Dunn GP: The surgeon's role in palliative care. Bull Am Coll Surg 82:15–17, 48, 1997.

10. Orringer M: Transhiatal oesophogectomy without thoracotomy for carcinoma of the thoracic oesophagus. Ann Surg 200:282–288, 1984.
11. Osteen RT, Guyton S, Steele G, Wilson R: Malignant intestinal obstruction. Surgery 87:611–615, 1980.
12. Petrou M, Kaplan D, Goldstraw P: Bronchoscopic diathermy resection and stent insertion: A cost effective treatment for tracheobronchial obstruction. Thorax 48:1156–1159, 1993.
13. Petrou M, Kaplan D, Goldstraw P: The management of recurrent malignant pleural effusion: The complementary role of talc pleurodesis and pleuroperitoneal shunting. Cancer 75:801–805, 1995.
14. Rubin SC, Hoskins WJ, Benjamin I, Lewis JL: Palliative surgery for intestinal obstruction in advanced ovarian cancer. Gynecol Oncol 34:16–19, 1989.
15. Schwartz SI, Shires GT, Spencer FC: Principles of Surgery, 6th ed. New York, McGraw-Hill, 1994.
16. Turnbull ADM, Guerra J, Starners HF: Results of surgery for obstructing carcinomatosis of gastrointestinal, pancreatic, or biliary origin. J Clin Oncol 7:381–386, 1989.
17. Walsh HPJ, Schofield PE: Is laparotomy for bowel obstruction justified for patients with previously treated malignancy? Br J Surg 71:933–935, 1984.
18. Webb WR, Ozmen V, Moulder PV, et al: Iodized talc pleurodesis for the treatment of pleural effusions. J Thorac Cardiovasc Surg 103:881–886, 1993.
19. Welch JP: Bowel Obstruction. Philadelphia, W.B. Saunders, 1990.

24. PEDIATRIC PALLIATIVE CARE

Gerri Frager, R.N., M.D., F.R.C.P.C.

1. When is the best time to involve palliative care when caring for a child?

Palliative care traditionally developed as a response to the unmet needs of dying adults, particularly adults with cancer, and their families. The management principles of palliative care include comprehensive care of physical symptoms and addressing the emotional, psychological, and spiritual needs of patients and their family members.

Children with a life-threatening illness who are enrolled in palliative care services will equally benefit. The best time to introduce the concept of palliative care is early, when a child is diagnosed with an illness likely to end in premature death.

The figures below compare the traditional model of palliative care with a model that enables the child to receive care that may be directed toward cure as well as the components of palliative care. Such a scenario would provide for appropriate pain and symptom management at any time during the child's illness, not solely at the end of life.

Traditional Palliative Care Services

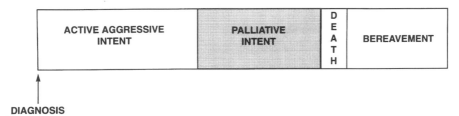

Traditional palliative care services.(Adapted from Palliative Care Services Guidelines: Health Canada, 1989, with permission of the Minister of Public Works and Government Services, Canada, 1998.)

Proposed Palliative Care Services

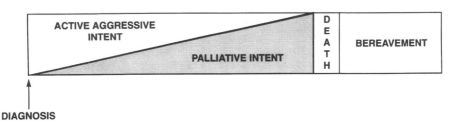

Proposed palliative care services. (Adapted from Palliative Care Services Guidelines: Health Canada, 1989, with permission of the Minister of Public Works and Government Services, Canada, 1998.)

2. What are the examples of terminal diseases in children appropriate for palliative care services?

- Congenital syndromes and anomalies likely to end in premature death, including trisomy 18 and Smith-Lemli-Opitz syndrome
- Progressive neurodegenerative disease from inborn errors of metabolism, including leukodystrophies and Tay-Sachs disease
- HIV or AIDS

- Neuromuscular disorders such as Duchenne muscular dystrophy and Werdnig-Hoffmann paralysis
- Malignancies with poor or unclear prognoses or relapses, such as neuroblastoma, metastatic rhabdomyosarcoma, and brainstem gliomas
- Disorders of mucopolysaccharide metabolism, such as Hunter, Hurler, and Sanfillipo syndromes
- Cardiac conditions likely to end in premature death
- Cystic fibrosis

3. How is this early approach of benefit later?

Early introduction of palliative care can help prevent crisis-oriented management and provides a framework for discussion of balancing the benefits and risks of any intervention. This approach can facilitate subsequent decision-making in the complex care of children living with chronic and critical illness. It also is of value early in the course of illness because the goals of palliative care are to diminish suffering and to enhance life.

4. Who is best suited to deliver pediatric palliative care?

Care is delivered by a multidisciplinary team working collaboratively to meet various complex needs. Both the child and family generally wish to continue to receive care from the health professionals (the pediatrician or family doctor as well as other "front-line" health care providers, such as the nurse or social worker) who know them best. These individuals have shared the previous trials of the child's illness and are well aware of the course of the disease, the existing and developing coping strategies, and the most difficult issues faced. However, the primary care provider may not have expertise in the care of a terminally ill child. Liaison with health professionals who have more experience in palliative care can be helpful, allowing continuity of care as well as best overall support. The health professionals who provide front line care for the child must engage in continual assessment and discussion of the goals of care. The appropriateness of various proposed interventions needs to be reexamined in light of the changing status of the child. The health professional needs to know when and how to consult palliative care experts and how to work collaboratively with them.

Similarly, palliative care services may be called upon to provide care for a dying child. In some instances, the palliative care health professional may not have skills relating to pediatrics. Working together, the pediatrician and palliative care expert can develop a plan of care that defines expectations and defines the role of each in meeting the child's and family's needs.

5. What is pediatric hospice?

Hospice traditionally has been defined as free-standing buildings or home care programs that provide care for the terminally ill. However, in North America, hospice has been applied more broadly to the same philosophy of care defined by palliative care. Hospice or palliative care can be involved early in the stage of a child's illness likely to end in premature death. One of the obstacles to involvement is the designation of criteria by some programs for a life expectancy of less than 6 months. Other programs exclude children continuing with interventions directed to cure. Such restrictions are unrealistic and inappropriate when facing the prognostic uncertainty of various childhood conditions and when children and families wish to pursue cure and palliative care. We should not force these families to choose between care or cure.

Once such barriers are overcome, hospice and palliative care programs would be able to provide much support to the child, family, and health professionals caring for them. Generally, palliative care health professionals have expertise meeting needs in pain and symptom management; the emotional, social, and spiritual realms; and grief and bereavement support. Although generally willing, most programs lack the experience to care for children. Hospice and palliative care professionals and volunteers need to acquire some basic knowledge of pediatrics if they want to be able to best support the child and family through this process. Some of the specific skills include knowing about the differences in the assessment of pain in the nonverbal and young verbal child, the variations in pain management techniques, the child's understanding of illness and death, how to talk with an ill child, and how to support others affected by a terminally ill child.

6. Who is affected by a terminally ill child other than the child, parents, and siblings?

The extended family, the child's and sibling's peers, schoolmates, teachers, and the broader social and religious community. Their needs may best be met through a collaborative plan with the health professionals who have worked with the child and family.

7. How do you tell a child and the family that the child's illness is terminal?

- If you are not the child's primary health provider, first find out what the child and family understand about the illness. A good way to start may be, "Tell me in your own words what you know about your/your child's illness."
- It is important to know how the family generally shares information. You can state that you have some test results and ask if they want to include the child in the discussion now or later. Clarify if the family would like to share the information with the child or if they would prefer that you do this. Do they want someone with them when they talk with the child?
- If the child is participating in the discussion, the words should be appropriate to the child's developmental level. Everyone benefits from a warning that difficult news is going to be discussed. Use whatever words feel right to you and are easily understood by the people with whom you are speaking. Saying "This is hard for me but I have to talk with you about Jamie's test results" announces that bad news is on the way. It is acceptable to show the child and family you are upset as long as you are able to offer them support throughout. Problems with communication are compounded when a health professional appears uncaring. Feedback from families and experience with litigation support this approach; communications difficulties are among the most frequent reasons health professionals are sued.
- Continue to offer pieces of information in manageable sizes. Pace the information according to how the child paces you. Children will ask for bits of information and clarification in amounts that they are best able to assimilate. If no further questions come from the child, assure them that you are available to talk if they think of something else and ask at intervals if they have thought of any other questions. It is often beneficial to tell the child that you have spoken with other children with the same condition who said they were worried about issues such as how they might feel if they got sicker or worried about how their parents would feel. If the child has no initial response you might ask if he or she has similar concerns. Continue to gauge how much to share with the child by taking the child's lead on the questions he or she asks. Provide updates regularly. Check with the child and family on what they have heard and understood. The use of art can help to enhance communication.
- Remember to include siblings and the child's schoolmates and friends. Some hospitals have a school visitation program to include the child's peers in the information process. One individual cannot do it all, but you need to ensure that a process is in place to cover all the bases.

8. Are children's symptoms in the terminal phase different from those that occur in adults?

Children with chronic illnesses such as cancer and AIDS frequently experience more pain from procedures and treatments than from the disease itself. Disease-related pain associated with cancer in childhood tends to resolve quickly with primary treatment of the malignancy. Leukemias and lymphomas represent most pediatric malignancies. They are diffuse diseases that, if unresponsive to curative therapy, frequently cause pain that is similarly widely disseminated. Compared to adults with advanced malignancies such as metastatic breast or prostate cancer, children with advanced disease tend to run a relatively rapid course to death.

Other predominant symptoms in endstage childhood illness correspond to the pathophysiologic process. For example, breathlessness may be prominent if the lungs have been affected by the disease process, as in cancer metastatic to the lungs, cystic fibrosis, or cardiac failure.

9. In what ways is the assessment of pain different in children?

As in adults, the gold standard of pain measurement is patient report. Children require modified measurement tools appropriate for their developmental capacity. In addition to variations in development, significant illness can cause children to regress or, at times, to advance beyond their expected stage of cognitive development. Health professionals should be aware that children may not express their pain if they believe it may lead to a painful intervention.

Children at a developmental age of at least 7 years should be able to understand the concept of the standard 0–10 numeric scale used for adults. For younger verbal children, there are a variety of modifications to the usual numeric scale. One example is Bieri's Faces Scale.

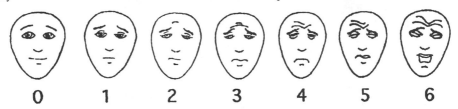

Bieri Faces Scale (Scale 0–6). (From Bieri D, Reeve RA, Champion GD, et al: The Faces Pain Scale for the self-assessment of the severity of pain experienced by children: Development, initial validation, and preliminary investigation for ratio scale properties. Pain 41:139–150, 1990; with permission.)

Use whatever word the child uses for pain, such as "hurt" or "owie." It is helpful to anchor the endpoints of the scale for the child by saying that "this face [Face 0] shows someone who has no pain and this face [Face 6] shows someone with the worst pain possible." Then ask the child which picture shows the way his pain makes him feel.

Questions That Should Be Included in the Child's Pain History

CHILD FORM	PARENT FORM
Tell me what pain is.	What word(s) does your child use in regard to pain?
Tell me about hurt you have had before.	Describe the pain experience your child has had before.
Do you tell others when you hurt? If yes, who?	Does your child tell you or others when he or she is hurting?
What do you do for yourself when you are hurting?	How do you know when your child is in pain?
What do you want others to do for you when you hurt?	How does your child usually react to pain?
What don't you want others to do for you when you hurt?	What do you do for child when he or she is hurting?
What helps the most to take your hurt away?	What does your child do for himself or herself when he or she is hurting?
Is there anything special that you want me to know about you when you hurt? (If yes, have child describe.)	What works best to decrease or take away your child's pain?
	Is there anything special that you would like me to know about your child and pain? (If yes, describe.)

Adapted from Hester NO, Barcus CS: Assessment and management of pain in children. Pediatrics: Nursing Update 1:2–8, 1986.

10. How do you assess pain in children who cannot voice their complaints?

When the child is nonverbal or cognitively impaired, pain assessment is based on behavioral observations, preferably by someone who knows the child well. Parameters include how the child is behaving compared with usual, degree of interaction and interest in surroundings, amount of sleep, ability to be comforted, body position, and tone. Two assessment tools are the CHEOP

(Children's Hospital of Eastern Ontario Pain Scale) and the Gauvin-Piquard Rating Scale. Physiologic parameters, such as changes in pulse and blood pressure, and other indicators, such as facial expressions, are unreliable in chronic pain or in ill children.

11. Are there any major differences in the pharmacologic management of pain in children versus adults?

The basic principles of pharmacologic pain management in adults, such as the World Health Organization's analgesic ladder, are appropriate to children regardless of the cause of the pain. However, for the first step of the ladder, nonsteroidal antiinflammatory agents are generally replaced with acetaminophen in children, because the chronic childhood illnesses that cause significant pain often result in low or dysfunctional platelets.

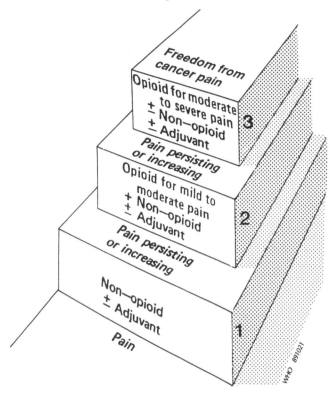

World Health Organization three-step analgesic ladder. (From Cancer Pain Relief and Palliative Care. Geneva, World Health Organization, 1990, technical report series 804; with permission.)

12. Are children at greater risk than adults of opioid-induced respiratory depression?

No. In general, the fear about respiratory depression and opioids is grossly disproportionate to the true degree of risk. This fear is even more exaggerated with respect to children. The risk of significant opioid-induced respiratory depression in adults is approximately 0.09%. Opioid pharmacokinetics are really no different in children older than 3 months.

For infants, particularly newborns, the following factors may increase their sensitivity to opioid-related respiratory depression:
1. Delayed liver enzyme function
2. Decreased renal clearance
3. High body water:fat ratio
4. High ratio of brain and viscera to muscle and fat

5. Reduced albumin and glycoprotein
6. Reduced ventilatory response to hypoxemia and hypercapnia

The presence of these factors does not mean that pain in a neonate should not be treated. Rather, analgesia can be given at a reduced starting dose, which is then judiciously titrated and monitored. To be cautious, children 6 months of age and younger are treated at approximately a quarter of the usual childhood dosing regimen on a mg/kg basis and then titrated to effect.

13. What is the pharmacologic management if the child's pain is unrelieved with regular acetaminophen or an NSAID, and what is the correct starting dose of opioid for a child with moderate to severe pain?

If dosing at regular intervals does not provide relief, then an opioid for mild to moderate pain can be added. Codeine is commonly used in pediatrics at 0.5–1.0 mg/kg per dose every 4 hours. Nothing is gained by giving more than 1 mg/kg per dose of codeine.

If pain is unrelieved, the codeine should be replaced by an opioid for moderate to severe pain, as indicated by the third step of the ladder. In an adolescent weighing 50 kg or more, the usual adult dose would be used rather than a mg/kg basis. (See table on facing page.)

14. What is an appropriate hourly rate for starting an opioid infusion in a child?

In an opioid-naive child, a starting infusion rate could be 0.02 mg/kg/hr of morphine with breakthrough doses as needed (refer to question 13). There are several options for calculating the infusion for a child already taking opioids. The rate could be based on the total previous 24-hour opioid requirements (around-the-clock doses with additional breakthrough doses). With an infusion, usually less is needed than with bolus dosing every 3–4 hours. It would be safe to give 75% of the previous 24-hour opioid requirements divided as the hourly infusion. Provide with breakthrough doses as needed.

A second option is to consider the bolus dose that gave adequate relief as the loading dose. A basic rule of thumb to calculate the hourly infusion rate for short halflife opioids is to multiply the load by the steady-state constant of 0.69 and then divide this number by the halflife of the opioid. Alternatively the load can be divided by twice the opioid's halflife. For example, if 5 mg of morphine was required to give adequate relief, the infusion rate would be 0.83 mg/hr. The calculation is $5 \div (2 \times 3)$; where 3 is the approximate halflife of morphine. This could be approximated to 1 mg/hr with breakthrough doses as needed.

15. What would be an appropriate rescue dose for breakthrough pain in a child?

Even though the child is provided with a background dose, an additional or "rescue" dose should be available for pain that "breaks through" the scheduled dosing. Because the principles of rescue doses for breakthrough pain are calculated on a proportion of the daily opioid requirements or the hourly dose, the guidelines are the same regardless of the child's weight. Once the background or hourly rate has been calculated on a mg/kg basis, the rescue dose is 5–10% of the 24-hour opioid requirement. Alternatively, and somewhat easier, the rescue dose is about 50–200% of the hourly dose. For example, if a 20-kg child is treated with 0.05 mg/kg/hr (1 mg/hr) of morphine by infusion, an appropriate breakthrough dose would be 0.025–0.1 mg/kg (0.5–2 mg) offered every 30–60 minutes. For a child with persistent pain, it is inappropriate to give repeated boluses at frequent as-needed intervals to obtain relief. In these situations, a requirement of more than four to six additional boluses in 24 hours is an indication to increase the basal rate. This is a different approach from that used for the child with acute, postoperative pain.

16. Is opioid titration any different for a child?

Essentially, no. Because the principles of titration are based on a proportion of the daily opioid requirements rather than on any given dose, the guidelines are the same. For example, if a 20-kg child is receiving 0.05 mg/kg/hr or 1 mg/hr of morphine by continuous infusion and in the preceding 24 hours required 10 additional bolus doses of 0.05 mg/kg (1 mg) for breakthrough pain with no adverse effects, the hourly infusion could be increased by at least 50% to 0.075

Short Halflife Opioids Used in Pediatric Palliative Care

DRUG	EQUIANALGESIC DOSE PARENTERAL	IV/SC:PO RATIO	EQUIANALGESIC DOSE ORAL	USUAL STARTING DOSE IV/SC		USUAL STARTING DOSE PO		BIOLOGIC T1/2 HALFLIFE
				< 50 KG	> 50 KG	< 50 KG	> 50 KG	
Codeine	130 mg	1:1.5	190 mg	0.5 mg/kg q 3–4 hr SC Not to be given IV	130 mg q 3–4 hr	0.5–1 mg/kg q 3–4 hr	15–30 mg q 3–4 hr	2.5–3 hr
Hydrocodone	N/A	1:1.5	30 mg	N/A	N/A	0.1 mg/kg q 3–4 hr	5–10 mg q 3–4 hr	3–4 hr
Oxycodone	N/A IV PO form Equianalgesic 1:1 with PO morphine	N/A	30 mg	N/A	N/A	0.1–0.2 mg/kg q 3–4 hr	5–10 mg q 3–4 hr	2–3 hr
Morphine	10 mg	1:3	30 mg	0.05–0.1 mg/kg q 3–4 hr	5–10 mg q 3–4 hr	0.15–0.3 mg/kg q 3–4 hr	5–10 mg q 3–4 hr	2.5–3 hr
Hydromorphone (Dilaudid)	1.5 mg	1:5	7.5 mg	0.01 mg/kg q 3–4 hr	1–1.5 mg q 3–4 hr	0.05 mg/kg q 3–4 hr	1–2 mg q 3–4 hr	2–3 hr
Oxymorphone (Numorphan)	1 mg	N/A	N/A	0.02 mg/kg q 3–4 hr	1 mg q 3–4 hr	N/A	N/A PO 5 mg PR equianalgesic with 1 mg IV	1.5 hr
Fentanyl *Caution:* rapid infusion may cause chest wall rigidity	Single dose 100 µg By infusion: 100 µg/hr = 2.5 mg/hr morphine	N/A	N/A	0.5–1.5 µg/kg q 30 min	25–75 µg q 30 min	N/A	N/A	IV: 3–12 hr TD: 18–24 hr (elimination halflife) TD:IV ratio = 1:1 based on clinical experience

N/A = not available; IV = intravenous; PO = oral; SC = subcutaneous; PR = per rectum; TD = transdermal.

Note: "Usual" starting doses are often empiric and not necessarily calculated according to equianalgesic principles, i.e., the usual dose for hydromorphone may be 2 mg PO even though the parenteral:PO ratio = 1:5. For infants ≤ 6 months of age, use 1/4 of the usual starting dose; then titrate to effect.

When converting from one short halflife opioid to another, reduce by 25–50% of the equianalgesic dose (because of incomplete cross-tolerance). Then titrate as required.

Meperidine (Demerol or pethidine) not recommended if opioids required for approximately > 3 days or if high doses needed (because of toxic metabolite, nor-meperidine).

mg/kg/hr (1.5 mg/hr) or at least by the amount that was taken in the previous 24 hours as break-through doses. This amount would then be divided by 24 and added to the hourly rate ([10×1] ÷ 24 = 0.4 added to the basal rate of 1 mg = at least 1.4 mg/hr).

17. Do the side effects of opioids differ between children and adults?

The importance of managing opioid-related side effects in children is that they may refuse analgesia if they dislike the feeling that is induced even if they are benefiting from pain relief. Adults are often more willing to tolerate side effects, because they understand that the effects are sometimes a trade-off for analgesia and that the side effects may be treated or resolve spontaneously.

Pruritus seems to be more bothersome to children and seems to occur with greater frequency than in adults. Sometimes children are less willing to take another medicine to treat the itch or to counteract other side effects. In such cases, particularly when ill children are already taking many medications, a change to an alternate opioid is an appropriate option rather than the addition of another medication.

The trust of the child must be established and maintained. Therefore, it is important to anticipate and ask about side effects and aggressively manage them. In addition to pain relief, what threatens to be lost is the child's trust in you and in your capacity to help him or her feel better. Because pain management often requires trial and error with a variety of agents, trust is critical.

18. Because the incidence of addiction is extremely low, why should this issue be raised with families and health professionals?

Many people associate the use of opioids with addiction. Health professionals often attempt to reassure each other and the families of a terminally ill child by expressing the idea that addiction is not really a concern because of the advanced stage of the child's disease. This is inappropriate. The reality is that both the child and family want to continue to live as they have lived even up to the point of death. They do not find such platitudes reassuring. Instead, health professionals should be knowledgeable about opioid use and, in turn, teach the older child and family about those truths. When starting opioid therapy, it is helpful to start the discussion by stating that many people have concerns and then list some of the common worries, such as addiction and the need to save the stronger medications for later.

19. Name ten facts, or myth busters, about opioid addiction.

1. The incidence of addiction in patients receiving opioid therapy for pain relief is no different than that of the general population—less than 1%.

2. The "just say no to drugs" movement does not apply to the child who is taking prescribed opioids for pain relief.

3. Taking drugs for pain management is different from taking them for pleasure.

4. The body will become physically dependent when treated with opioids for a time.

5. The body will have effects of withdrawal if the opioid is stopped suddenly.

6. Physical dependency is not synonymous with addiction.

7. Physical dependency is easily managed by a slow taper of the opioid when the pain has resolved.

8. Addiction is a psychological problem, not a physical one.

9. Individuals who are addicted use opioids for reasons other than pain.

10. Individual who are addicted will engage in all manner of manipulations, including illicit ones, to secure drugs.

20. Discuss the use of adjuvants in children.

As in adults, adjuvants are helpful in pain management in three ways. They can be used as coanalgesics, particularly for certain types of pain syndromes, such as neuropathic pain. As coanalgesics, adjuvants allow widening of the therapeutic window, enabling less opioid to be given. They can be used to help counteract side effects of opioid therapy, such as nausea or pruritus. They can be of benefit for a second symptom, such as pain, when used for their primary purpose. An example would be the use of a benzodiazepine for anxiety in a patient with muscle spasm. Relatively few data exist on the use of adjuvants for particular pain syndromes in terminally ill children. However, information gained from the adult experience has been of benefit for similar types of pain.

As with opioid dosing in children, starting doses for adjuvants should be determined on a mg/kg basis unless caring for a child weighing more than 50 kg. At that point, the maximum initial starting dose or usual adult dose would be prescribed. Adjuvants are then titrated to effect.

Adjuvants

CLASS OF DRUGS	ROUTE	HOW MUCH (INITIAL DOSE)	HOW OFTEN	COMMENT
TCAs				
Amitritpyline Despiramine	PO	0.2 mg/kg 0.2–3 days ↑ by 0.2–0.4 mg/kg	Nightly	Useful for neuropathic pain, particularly the dysesthetic variety Can enhance sleep Monitor blood levels, EKG Other antidepressants may be tried if these fail at maximum dose or toxicity
Anticonvulsants				
Carbamazepine	PO	2 mg/kg/dose ↑ as tolerated to relief	BID-TID	Useful for neuropathic pain, particularly the lancinating variety
Phenytoin	PO-IV	"Load" = 15 mg/kg (if PO ÷ in 3 doses)		Phenytoin useful in pain crisis; patient can be rapidly "loaded" IV-PO (max =1 gm) Cardiac monitor and care with IV load
		Maintenance 5 mg/kg/dose	BID	Other anticonvulsants may be tried if these fail at maximum dose or toxicity
Corticosteroids				
Dexamethasone	PO-IV	"Load" = 1 mg/kg Maintenance varies 0.1+ mg/kg/dose	BID-TID	In acute pain crisis, may "load" and then decrease to maintenance dose May stimulate appetite, improve mood (also dysphoria) Timing important as + + long-term adverse effects
Local anesthetics				
Mexiletine	PO	1 mg/kg every 2–3 days ↑ as tolerated to relief	BID-TID	Monitor blood levels GI side effects
Benzodiazepines				
Lorazepam SL (sublingual tabs available)	IV-PR-PO-SL	0.02–0.05 mg/kg	Every 6–8 hr	May be helpful width musculoskeletal spasm, anxiety, nausea (particularly anticipatory)
Diazepam (irritating via- peripheral IV)	IV-PO PR	0.05–0.1 mg/kg/ dose 0.3 mg/kg/dose		
Psychostimulants				
Methylphenidate Dextroamphetamine	PO	0.1 mg/kg ↑ gently as tolerated by 0.05–0.1 mg/kg	Every morning and noon	Helpful to counteract opioid-induced sedation Caution: can exacerbate dysphoria, agitation
Neuroleptics				
Methotrimeprazine (can be irritating SC)	PO-IV-SC	0.1 mg/kg/dose	Every 8 hr	Sedative properties vary within class Caution: can cause dystonia (reversible with diphenhydramine 1 mg/kg)

(Table continued on following page.)

Adjuvants (Continued)

CLASS OF DRUGS	ROUTE	HOW MUCH (INITIAL DOSE)	HOW OFTEN	COMMENT
Neuroleptics *(cont.)*				
Haloperidol	PO-IV	0.01 mg/kg/dose		Check haloperidol preparation for IV use
Miscellaneous				
Baclofen	PO	5 mg/dose ↑ by 5 mg/dose as tolerated	BID– TID	Can be helpful in neuropathic pain, spasticity Can cause sedation, may improve with time Caution: avoid abrupt withdrawal

These dosing guidelines include an initial starting dose. From this starting point, doses can be increased (↑) gradually until relief is achieved or toxicity is reached.
TCAs = tricyclic antidepressants; IV = intravenous; PO = oral; SC = subcutaneous; PR = per rectum; SL = sublingual; BID = twice daily; TID = thrice daily.

21. Is there a class of adjuvant that should not be used in children?

Concern has been expressed about the increased risk of dystonic or extrapyramidal reactions with the use of neuroleptics such as haloperidol or chlorpromazine in children. For this reason, some clinicians routinely order diphenhydramine (Benadryl) in combination with a neuroleptic. The author has three comments about this practice:

1. The fear of increased incidence in young children is probably overrated. Despite extensive use of these agents, the only instance of dystonia witnessed by the author was in a child who had overdosed on his mother's haloperidol.

2. There is no evidence that using these agents in combination prevents the onset of dystonic reactions.

3. If such a reaction were to occur, acute drug-induced dystonia is readily reversible with diphenhydramine (1 mg/kg IV) or benzotropine (0.5 mg/kg IV).

22. Is there any role for nonpharmacologic approaches in managing pain in children?

It is always important in managing pain to include nonpharmacologic measures directed to management of anxiety and fostering of positive coping techniques. Pain in children can be exacerbated by fear as procedural pain assumes increasing importance. Communication difficulties relating to their capacity to understand why certain things are being "done to them" compounds their vulnerability for associated pain. Cognitive and behavioral interventions for pain relief and pharmacologic management work better together than alone.

Simple measures include giving the child some choice and, in turn, a sense of control in a situation over which they have little control. Wherever possible, include the child in decision-making, but tailor this inclusion to the child's degree of willingness to participate. Having a pocket or examining bag filled with distracters such as a small pop-up book, a magic wand, or a small container of bubbles can help immeasurably.

Children report that what helps them the most to deal with pain is having a parent with them. The parent is generally frightened and made less effective by their own fear. Therefore, the health professional must show the parent how to support the child. Having the parent interact with the child over a favorite story, listening to music together, or using structured relaxation techniques often brings far more relief than might be anticipated through such simple measures. It also helps to have something to do while the medication takes effect.

More formal techniques such as hypnotherapy and advanced guided imagery can be learned by health care providers. These techniques are then taught to the child so that he can learn to help himself. This promotes self-confidence.

23. How do you address physical symptoms other than pain in children at the end of life?

The pattern of nonpain symptoms largely depends on the disease process. It helps to discuss with the child and family the anticipated course and support that is available to them.

Progressive neurodegenerative diseases and some metabolic disorders of childhood have a propensity to cause seizures. Similarly, seizures may distinguish certain cancers of the central nervous system and cardiac or respiratory conditions associated with hypoxemia.

Seizure management in the terminal phase should be proactive. The child may already be receiving anticonvulsant therapy. However, he or she may experience breakthrough seizures, particularly as they become more ill. It helps to instruct the family on measures that can be taken during a seizure so that they can meet this distressing situation with an action plan and a sense of control. The plan will include knowing what medication to give and whom to call. The family benefits from hands-on practice in administering the medication.

Opioid therapy and anxiolytics form the primary symptomatic management for terminal breathlessness. It is important to consider only interventions directed at the cause of the breathlessness in terms of potential provision of relief without causing further distress to the patient. An example would be the use of antibiotics in a terminally ill child with pneumonia. This would be reasonable if it would not place an undue burden on the child, such as causing difficulty with oral administration or intravenous access. Similarly, oxygen can be helpful if it makes the child feel less breathless or the child seems more comfortable with its administration. However, for the terminally ill child, checking the degree of oxygen saturation and administering oxygen according to such parameters should be discouraged.

It is important to ask the child how he or she feels as well as to listen to the parents' concerns. This process is usually time-consuming, but the rewards are substantial, even following the death of the child. Parents and friends will forever remember how their child was cared for and how the child felt through this time.

24. Do psychiatric emergencies occur in children receiving palliative care?

Facing a life-limiting or significant life-threatening illness can lead to emotional upset, which can manifest as anxiety and depression. Illness can cause children to be isolated from their familiar environment, activities, and peers at home, school, and play. They may be experiencing loss of body image, such as hair loss with chemotherapy, a cushingoid appearance from steroids, hirsutism with immunosuppressive agents, or more dramatic losses, such as the loss of limb.

It is helpful to have a psychologist or a psychiatrist work with the staff, family, and child from the time of diagnosis. Existing coping techniques are explored and strategies put in place to enhance and build on the positive ones. It is much more helpful to incorporate these techniques at the outset rather than to hold these resources in reserve for crisis intervention.

A child with problematic symptoms can be depressed. Managing the symptom, such as providing pain relief, can help to relieve the depression. Some of the medications used in pain management as adjuvants, such as the tricyclic antidepressants, can help with improved sleep and mood. Although of potential benefit for pain relief primarily for neuropathic pain at lower doses than that needed primarily for depression, a secondary positive effect may be on mood.

Disturbances in sensorium may occur in children with various medical problems, who usually are taking a variety of medications. If hepatic or renal compromise develops, a previously well-tolerated medication such as an opioid may cause the child to become delirious with a sedated or agitated delirium. The latter is usually much more difficult for staff and families to witness. Such a presentation should be investigated as appropriate for possible treatable medical causes, such as electrolyte abnormalities or hypoglycemia. It may be the result of worsening of the child's medical condition, such as central nervous system involvement by cancer. With new onset of hepatic or renal insufficiency, medications will need to be reviewed and the dosing interval and dose adjusted. As much as possible, centrally acting medications should be decreased or stopped. Opioids may require adjustment. In some instances, if a patient who is taking morphine develops renal compromise, a change to another opioid may provide amelioration of the delirium. This relates to the active and toxic metabolites of some of the opioids, including morphine. Meperidine would not be an option because it has a known toxic metabolite, nor-meperidine.

While the delirium is worked on and medications are adjusted, the child may benefit from a neuroleptic to relieve some of the agitation. If particularly agitated, the neuroleptic should have sedative properties, such as methotrimeprazine (starting with 0.1 mg/kg/dose intravenously/subcutaneously/orally every 8 hours). The option of using a benzodiazepine should be carefully considered in the face of confusion or agitation, because sometimes benzodiazepines have had the paradoxical effect of exacerbating the delirium. It may be helpful to consult the psychiatrist at such times.

25. What can be done when the child's pain or other distressing symptom, such as breathlessness, is uncontrollable?

Most symptoms in children are amenable to standard therapeutic interventions. In exceptional cases, refractory symptoms may present in a dying child.

When pain, breathlessness, or some other symptom is refractory, the goal of symptomatic relief cannot be achieved with maintenance of cognitive function. Extensive and thoughtful consultation with an expert in symptom management at the end of life should first be pursued as detailed by Cherny and Portenoy. It can be difficult to assess a refractory symptom in a child with limited capacity to describe the symptom and level of distress. The child's preferences or capacity to tolerate the symptom may differ from the family or caregiver's preference or capacity to tolerate perceived distress. The treatment of refractory symptoms at the end of life in children, including the use of terminal sedation, is detailed by Kenny and Frager.

Once it is clear that the symptom is truly refractory, the option of being able "to sleep through their breathlessness" or other symptom is discussed and all concerns gently but thoroughly explored. The family needs to be aware that with medication the child will be sedated and not usually arousable. However, the family should be encouraged to talk to and hold their child in keeping with their wishes.

26. How can it be ensured that aggressive symptom management is not misunderstood as euthanasia?

Health professionals need to have a thorough understanding of the medical, ethical, and legal aspects of symptom management at the end of life, including the provision of terminal sedation.

Confusion persists about the distinction between aggressive symptom management, especially terminal sedation, and euthanasia. Terminal sedation is the titration of sedating and analgesic mediations in patients who are terminally ill, with the primary goal of symptom relief. The clinician adjusts the medication to achieve relief of the symptom even if cognitive, respiratory, or cardiac function becomes secondarily compromised. This principle of "double effect" is medically, ethically, and legally accepted. On the other hand, euthanasia is the deliberate act of ending life to end suffering and is not generally medically, legally, or ethically sanctioned.

All members of the caregiving team need to discuss their concepts of terminal sedation and have any concerns validated and misperceptions clarified. With a full understanding of the principles, no one will feel guilty if the child's death had a temporal association with a dose of medication given for refractory distress.

It is always helpful to document the discussion and the plan of care, including the primary goal of symptom relief, even if this causes a secondary consequence of respiratory depression or cardiovascular instability.

27. Summarize some guidelines for symptom management, including sedation at the end of life.

- Care must be intended solely to relieve suffering.
- Sedation must be administered in response to suffering or the signs of suffering.
- It must be commensurate with the suffering.
- It cannot be a deliberate infliction of death.
- Doses must be increased progressively.
- Documentation is required.

28. How is terminal sedation provided once expert help for the symptom has been sought and the child, family, and health care team have been consulted?

The primary determinants guiding the choice of pharmacologic agent are the child's current and past medication history and the physician's preferences. The basic principles are the same regardless of the class of drug used singly or in combination.

Although the usual approach is to increase the dose of the opioid if the child is already being treated with opioids, sedation may be elusive as a result of significant opioid tolerance in the face of great symptom distress. Side effects such as central nervous system toxicity may be exacerbated with opioid escalation. Opioid therapy is continued with the addition of a second agent. Options for second agents include a neuroleptic, benzodiazepine, or barbiturate. Because meperidine has a toxic metabolite, nor-meperidine, meperidine should not be used in chronic pain management or terminal sedation.

29. When it is emotionally difficult to care for such ill children, how can one ensure that the interventions chosen are the most appropriate?

The availability of life-sustaining technologic advances has tipped the balance of decisions made by both parents and health professionals toward active intervention. Children hold a special place in our hearts and souls. Not doing something for critically ill children even though they are likely to die is profoundly difficult for us as individuals and as a society. The options of withholding or withdrawing treatments need to to be integrated more often into discussions about treatment possibilities. Offering a treatment implies that the treatment is reasonable and viable. If death occurs following such an intervention, family and health professionals often find helpful ways of framing the situation, such as, "They tried everything, they gave it their all, she died fighting." Virtually no one considers that the intervention may have presented no realistic possibility of a positive outcome.

It is incumbent upon us to evaluate every intervention that we propose for critically ill children. The potential benefit to the patient must always be balanced with how he or she may be expected to feel as a result.

30. What questions should be asked when considering, evaluating, and discussing treatment options?

1. How realistic is it that the intervention will cure the disease?
2. If not able to cure the disease, will it prevent progression of the disease?
3. Will the intervention improve the way the child feels?
4. Could the intervention make the child feel worse? If so, for how long?
5. What will it be like for this child to go through this treatment?
6. What is likely to happen without the intervention?
7. Will the intervention change the outcome for the child?[19]

If these questions are asked and answered honestly, the child will have the best chance of receiving optimal care that is truly in his or her best interest. Health professionals could carry a copy of these questions in their pockets and give a copy to other members of the team and to the child (modified as developmentally appropriate) and family to help remind one another about critical points for discussion.

31. Is addressing do-not-resuscitate (DNR) orders in children more difficult than with adults?

Generally, DNR discussions are more difficult when the patient is a child. Important life decisions are the responsibility of a surrogate for the child, usually the parents. Anytime someone other than the patient is making such critical decisions, the complexity of the discussion increases. The child should have a part to play that is appropriately tailored to his or her stage of development and capacity to understand the situation. Such involvement may be as basic as taking into account the child's level of distress with having procedures performed relative to the well-being achieved. Older children and adolescents have more to contribute concerning their wishes for future care.

When posing the options of resuscitation or no resuscitation to families, the physician should take the lead. It is nearly impossible for most parents to say, "Do not make the attempt." Even if they do choose DNR, some families have reported feeling guilty following the death of the child, even years later. The issue of DNR is generally raised in the context of a progressive deterioration or a profound acute insult. Too often the options of resuscitation versus no resuscitation are offered as equally weighted choices, as if simply choosing resuscitation means there is a reasonable chance of the desired outcome. It is more reasonable and ultimately more acceptable to the family for the physician to propose a plan as to what may occur along with a rationale for the direction proposed.

32. Cite an example of when resuscitation is futile.

Offering resuscitation to a family whose child has a platelet count of 7,000 from multiply re-lapsed, refractory leukemia is not truly an option because a resuscitative effort would be futile in such a context, unsuccessful, and unable to restore the child to a state of health in any capacity. Instead, not pursuing attempts at resuscitation is offered as part of the plan along with a clear expla-nation as to what interventions will be taken to ensure that the child is not in pain or breathless. The discussion can be framed by the health care provider asking the family how they feel their child is doing. Following clarification about the child's status, the physician could say that he believes that nothing would be able to reverse the child's condition, including any attempts at resuscitation.

Pacing the discussion by the cues received from the family helps the physician to move through the discussion in steps. Such discussions should take place before the child is in crisis. When death is anticipated, even if death may be months away, an early discussion along such lines can be helpful for the later time when the crisis arises. There may be instances in which, de-spite gentle direction and explanation as to what you feel is the best choice for the child, the family continues to prefer resuscitation. The family's wishes are followed unless resuscitation is documented as medically futile (stipulations may vary according to state and province).

33. What does a child understand about death?

Children's concepts of illness and death evolve as they grow and develop.

Children's Concepts of Death

STAGE OF DEVELOPMENT	KEY CONCEPTS	EXAMPLE	PRACTICAL IMPLICATIONS
Infancy (0–2 yr)	Experience the world through sensory information	Aware of tension, the unfami-liar, and separation	Comfort by sensory input (touch, rocking, sucking) and familiar people as well as transitional ob-jects (toys)
Early verbal childhood (2–6 yr)	See death as reversible Death is not personalized Magical thinking	May play with stuffed animal, repetitively alternate lying it down "dead" and standing it up "alive" Do not believe death could hap-pen to them May equate death with sleep May believe they can cause death by their thoughts, such as wishing someone would go away	Provide concrete informa-tion about state of being dead, e.g., "A dead person no longer breathes or eats." Need to dispel concept of being responsible and therefore guilty because of thoughts
Middle childhood (7–12 yr)	Personalize death Aware that death is final Earlier stage: understand causality by external causes Later stage: understand causality by internal causes	Aware that death can happen to them Believe that death is caused by event such as an accident Understand that death also can be caused by an illness	Child may request graphic details about death, including burial and decomposition May benefit from specifics about an illness

(Table continued on following page.)

Children's Concepts of Death (Continued)

STAGE OF DEVELOPMENT	KEY CONCEPTS	EXAMPLE	PRACTICAL IMPLICATIONS
Adolescence (older than 12 yr)	Appreciate universality of death but may feel distanced from it	May engage in risky behavior, stating "it can't happen to me" or "everyone dies anyway"	May have a need to speak about unrealized plans, such as schooling and marriage

34. How do we support the child through this experience?

Emotional support of the child often hinges indirectly on supporting the family members, who in turn support the child. Children derive a great deal of support from being able to participate in activities that promote their role as a child. Relationships with peers, maintaining school contacts, and maintaining modified play are crucial for well-being throughout illness.

How children perceive spirituality is highly individual, although the social, religious, and spiritual environment of the family and community influences the child's perceptions. Terminally ill children will talk of spiritual concepts in ways that belie their stage of development. While listening and encouraging the child's thoughts in this area, it helps to defer to family members so that discussion can take place openly among them. This also avoids contradictory views linking religious ideology with those that are spiritually rooted.

35. Can any other measures help the family through this tragic time?

Part of the care provided to the child and family includes proactive planning. It is most helpful to discuss and plan for what measures will be taken to manage events such as increased pain or breathlessness. In this way, both the child and family will be assured of an action directed to relieve the distress. The child benefits from decreased anxiety among family members, which is eased by their knowing the planned path and sequence of action. An example is to make the family aware of the next incremental dose of opioid that is required if pain relief becomes inadequate with the current regimen. Another example is to have a prescription for an antiemetic or a few doses available in the home. This provides a strategy if the child develops a new symptom, such as vomiting, and the family avoids needing to contact someone for a prescription and not having access to required medications after hours.

It is important to clarify with the family any fears or misperceptions they may harbor about the dying process. Although most families have never experienced the death of a child, they often have a particular memory from another event or imagine what the process will be like for their child. It is generally helpful to address these concerns, including their wishes concerning autopsy, organ and tissue donation, and funeral arrangements, ahead of time and make some arrangements in anticipation of the child's death.

Treatment measures for the child sometimes are directed toward relief of the family's distress, e.g., the use of an anticholinergic for the noisy breathing, or "death rattle," at the end of life. Having a quiet child in quiet surroundings can help ease some of the distress of staying with the child.

A parent who has experienced the death of a child can be a tremendous source of support for another family with a dying child. Bereaved parents who have made progress in dealing with their own grief can provide invaluable guidance for the family.

36. What modifications are required to provide care closer to the child's home?

Terminal care for children is often more technologically complex than for adults. The hydration-nutrition discussion has not yet reached pediatrics to the same degree that it has for adults. Dying children in North America usually receive hydration if not nutritional support. For many children with progressive life-limiting illnesses, much of their ongoing care has been focused on optimization of function through active and aggressive supportive care. A child with cystic fibrosis, for example, would receive supplemental oxygen, physiotherapy, and systemic and aerosolized antibiotic therapy both at home and in the hospital. The mental association with being cared about is integrally linked to this mode of intervention. Withdrawal of such treatments is more likely to be interpreted as abandonment. In children, it is not unusual to continue such interventions while simultaneously treating terminal symptoms and discussing death. For these reasons, providing care for dying children at home and in smaller community hospitals can require more human and technical services and more funding.

The other potential barrier to providing care for dying children close to or within their own home is the shortage of trained health professionals with expertise in both palliative care and the care of children. Illnesses causing death in childhood are infrequent, diverse in etiology, and present tremendous variability relative to a child's stage of growth and development. These factors make it difficult for clinicians to have enough exposure to gain expertise.

37. What is anticipatory grief, and how is bereavement support provided following the child's death?

In caring for a child with a progressive life-limiting illness, bereavement occurs early and is ongoing. Children and their families experience multiple losses over the course of the illness. Parents mourn the loss of a well child and need to frequently modify their hopes and aspirations for the child. The child with an altered body image may be grieving over changes such as living with a nasogastric tube, hair loss, or loss of a limb. Before the child's death, those close to the child reflect on what their life may feel like without the child. These are all forms of anticipatory grief.

A child's death has been described as one of the most profound losses humans are capable of experiencing. Ongoing bereavement follow-up should include parents, siblings, extended family, and the child's schoolmates, peers, friends, and fellow patients on the ward. The primary health providers who cared for the child prior to death may not be the actual providers of bereavement services, but should ensure that this ongoing need is addressed.

38. How may the health professional best be supported while caring for the child and family?

Caring for a critically ill child is a particular challenge to personal and professional issues relating to death and loss. Many individuals feel significantly more emotionally distressed in caring for a terminally ill child than for an adult. Children tend to move us in ways that are rare in adult encounters. Although it is important to acknowledge the difficult emotional aspect of this care, it does not have to detract from the services provided. Measures must be taken so that staff members feel supported and are not left with a sense of isolation. The sense of futility in not being able to "save" the child can be profound. Staff members need to take and be offered solace in knowing in what ways they helped the child, family, and friends. The loss of a patient may affect health professionals in different ways based on their own history and life experience with loss. A meeting for all involved staff members is helpful to provide an opportunity to share their feelings and acknowledge one another's contribution. It is also important for other resources to be made available and funds allocated for them. Such options include one-on-one counseling support for individuals whose needs may be better met through a more private format.

In a pediatric hospital, ward, or agency providing for home care, a process should exist for how staff members support each other throughout the caregiving process. Some administrators call in extra staff either to care for the other patients or to support work in tandem with the staff involved with a dying child. Although the major responsibilities for care often fall to a small group of individuals, staff members need to be supported by their colleagues to avoid feeling that they are shouldering the situation on their own.

ACKNOWLEDGMENT

Dr. Frager is supported by the Open Society Institute's Project on Death in American Faculty Scholars Program.

BIBLIOGRAPHY

1. Armstrong-Dailey A, Goltzer S: Hospice Care for Children. New York, Oxford University Press, 1993.
2. Berde C, Albin A, Glazer J, et al: Report of the Subcommittee on Disease-Related Pain in Childhood Cancer. Pediatrics 86:818–825, 1990.

3. Bieri D, Reeve RA, Champion GD, et al: The Faces Pain Scale for the self-assessment of the severity of pain experienced by children: Development, initial validation, and preliminary investigation for ratio scale properties. Pain 41:139–150, 1990.
4. Cancer Pain Relief and Palliative Care. Geneva, World Health Organization, 1990, technical report series 804.
5. Cherny NI, Portenoy RK: Sedation in the management of refractory symptoms: Guidelines for evaluation and treatment. J Palliat Care 10:31–38, 1994.
6. Corr CA, Corr DM: Hospice Approaches to Pediatric Care. New York, Springer Publishing, 1985.
7. deVeber LL, Jacobson SJ, Koren G, et al: Symptom management. In Doyle D, Hanks GWC, MacDonald N (eds): Oxford Textbook of Palliative Medicine. New York, Oxford University Press, 1993, pp 691–699.
8. Frager G: Palliative care and terminal care of children. Child Adolesc Psychiatric Clin North Am 6:889–909, 1997.
9. Goldman A: Care of the Dying Child. Oxford, Oxford University Press, 1994.
10. Hester NO, Barcus CS: Assessment and management of pain in children. Pediatrics: Nursing Update 1:2–8, 1986.
11. Howell DA: Special services for children. In Doyle D, Hanks GWC, MaDonald N (eds): Oxford Textbook of Palliative Medicine. New York, Oxford University Press, 1993, pp 718–725.
12. Kenny N, Frager G: Refractory symptoms and terminal sedation in children: Ethical issues and practical management. J Palliat Care 12:40–45, 1996.
13. Kuttner L: Management of young children's acute pain and anxiety during invasive medical procedures. Pediatrician 16:39–44, 1989.
14. McGrath PJ, Finley GA, Turner CJ: Making Cancer Less Painful. A Handbook for Parents. U.S.A. ed. Halifax, Nova Scotia, 1992.
15. Olness K, Gardner GG: Hypnosis and Hypnotherapy with Children. 2nd ed. Philadelphia, Grune & Stratton, 1988.
16. Palliative-Care Services, Report of the Subcommittee on Institutional Program Guidelines. Health Services and Promotion Branch, Health and Welfare, Ottawa, Canada, 1989.
17. Pediatric Pain, an electronic mailing list, is an Internet forum for informal discussion of any topic related to children's pain management. To subscribe, send an e-mail message to MAILSERV@ac.dal.ca. The first line of the message should read: subscribe PEDIATRIC-PAIN.
17a. Roy D (ed): When Children Have to Die: Pediatric Palliative Care. [Special issue] J Palliat Care 12(3):3–59, 1996.
18. Schechter NL, Berde CB, Yaster M: Pain in Infants, Children, and Adolescents. Baltimore, Williams & Wilkins, 1993.
19. Smith TJ: Commentary: Talking to patients about treatment realities. Knowing when to bow out gracefully. Oncol News 5(9):4, 1996.
20. Solomon R, Saylor CD: National Cancer Institute's Pediatric Pain Management: A Professional Course. East Lansing, MI, Michigan State University, 1995.
21. Sourkes BM: Armfuls of Time: The Psychological Experience of the Child with a Life-Threatening Illness. Pittsburgh, University of Pittsburgh, 1995.
22. Steward DJ: Management of childhood pain: New approaches to procedure-related pain. J Pediatr 122(Pt 2):S1–S46, 1993.
23. U.S. Department of Health and Human Services: Acute Pain Management in Infants, Children, and Adolescents: Operative and Medical Procedures.Quick Reference Guide for Clinicians. Rockville, MD, Agency for Health Care Policy and Research, 1992, AHCPR publication 92-0020.
24. U.S. Department of Health and Human Services: Management of Cancer Pain, Clinical Practice Guideline No. 9. Rockville, MD, Agency for Health Care Policy and Research, 1994, AHCPR publication 94-0592.

25. FAMILY CAREGIVERS FOR PALLIATIVE CARE PATIENTS AT HOME

Suresh K. Joishy, M.D., F.A.C.P.

1. Who is a caregiver?

Any person participating in the health care of a patient is a caregiver. Health care given to the patient can be informal or professional. Several chapters in this book outline the roles of professional caregivers. The burdens and rewards of caring for patients with life-limiting illnesses are also shared by informal caregivers, including relatives, friends, and neighbors.

2. Describe the informal caregivers.

An informal caregiver is responsible for the physical comfort, emotional support, and supervision of the family member with life-limiting illness. About a third of cancer patients receive care from one close relative only. Nearly half are cared for by two or three relatives, typically a spouse and an adult child. Many studies have shown that primary caregivers are mostly women. The mean age of caregivers is 60. Less often, friends of patients willingly take on the role of informal caregivers.

3. How does a family member or friend become qualified as a caregiver?

Professional caregivers are required by law to have years of intensive training and pass examinations to become caregivers to treat patients with advanced diseases. A family member or friend needs no such training or formal examinations to become a caregiver. However, they do perform simple nursing procedures daily and need proper information and practical instructions on how to care for the patient. As the patient's illness progresses and performance status deteriorates, the patient becomes immobile. Nursing care increases, and the patient becomes totally dependent on the caregiver.

4. Is it easy for a family member or friend to assume the role of a caregiver for palliative care patients?

Given how overwhelming the task of taking care of palliative care patients can be even for the hospital nursing staff, it is amazing how often family members and friends willingly take on the role of informal caregivers. Studies that have examined the dynamics of caregiving identify the price of familial caregiving as high. Caregiving can affect the mentality and social life of the caregivers and their families and result in feelings of burden or unbearable stress. Studies have shown that more than half of caregivers find the caring "rewarding," 10% find it a burden, and the rest find it rewarding and burdensome in equal measures.

5. Does age or gender of the caregiver influence the care to the patient?

Studies have shown that male caregivers experience more difficulties managing care-related activities outside the home. Male caregivers had a low sense of purpose in life versus female caregivers. Older caregivers who perceived their caregiving experience as time-limited or purposeful coped better than younger caregivers. Female caregivers reported a greater number of demands than male caregivers.

6. Why is there such a tremendous interest in health care professionals working with families of patients with life-limiting illness?

The focus of care for cancer patients has moved from the hospital to the home as result of shortened acute care stays, early discharges, and shifting cancer therapy to outpatient clinics. Thus, treatment-related side effects also must be managed at home. During periods of active treatment, patients frequently depend on family members for self-care, transportation, assistance with medications, and symptom management. It is logical to seek the help of the family caregivers when curative treatments cease and palliative treatments begin. Most cancer patients in the U.S. and Europe receive some kind of formal nursing care by home health care agencies or home hospice. The health care systems taking care of patients with life-limiting illness have realized the importance of family caregivers as indispensable team members. Without the support of family or friends as caregivers, it would be impossible for many palliative care patients to remain at home.

7. Can a family caregiver function alone, or is assistance necessary?

Family caregivers usually receive assistance from another family member. If a spouse caregiver has underage children, other family members usually provide support. However, studies have shown that additional family member support does not extend when the caregiver and patient live alone; friends and neighbors do not appear to offer increased assistance. About a third of caregivers have no assistance at all.

8. Describe caregiving by family caregivers.

Caregiving to palliative care patients by family members involves more than providing physical care. Caregiving has two components: (1) the meaning and purpose of caregiving behavior and (2) the nature or demands of the behavior itself. For example, driving the patient to a physician's appointment, monitoring the side effects of treatment, or listening to the patient talk about the uncertainty of the illness may be considered as much a caregiving task as bathing the patient.

9. How do professional palliative care team members help family caregivers?

Education about how to care for the patient at home is the most important service provided to family members by the palliative care team. In the absence of such education, caregivers describe feeling useless and helpless. Being well informed seems to allay caregivers' anxiety provoked by uncertainties and fears. Adequate information about illness enables patients and caregivers to make informed decisions about medical care as well as broader personal and social issues.

10. What do caregivers need to know in terms of medical information and education?

Palliative care patients run a clinical course that is never static. Their needs may change daily as new symptoms or complications develop. The caregivers are challenged by multiple demands that occur throughout the course of the illness.

Information and Education Needed by Caregivers

INFORMATION	EDUCATION
Patient's diagnosis	Simple terms, easy to remember
Symptoms	Important causes/goals of treatment
Likely prognosis	What to look for: improvement or how the patient may be approaching death
Sudden changes in patient's condition	How to access emergency services
Patient's emotions	How to offer psychosocial, spiritual support
Community support agencies	How to access them

11. Summarize a caregiver's needs at home.

1. Personal needs: related to patient's self-care; bathing, hygiene, mobility.
2. Instrumental needs: preparing meals, light or heavy housework, shopping, transportation, home health care.
3. Administrative needs: forms, financial advice, legal advice.
4. Other: any other need not necessarily belonging to the above categories.

12. How might caregiving adversely affect the lives of caregivers?

Continuing and increasing responsibilities may affect their employment. Many take part-time work, which affects financial needs. Spouses of patients may develop concerns about their own health. Provision of emotional support has been perceived to be among the more difficult tasks of caregiving.

The stress of caregiving may lead to the caregivers' developing physical symptoms and psychosocial needs of their own.

13. Are there sources of support to help family caregivers provide care?

Many professional and community resources are available to support family caregivers, but many caregivers do not know how to access these services. Palliative care team members are a great source of help.

Sources of Support for Caregivers

AREAS OF SUPPORT NEEDED	SOURCES OF HELP
Diagnostic/medical treatment information, symptom control, course of illness, anticipatory guidance	Palliative care physician and nurses
Nursing care needs of patient	Home care, hospice nurse
Interpretation of patient's emotions	Spiritual counselor
Financial constraints, transportation	Social services, community services

14. Are there nonterminal illnesses that can serve as models for professional collaboration with family caregiving?

Family caregiving is not a new phenomenon. Family members have traditionally taken care of patients with serious chronic mental illness that can drastically limit self-care. The enormous emotional, financial, and interpersonal impact on a caregiver whose family member has serious mental illness is well documented in psychiatric literature. The stress of caregiving may lead to the caregivers developing physical symptoms and psychosocial needs of their own.

Bernheim described eight generic principles for professional and family collaboration for caregiving at home. The following questions are adapted for palliative care professionals.

15. Why is it important to maintain respect toward family members?

Family members may have knowledge about the patient that palliative care team members lack. The patient's temperament, needs, aspirations, values, and interests are known to family members only, and these factors have an impact on the patient's response to palliative care measures. This implies empowering relatives and mutual decision-making. When difficulties are encountered in patient care, palliative team members should refrain from using pejorative language or concepts, because such attitudes are counterproductive to genuine collaboration.

Procedures for orientation should be constantly revised and updated to include a module on family-professional collaboration.

16. How can one provide orientation and education on the role of each palliative care team member?

Family members are likely to interact with multiple health care providers simultaneously. Inadequate orientation may cause or contribute to friction among staff, the patient, and family members. Verbal and written information should be given to family members, including names and roles of staff members and mechanisms for ongoing information exchange between staff and family.

17. What are some ways to communicate with the family?

Regular phone calls inviting relatives to treatment planning sessions is one useful way to communicate with the family. Not generally considered in the palliative care setting are social gatherings for patients, relatives, and the palliative care team when patients have good relief from symptoms.

18. How can one help to reduce the family's burden?

Reducing stress and tension within the family will benefit the patient. Emotional support, information, education, advice, skills training, crisis intervention, and respite care are extremely important.

19. Why is it important to develop individualized palliative care service plans?

Numerous intra- and interfamilial differences contribute to the need for an individualized approach to families. Cultural background, educational level, density of social networks, previous experience with life-limiting illness in relatives, and each relative's own typical response to hardship and grief are variables that must be considered in designing services. Caregivers who are parents are likely to require different services than the patient's siblings or children.

The service plan for each family caregiver should be developed in the context of an initial consultation phase in which relatives and staff can make a joint assessment of the family's needs and wishes.

20. How can one respond flexibly to the changing needs of family caregivers over time?

Just as palliative care treatment plans are reviewed regularly, plans for family involvement also need to be updated. This requires a mechanism for feedback about the family's changing perceptions and wishes. Regular informal sessions may be arranged to review the relatives' goals or objectives and to ask focused questions about their level of satisfaction.

21. How can one make the palliative care "family friendly"?

Palliative care team members may feel threatened, frightened, and angry about some families' assertiveness and may be unable or unwilling to develop an amicable alliance with some family members. Some palliative care team members may initially require sensitization to the needs of families, updates on new theories of dealing with families, or skills training followed by regular supervision. Continuing care programs are needed in the community for family caregiver education, health professional education, and caregiver group intervention programs. All of these programs should include an evaluation component.

22. Describe role stress, role overload, role conflict, and role strain.

Role stress is a social structural condition in which role obligations are vague, irritating, difficult, conflicting, or impossible to meet. Poorly educated family caregivers may feel considerable role stress.

Role overload refers to an individual's perception that he or she lacks the time and energy to fulfill the obligations of all of their roles.

Role conflict is a condition in which existing role expectations are contradictory or mutually exclusive.

Role strain is the subjective state of distress experienced by a caregiver who is exposed to role stress. Role stress and strain may manifest in caregiver fatigue, irritability, insomnia, and other physical symptoms. Palliative care team members have a great role to play in preventing caregiver stress and strain.

23. What improvements are envisioned for palliative care team collaboration in the future?

More experience is needed to examine how caregivers need change over the course of a patient's illness. Information regarding the caregiver's satisfaction with the palliative care team needs to be incorporated into training programs. Caregiving-related variables such as nature of caretaking, time required for caretaking, and which family member becomes involved and under what circumstances are important considerations.

BIBLIOGRAPHY

1. Bernheim KF: Principles of professional and family collaboration. Hosp Community Psychiatry 41:1353–1355, 1990.
2. Francell CG, Conn VS, Gray DP: Families' perceptions of burden of care for chronic mentally ill relatives. Hosp Community Psychiatry 39:1296–1300, 1988.
3. Laizner AM, Shegda Yost LM, Barg K, McKorkle R: Needs of family caregivers of persons with cancer: A review. Semin Oncol Nurs 9:114–120, 1993.
4. Longman AJ, Atwood JR, Sherman JB, et al: Care needs of home based cancer patients and their caregivers. Cancer Nurs 15:182–190, 1992.
5. Oberst MT, Thomas SE, Gass KA, et al: Caregiver demands and appraisal of stress among family caregivers. Cancer Nurs 12:209–215, 1989.
6. Stoller EP: Males as helpers: Role of sons, relatives, and friends. Gerontologist 30:228–235, 1990.
7. Temple A, Fawdry K: King's theory of goal attainment. Resolving filial caregiver role strain. J Gerontol Nurs 18:11–15, 1992.

26. DEPRESSION IN THE TERMINALLY ILL

Mark Lander, M.D., F.R.C.P.C., and
Harvey Max Chochinov, M.D., Ph.D., F.R.C.P.C.

1. Are all dying patients depressed?

All dying patients can be expected to express sadness as part of their grieving process. However, most patients do not develop what psychiatrists call major depression, a syndrome characterized by a persistent, prominent depressed mood or loss of interest and associated neurovegetative symptoms, including sleep or appetite disturbance, inability to concentrate, loss of energy, and reduced libido. Major depression also is associated with a number of psychological symptoms, including preoccupation with death, suicidal ideation, anhedonia, hopelessness, excessive guilt, and feelings of worthlessness.

2. How common is clinical depression?

The prevalence of depression among the general population is 3–5%; the lifetime incidence is 7–10% for men and 15–20% for women. The prevalence of depression among the medically ill ranges widely in studies, from 10% to as high as 70%. It is perhaps realistic to expect that 10–25% of dying patients fall within this classification.

3. What are the risk factors for developing major depression?

The most important risk factor for any given individual patient is a personal past history of major depression. Other risk factors include a family history of mood disorder, substance abuse, particular types of malignancies (e.g., retroperitoneal cancers, brain tumors, head and neck cancers), and exposure to certain types of medications (e.g., steroids, vincristine, vinblastine, interferon, interleukin, intrathecal methotrexate).

4. How does one differentiate between clinical depression and the normal consequences of advanced illness?

This question has been widely debated and presents a challenge for clinicians working with dying patients. Many of the vegetative symptoms of depression overlap with the symptoms of advanced physical disease. The nonspecificity of symptoms such as loss of appetite, energy, and libido often leads to the diagnosis of depression being overlooked. As such, clinical wisdom and experience suggest that greater emphasis should be placed on psychological symptoms—depressed mood and loss of interest, helplessness, hopelessness, excessive guilt, feelings of worthlessness, and desire for death—than on physical symptoms.

5. When should one consult a psychiatrist?

1. When there is uncertainty about the diagnosis of depression.
2. When assistance is required in choosing a suitable antidepressant.
3. When there are concerns regarding suicide risk.
4. When depression is nonresponsive to an adequate trial of medications.

6. What psychosocial stressors are associated with clinical depression in the terminally ill?

Inadequately controlled pain can present with many symptoms consistent with major depression. In fact, aggressive pain management should be considered concomitantly when initiating treatment for clinical depression. Perceived lack of social support also been shown to be associated with significant mood disturbance. This suggests possible strategies for psychosocial intervention, such as optimizing social contact and availability, individual and group psychotherapy, and spiritual counseling.

7. What are the consequences of underdiagnosing and undertreating depression in these patients?

Underdiagnosing and undertreating depression can impair the quality of life and thus add to the burden of suffering. Negativistic thinking, commonly associated with depression, can lead to a lack of compliance, treatment refusal, and profound social withdrawal. Depression can accelerate a patient's social withdrawal and heighten his or her sense of isolation. The patient's support network can become unavailable. Care providers frequently dismiss these behaviors and mood states as normal reactions to illness, even in the face of severe affective disturbances. Such inaction, what some have referred to as "therapeutic nihilism," further compounds patients' suffering.

Misdiagnosing depression as conditions such as anxiety or delirium can lead to inappropriate therapy, which can further reduce the patient's quality of life. For instance, tranquilizing medications are commonly associated with side effects such as sedation, confusion, or generalized cognitive slowing. Patients may appear calmer, but their depression remains unabated.

8. What investigations should be carried out on depressed dying patients?

In keeping with palliative care principles, diagnostic testing should be kept to a minimum and guided by the principle of confining tests to those that will directly lead to effective interventions. Because there are no specific diagnostic tests for major depression, investigations are performed to exclude organic causes for the mood disturbance. Specialized serum analyses should be used to rule out metabolic dysfunctions. Careful examination of medications prescribed for the patient may reveal that some are prone to cause depression as a side effect.

9. How do you treat depression in the terminally ill?

Psychological and psychopharmacologic treatments have proven effective for patients with major depression, and they should be undertaken simultaneously. Both may serve a critical function. The physician needs to supply psychoeducation to enhance compliance, offer encouragement, and maintain hope. Medication without ongoing contact with a clinician is often seen by the patient as abandonment and thus is never an acceptable approach.

10. What are the critical components of psychotherapy?

The relationship with the primary medical caregiver is the most important component of psychotherapeutic support for many patients with serious illness. These relationships work best if they are based on mutual trust, respect, and sensitivity. In particular, the ability to acknowledge patients as whole persons and to respond to them on the basis of their individual personal style and needs—rather than an unwavering standardized approach—tends to work best.

Most psychotherapeutic approaches in terminally ill patients combine (1) promotion of active coping strategies to maintain their level of functioning and (2) assistance for patients to understand, manage, and work through their feelings related to their disease. Active coping and regaining a sense of mastery and control can sometimes be achieved with group or mutual supportive therapy. These modalities offer the ability to share common experiences with similarly afflicted patients, thus reducing the sense of emotional isolation that often accompanies illness. These approaches can be augmented with other techniques, including relaxation, biofeedback, guided imagery, or hypnosis.

Other psychodynamic approaches, which focus on the development of new psychological understanding and coping strategies, are less practical. Interpersonal therapy is a short-term psychotherapeutic treatment that focuses on discrete, manageable psychological and interpersonal issues. It has shown promise in research pertaining to HIV-positive patients and patients with breast cancer.

11. What antidepressant medications are best suited for depressed terminally ill patients?

Treatment with antidepressant medication should follow the same guidelines as for anyone who is medically ill. The key is to minimize side effects and to avoid drug interactions. Thus, the old dictum, "Start low and go slow," is particularly appropriate.

Although there is more experience and literature on the use of tricyclic antidepressants in terminally ill patients, serotonin-specific reuptake inhibitors (SSRIs), serotonin norepinephrine reuptake inhibitors (SNRIs), and reversible inhibitors of monoamine oxidase A (RIMAs) are probably the most appropriate classes of medications to use because they have a more tolerable side effect profile. Seriously ill patients are particularly sensitive to the anticholinergic side effects common with tricyclics, which may be additive to the anticholinergic effects of other medications they are taking.

Although it is less cardiotoxic and anticholinergic than the tricyclics, fluoxetine's long halflife and its potential for interaction with other drugs (because of its impact on the cytochrome P 450 system) makes its use somewhat problematic. It also may cause a transient decrease in appetite, some initial anxiety, and nausea, all of which limit its use in the terminally ill. Other SSRIs, such as sertraline, fluvoxamine, paroxetine, and nefazodone, appear to be useful, but there is little clinical experience and research on the use of these drugs in this population. Venlafaxine also appears to have a relatively mild side effect profile (nausea, somnolence, and mildly elevated blood pressure) and may prove useful.

12. What is the role of psychostimulants?

Psychostimulants are an alternative and effective treatment for depression in the terminally ill. They have the advantages of rapid onset of action—often 24–48 hours—and are energizing, well tolerated, and may even be helpful for mild cognitive impairment (with improved attention and concentration). Their rapid action makes them especially appropriate for patients with days to a few weeks to live. They also improve appetite, fatigue, and promote a sense of well being. Dextroamphetamine or methylphenidate treatment can begin with 2.5 mg at 8:00 a.m. and at noon and slowly be increased over several days. Typical doses are in the range of 20–30 mg per day; doses as high as 60–90 mg per day have been used in some patients with AIDS. The medication often can be withdrawn after 1–2 months. Side effects may include nervousness, insomnia, mild increases in pulse and blood pressure, tremor, and confusion.

Pemoline is another stimulant that may be used. For patients in whom oral access is limited, pemoline, given sublingually, is well absorbed through the buccal mucosa. It can be started at a dose of 18.75 mg in the morning and at noon and gradually increased up to a maximum of 75 mg per day. Patients taking pemoline should have periodic liver function testing because it has been associated with increased liver enzymes.

13. What course should be taken in patients who do not respond to antidepressants?

If a patient does not respond to one of the newer antidepressants or the patient has a history of good past response, a tricyclic/heterocyclic should be considered. However, the medication should be started at low doses (10–25 mg) and increased slowly in increments of 10–25 mg. Doses in the ranges of 25–150 mg per day are often adequate. Nortriptyline and desipramine are less anticholinergic—which is particularly important if the patient is taking other anticholinergic drugs—and generally better tolerated. They also have the advantage of having well-established plasma levels, which can be monitored to ensure that even patients who are taking a low dose are in the therapeutic range. If patients are very anxious or have insomnia, sedating tricyclics such as amitriptyline or doxepin may be useful (see table on following page).

Electroconvulsive therapy (ECT) would rarely be used in terminally ill patients. However, for patients who have psychotic depression or who are refusing to eat or drink because of their depressive illness, it may be the treatment of choice. A consultation with an anesthetist would be mandatory to ensure that the patient is able to tolerate the anesthetic.

14. How can we gauge a successful outcome in these patients?

It would be unrealistic and not necessarily desirable to think that all sadness in the face of terminal illness could be eliminated. However, patients whose depression is treated often recover the ability to enjoy social discourse, which may rekindle some prior interests. Successful treatment can often improve energy, sleep, and appetite. Perhaps most critical is patients' renewed ability to find meaning in their lives despite their impending death.

Antidepressants Used in Patients with Advanced Disease

DRUG	THERAPEUTIC ORAL DAILY DOSAGE (MG)
Heterocyclic antidepressants	
Amoxapine	100–150
Maprotiline	100–200
Monoamine oxidase inhibitors	
Isocarboxazid	20–40
Phenelzine	30–60
Tranylcypromine	20–40
Psychostimulants	
Dextroamphetamine	5–30
Methylphenidate	5–30
Pemoline	37.5–75
Second-generation antidepressants	
Bupropion	200–300
Trazodone	50–200
Selective serotonin reuptake inhibitors	
Fluoxetine	10–60
Fluvoxamine	50–300
Paroxetine	10–60
Sertraline	25–200
Nefazodone	50–600
Tricyclic antidepressants	
Amitriptyline	25–125
Clomipramine	25–125
Desipramine	25–125
Doxepin	25–125
Imipramine	25–125
Nortriptyline	25–125
Other	
Moclobemide	100–600
Venlafaxine	37.5–225

Adapted from Massie MJ, Holland JC: Depression and the cancer patient. Psychiatry 51:12–17, 1990.

BIBLIOGRAPHY

1. Chochinov HM, Wilson KG, Enns M, et al: Prevalence of depression in the terminally ill: Effects of diagnostic criteria and symptom threshold judgements. Am J Psychiatry 151:537–540, 1994.
2. Cohen-Cole S: Major depression and physical illness. Psychiatr Clin North Am 10:1–17, 1987.
3. Derogatis LR, Morrow GR, et al: The prevalence of psychiatric disorders among cancer patients. JAMA 249:751–757, 1983.
4. Lynch ME: The assessment and prevalence of affective disorders in advanced cancer. J Palliat Care 11:10–18, 1995.
5. Massie MJ: Depression. In Holland JC, Rowland JH (eds): Handbook of Psychooncology. Oxford, Oxford University Press, 1989, pp 283–290.
6. Rodin G, Craven J, Littlefield C: Depression in the Medically Ill. New York, Brunner/Mazel, 1991.

27. DESIRE FOR DEATH IN THE TERMINALLY ILL

Harvey Max Chochinov, M.D., Ph.D., F.R.C.P.C.,
and Mark Lander, M.D., F.R.C.P.C.

1. How common is a desire for death among the terminally ill?

Intermittent or fleeting thoughts of death may occur in up to 50% of patients. However, a persistent, prominent, genuine desire for hastened death, which is consistently held over time, is far less common, affecting 8–10% of patients.

2. What is the incidence of suicide among the terminally ill?

Completed suicides appear to be no more common in the terminally ill than other general medical populations. However, certain conditions, such as head and neck malignancies, gynecologic cancers, and AIDS, appear to have a higher rate of completed suicide. It would thus seem that conditions that highly disfigure the body, confer a particularly hopeless prognosis, and have a relentless course are associated with a higher prominence of completed suicide.

3. Does desire for death mean that the patient has a mood disorder?

No. However, the prevalence of major depression among patients expressing a genuine and persistent desire for death appears to be exceedingly high. About 65% of this group but fewer than 8% of the terminally ill not endorsing a desire for death will meet diagnostic criteria for major depression.

4. What clinical factors correlate with a desire for death?

Poor pain control, social isolation, and clinical depression. Depression appears to be the most important, although one cannot underestimate the importance of good pain control. Psychiatric morbidity among patients with poorly controlled pain is significantly higher than in patients whose pain is well managed.

5. How stable is a desire for death in the terminally ill over time?

Desire for death is quite unstable. When good palliative interventions are made available, patients who initially might endorse a desire for hastened death often change their minds.

6. Is there ever a case to be made for euthanasia or physician-assisted suicide?

This question has come to preoccupy medical ethicists, moral philosophers, clinicians, and various advocacy groups. There is a great deal of passion on both sides of the euthanasia/physician-assisted suicide debate. Some argue that respecting a patient's expressed wish for hastened death is necessary because the patient's autonomy must supersede all other concerns. Others raise the "slippery slope argument," indicating that one patient's right to assisted suicide becomes another patient's obligation. Others cite the absolute prohibition against physicians expediting death under any circumstances and express concern that taking on this role will fundamentally change the fiduciary nature of the physician-patient relationship.

7. How do you avert conflict with a patient who requests euthanasia or physician-assisted suicide?

Rather than becoming too preoccupied with the moral and legal issues, it is critical that clinicians remain attuned to the demanding clinical challenges that such requests invariably create. Preoccupation with whether the patient has the "right to assisted suicide" can sometimes interfere with focusing on the clinical imperatives and create an unnecessary standoff between the patient and care provider. If the care provider's personal position leaves patients feeling that they are not free to express their opinion or discuss the fact that sometimes death seems a preferable option to what life has become, patient care will be compromised. Patients need to be given implicit or, if necessary, explicit permission to discuss their every fear, concern, or wish, even should that include the wish for hastened death. Inviting such a dialogue will decrease their sense of isolation and allow them an opportunity to explore their concerns. These discussions can provide an opportunity to give reassurance when the wish for hastened death is spawned by concerns around remediable sources of suffering such as pain or dyspnea. The ability to skillfully attend to distressing symptoms demonstrates to patients that their dying need not be accompanied by unnecessary distress.

8. How do you reassure a patient suffering from fear of abandonment?

Some sources of suffering are not so easily reversible. Existential angst, fear of being a burden, or the inability to accommodate a life that has become truncated by an advancing disease are often deeply held concerns that are not easily shifted. One must bear in mind that these feelings are often underpinned by a fear of abandonment—a fear that is almost universal among dying patients. An unwavering commitment to remain involved and attentive to patients throughout their course directly and tangibly addresses this fear. In most instances, this will lead to a workable collaboration that is far preferable to an irreconcilable clashing of philosophies between patient and care provider.

9. What happens if the patient maintains his desire for hastened death?

This will almost always engender a sense of helplessness and impotence within the health care provider, neither of which is easy to bear. Such a scenario begs the question, "If we acquiesce to these requests, are we responding to our patients' hopelessness or our own?" Studies have shown that clinicians who feel more skilled at palliative interventions are less likely to endorse death-hastening measures. Clearly then, a clinician's attitude and sense of competence are as important in these decisions as patient-mediated factors. Therefore, it is critical to evaluate how both the care provider and the patient are coping with the impending death.

Despite the clinician's adopting a therapeutic stance and attending to the clinical issues, the occasional patient will still advocate a "hastened death" agenda. In these instances, explicitly stating one's positions may be helpful, but is not done without certain risks.

10. What role should a physician's personal belief system play in responding to death-hastening requests?

A physician's personal beliefs and values should occupy the background. Conveying a dogmatic stance can make patients feel that expressing their wish for death is simply not acceptable. This can deepen their sense of isolation and cause them to withhold information that might have proven helpful in meeting their palliative care needs.

On the other hand, sharing a pro-euthanasia stance and an accompanying willingness to assist the patient may erroneously be interpreted by patients as validating their fear that life is devoid of meaning, purpose, or any value whatsoever. By indicating that assisted suicide is a reasonable option, the care provider may at some level be colluding with the patient's sense of hopelessness, thereby accelerating the patient toward the option of hastened death.

11. What is the role of the multidisciplinary team in managing patients who request that death be hastened?

The multidisciplinary team allows people with diverse skills and areas of expertise to provide patient care. Social workers often work with families concerning issues of grief and can assist in the management of practical issues such as financial matters and housing. Members of the clergy are best qualified to discuss spiritual matters that may arise in the palliative care setting.

Psychiatrists should be consulted if there is a suspected underlying psychiatric disorder that may account for the desire for death. When concerns exist about the patient's competence, psychiatric opinion can be helpful. Palliative care specialists may become involved when there are distressing symptoms that have been difficult to control. The task of providing excellent nursing care is never more critical than among patients with advanced disease. They are most often the front-line workers who carry out the treatments recommended by the various consultants. Some programs involve practitioners of various complementary treatments, such as therapeutic touch practitioners, herbalists, acupuncturists, music therapists, and massage therapists.

12. What basic clinical interventions should be initiated with patients requesting hastened death?

It is most important to understand the patient's motivation. While suicide occasionally has been described as a rational act, it is most often encumbered by psychiatric disturbance. One must ensure that (1) the patient's mental processes are unimpaired by psychiatric illness, cognitive impairment, or severe emotional distress that might result in an impulsive request that quickly changes as circumstances change; (2) the patient has a realistic assessment of his or her situation, and (3) the motives for the decision are understandable to other observers.

The physician must establish rapport with the individual, try to talk openly about the patient's wishes, convey the message that it is acceptable to talk about these matters, and not appear critical. Talking about suicide does not "put ideas into a patient's head" but often makes such ideas and impulses less distressing. Allowing a patient to maintain a "suicide option"—by not adopting or demonstrating a rigid oppositional stance—often allows patients a greater sense of control and seems to help them tolerate their deteriorating circumstances.

It is important to mobilize as much support for the patient as possible. Involving close family members or friends is helpful. Ultimately, the physician must take sufficient time to understand the patient's wishes. How does the patient view his future? What are his values? Does the family understand the patient's request? Is there any aspect of the patient's life that he experiences as being meaningful? Is he concerned about being an undue financial or care burden on his family? Is there family conflict that contributes to the request? The palliative care team should help patients examine their personal needs to help them shape their death, and live the rest of their life, with as much grace and meaning as possible.

BIBLIOGRAPHY

1. Chochinov HM, Wilson KG: The euthanasia debate: Attitudes, practices and psychiatric considerations. Can J Psychiatry 40:593–602, 1995.
2. Brown JH, Henteleff P, Barakat S, et al: Is it normal for terminally ill patients to desire death? Am J Psychiatry 143:208–211, 1986.
3. Chochinov HM, Wilson KG, Enns M, et al: Desire for death in the terminally ill. Am J Psychiatry 152:1185–1191, 1995.
4. van der Mass PJ, van Delden JJM, Pijnenborg L, et al: Euthanasia and other medical decisions concerning the end of life. Lancet 338:669–674, 1991.
5. Foley KM: Competent care for the dying instead of physician-assisted suicide. N Engl J Med 336:54–58, 1997.

28. THE LAST HOURS OF LIVING

Martha L. Twaddle, M.D.

1. Does revealing or discussing a terminal diagnosis cause patients to lose hope?

Physicians often fear that telling patients "the bad news" will "take away their hope." Historically, physicians did not reveal the complete diagnosis to patients and families because there was not much that could be done to treat many terminal illnesses. In Asian cultures, the withholding of information is preferred. In the United States, patients and families most often take an active role in decisions regarding treatment options; thus, it is inconsistent to withhold information with respect to prognosis. Additionally, to do so would potentially risk a loss of trust between patient, family, and physician. In the hospice experience, hope is not lost, but redefined. One hopes for cure at the time of a diagnosis. If the disease cannot be cured, one hopes for more time. If time is limited, patients hope for relief of pain and a more comfortable death.

2. What are the most common fears of patients at the end of life?

Fear of pain, abandonment, isolation, and suffering are often cited as the expressed fears of the dying patient. Hospitalized patients commonly experience a sense of loss of control, and thus feel that their integrity and autonomy are threatened. The spoken and unspoken fear of losing control has an impact on the patient's experience of pain. Conscious efforts to provide patients with choices, opportunities for expression, and time for explanation and education can do much to enhance their sense of comfort and security.

3. Do male and female patients, and patients in different age groups react differently to the diagnosis of life-limiting illness?

Generally, each person's response to life-changing news is unique and consistent with the manner in which that individual has coped with major stress and change on prior occasions. Some patients will become more isolated; others will verbalize their grief and anxiety. These coping mechanisms are not gender-specific; instead, they are consistent with the individual's personality. Generally, younger patients tend to be less accepting of approaching death given the length of their planned future. Many younger patients have very young families and are devastated emotionally at the prospect of that loss and its implications for their children. Thus, most young patients, male or female, pursue disease altering treatments for as long as possible, usually deferring hospice care until very late in the disease process or never accepting it at all. Middle-aged patients suddenly confronted by a terminal diagnosis represent a common and unfortunate group. Most of us have had the difficult task of breaking the bad news to a patient knowing that they had just taken early retirement with plans to "enjoy life." This unexpected interruption to future plans can be met with severe depression or anger; thus, intensive psychological and social support is imperative. Patients of advanced age are generally less surprised by a terminal diagnosis, although no less grieved. They may have experienced the death of several friends or siblings, and may see disease and death more in terms of "when" rather than "if." Their prior personal experiences with death may make it less frightening. The news and change that a terminal diagnosis implies is no less profound, but many older adults can see their approaching death in the context of a full life. They may have a sense of accomplishment and even completion relative to their personal history, something that would not be possible for a much younger person.

An interesting trend that I have observed is that younger women with children tend to prefer dying away from the home. They will stay home as long as possible, but verbalize a desire to be hospitalized (usually in the inpatient hospice unit) when death is more imminent. The most common reason given for this is their desire to spare their children the memory of them being comatose or unresponsive. It is critical for physicians to honor that choice and to make provisions for patients to die in a setting in which they feel secure and comfortable.

4. What are the most frequently asked questions at the end of life?

Patients and families are most often concerned with when death will occur (how much time do I have?) and what death will be like (what is going to happen?). Taking the time to discuss these concerns can greatly diminish the anxiety surrounding death. Physician training in internal medicine provides physiological insight into the visible changes manifested by the dying patient. The metabolic effects of declining end-organ function can be explained to patients and families so that they can better understand symptoms, signs, and their implications. This knowledge frequently helps families and patients cope with the changes and better anticipate the time frame of life. Assuring a professional vigilance to provide comfort and symptom relief for the dying patient can also relieve the anxiety for patients and their families regarding the potential for physical suffering. The opportunities to provide comfort to the individual patient are vast. Families and caregivers can focus on these, with the aid of the physician, through questions such as "what would comfort your (mother) at this time?" "What types of things did she enjoy?" "What smells, sounds, or feelings would reassure her?" Facilitating the emphasis on active caring can help the family cope with the dying process.

5. How does the physician determine how long a patient has to live?

Prognosticating is extremely difficult and is an area in which physicians do not excel. Data regarding prognostication comes primarily from population studies regarding patients receiving treatment. There is little information regarding patients receiving treatment based only on palliative care principles. It is also difficult to translate population-based information to the individual patient, as the issues of comorbidity and their emotional and physical status greatly affect prognosis.

Families and patients will seek a time frame in order to finalize business matters and for personal closure with family members; thus the physician is frequently called upon to predict the time course of the terminal illness. Explanation regarding the disease process may provide insight regarding the nearness of death. I often use the phrase "cadence of disease" to describe the current and expected rhythm of decline. Also helpful to families is to describe time in terms of hours to days, days to weeks, weeks to months, or months to years. We cannot be specific as to how many weeks or days, but based on the cadence of disease, we can put the time frame in those terms to provide patients and families with a benchmark of reference. Changes in respiration, mental status, and urinary output indicate decline and can be explained to families in terms that suggest a time course to death.

6. Are the perceptions of dying for physicians, families, and patients different in a noncancer illness such as neurodegenerative disorders?

The terminal diagnosis itself often provides insight to the physician and professional caregivers regarding the possible stresses that the patient and family have and will face. Progressive neurological conditions such as ALS, Huntington's disease, or Alzheimer's dementia are characterized by *years* of decline. The chronicity of caregiving can lead to physical, emotional, and even financial exhaustion for the spouse or defined family. Often, the grief experienced by the family literally occurs before the death; death itself is met with a certain amount of expressed relief ("He suffered so long, it's a relief that he's finally gone.") Access to supportive care for these individuals and their families is often challenged by the very chronicity of the illness. Hospice, as currently defined, is too time limited for the needs of these patients; many are discharged from traditional hospice programs for "extended prognosis," despite the need for supportive care. Physicians may need to work with families, community, and national organizations to facilitate this supportive care throughout the course of the illness, accessing traditional hospice care when patients enter the very end-stages of their disease.

7. How do the perceptions differ in heart disease and chronic obstructive lung disease?

The end stages of diseases such as heart disease and chronic obstructive lung disease differ from cancer only in that the patient's decline is generally not as predictable. Symptom management often allows the patient to plateau in a debilitated state for a period of weeks or even months. Death, when it occurs, is often abrupt—the result of an arrhythmia, a pulmonary embolism, or an acute myocardial infarction. Thus, even though the course of decline may have been gradual, if not slow, the swiftness of death may leave families feeling unprepared or shaken. The physician and palliative care team can do much to prepare families for the possibility of sudden change. It is critically important to have supportive care readily available at *all* times—families often panic in these situations and may activate emergency medical services despite this being contrary to their prior plan of care.

8. How do these perceptions differ in AIDS?

The majority of individuals who die as a result of AIDS are still young, and many have limited or nonexistent support. Often estranged from their family of origin, their chosen family may also be beleaguered with AIDS. It is not unusual in the homosexual population for both partners to have HIV disease, or for one individual to have lost several partners to the disease. Thus, the grief expressed by caregivers in the dying process may reflect not only the immediate loss but also past and future losses. The magnitude of this suffering will require intensive pyschological and social work support. The chaplaincy may also be beneficial and facilitate healing in a greater sense.

For the large population who have contracted AIDS through intravenous drug abuse and have lived their lives on the street, the possibility of compassionate supportive care at the end of life seems unfathomable. Their caregivers are usually not family members, but professionals or devoted friends. Many of these individuals die in the hospital, and some have the opportunity to be cared for in inpatient hospices or facilities designated for the supportive care of AIDS patients. Because there is often no long-term relationship with a physician, medical care will be challenged by a lack of follow-up as well as by ongoing substance abuse. Because of this, end of life care is often unable to enhance the quality of life for this population, but merely eases the dying phase.

Newer medications have changed the course of AIDS so that it is evolving into more of a chronic illness, characterized by exacerbations and remissions, and often managed over a period of many years. Given this, the youth of those afflicted, and the rapid development of disease-altering treatments that are becoming available, the desire to continue interventional care or wait for the "miracle cure" will be strong. Physicians must be keenly aware of the high risk of suicide among patients with AIDS—supportive care is truly critical from the time of diagnosis.

9. What can be done when the family and patient perceive the dying process as taking "too long?"

Patients who experience a prolonged dying state are typically sustained by intravenous fluids or other interventions that prolong the dying process. There can be tremendous ambivalence on the part of patients and their families to discontinue these modalities even as they plead for death to occur more quickly. This ambivalence is often stressful and even frustrating for the physician and palliative care team. Careful explanations regarding the burden and benefit of treatments must be reviewed frequently. Physicians can do much by presenting choices in a manner that minimizes a sense of perceived guilt for the survivors—stopping the treatment doesn't "kill" the patient, but allows the disease to more quickly run its course. At times, cultural or religious reasons will preclude a family from discontinuing nutritional support; however, with the aid of the palliative care team, families may choose not to treat infections or complications when they arise. Careful counsel of patients and families to avoid the introduction of futile treatments may avert the agony experienced by abruptly discontinuing them, such as in the case of mechanical ventilation. Even when life-prolonging measures are discontinued, some patients do not rapidly succumb. Those who have received intravenous fluids over time may be sustained for many days after these fluids are discontinued because of the gradual mobilization of third space fluid. Discontinuation of steroids in the circumstances of CNS tumors may not precipitate a rapid ending. Families will often require tremendous psychological support. *It is imperative that the caregiving team not abandon a patient and family at this time.* Traditionally, those patients who are "slowly dying" are visited infrequently by physicians. Whether in a home, hospital, or nursing home setting, the palliative care team's continued involvement can greatly ease the pain of waiting for the end to come.

10. Do patients progress through stages of coping as death approaches?

Kubler-Ross's notable work on death and dying is often utilized by physicians and laypersons to heighten insight regarding the dying process. However, not all patients move through the phases of denial, anger, bargaining, acceptance, etc. But, awareness of these potential modes of facing death may help caregivers facilitate the coping of the dying patient. It is imperative that physicians and caregivers do not impose their agenda and expectations on the patient, but rather strive to support the means of coping for the individual. We all have assumptions regarding the death process; it is best to remind ourselves whose needs take precedent.

11. How do you deal with the angry or bitter dying patient?

The psychological struggles of patients and families throughout the dying process can be as intense as the physical deterioration of progressive disease. Patients may become frustrated and depressed as their independence fades. They may withdraw socially or become bitterly depreciative of loved ones. Central nervous system impairment secondary to neoplastic invasion or stroke may result in significant personality changes and mood lability. These changes are usually unexpected by families, who tend to have a preconception of how the dying process will unfold. For family and others who gather for support, anger, and even fear will create great tension at the bedside, interfering with care delivery. Ideally, the physician will prompt early involvement of social work and chaplaincy to help ease these tensions and facilitate resolution of unspoken or unfinished personal issues. The end of life presents an opportunity for personal growth, spiritual expression, and emotional healing. Facilitating and supporting an environment conducive to these is crucial.

12. How can the palliative care team be proactive in dissipating anger and bitterness in family members?

Well developed skills in communication and active listening are imperative for the physician practicing end-of-life care. The manner in which information is shared with families can greatly affect their response to the news as well as their receptivity to ongoing supportive care. The simple practices of the physician sitting down, avoiding crossed arms and legs, and being attentive and mindful to the emotional reactions to breaking the bad news can avoid anger as the precipitated response. Allow patients and families time to react and time to re-discuss issues. A terminal diagnosis has a ripple effect—each family member and close friend will be affected. The physician and caregiving team may need to redirect the priorities of care to the patient as the impending death may raise "unfinished business" for family members and friends who feel compelled to seek reconciliation or resolution.

Often, a previously absent family member will appear, demanding more medical evaluations or "aggressive" treatments. This can be particularly challenging when this individual is another physician or lawyer; the caregiving team can become distracted by conflicting directions and lose sight of care goals. When these previously absent family members become threatening or hostile, care is even more difficult to deliver. It is important to recognize the common goal of caring while also acknowledging that anger and aggressiveness may have their roots in the desire to control or "fix" an uncontrollable or "unfixable" situation.

The palliative care team can help facilitate the coping of the family, and without judgment, provide support and direction for the members to discuss and resolve their issues as death approaches, acknowledging the dimension of their grief and loss. Whenever possible or appropriate, kind humor may dissipate some of the intensity and help foster a spirit of camaraderie between the family and the palliative care team.

13. Are loved ones usually present when the patient dies?

Death frequently occurs when neither the physician nor family is present. Occasionally, a spouse will be in close attendance, even in embrace when a loved one dies. This is, however, the exception, despite what Hollywood would have us believe. More typically, even for families in vigil, death often occurs when the child or spouse has even briefly left the room. Family member reaction to this occurrence can be intense: they may verbalize a sense of failure for not having been present. The physician can do much to relieve potential anguish by explaining this phenomena before the death occurs.

14. How can family and friends provide physical comfort in the last hours of living?

Involving family members, friends, and caregivers in the plan of comfort can often enhance the level of care. Oral swabbing with water or soda water provides hygiene and soothes dry membranes. Using juices or beverages that are favored by the patient is also appropriate; we have even utilized Guinness Stout for mouth care! Artificial tears or cool compresses to the eyes can also provide soothing relief. Gentle massage or limb movement may ease cramping or pressure on boney pressure points. Typically, family members welcome an opportunity for active care through the dying phase. A directed focus on the patient and discerning their individual means of comfort often helps families and friends recall pleasurable memories and previous enjoyments. The active participation of families and friends may also promote a sense of contribution to comfort and facilitate a healthy mourning process.

15. Is it necessary to treat high fevers in dying patients?

Fever may occur for a number of reasons as death approaches, including pneumonia or infections. Fever that is sometimes the result of brain or liver infiltration with tumor tends to be recalcitrant to treatment. Treatment for fever is optional; the fever may not be a discomfort to the patient. The use of cooling blankets or ice packs is contraindicated; they do not promote comfort and will not change the dying process. When indicated, acetaminophen via suppository may reduce a temperature elevation. Fever resulting from tumor infiltration tends to be best treated with non-steroidal anti-inflammatories or steroids. Again, restoring a normal body temperature is not necessarily imperative.

16. What are the random twitches and jerks sometimes displayed by patients on high-dose morphine?

Myoclonus appears as the random twitching or jerking of the extremities, which can often be confused with seizure activity or restlessness. Myoclonus is more common in the setting of high-dose opioids or in instances of hepatic or renal failure. It can exacerbate pain significantly in the setting of widespread bone metastases. Liberal dosing with benzodiazepines or barbiturates is usually necessary to quiet the movements; at times continuous infusion of these is required. Relieving restlessness, agitation, and severe myoclonus can profoundly influence the dying experience for families as much as for the patient. The results achieved in this area of symptom management may influence the survivors' memory of the death as either peaceful or painful.

17. How is restlessness and agitation managed prior to death?

The restlessness occurring as a result of encephalopathy and organ failure may be more difficult for families to observe than it is for patients to experience. Restlessness may indicate uncontrolled pain, unrelieved constipation, a distended bladder, or unresolved psychological distress. Safety issues can arise if restlessness is severe, but restraints should never be used in this situation. Rather, assessing for physical distress, enhancing pain control, or providing other forms of comfort are essential. At times, mild sedation to induce a light sleep is indicated.

Agitated delirium may also occur in some patients; these symptoms would manifest more intensely than simple restlessness. Frequently, the occurrence of delirium can jeopardize the ability of families to care for dying patients at home. Medications such as haloperidol are often used for this symptom, sometimes alternating with benzodiazepines. Delirium can also be the result of haloperidol or even morphine; therefore, thoughtful reassessments by the physician are critical.

For some patients, the apprehension surrounding death is profound. Perhaps they have not had the opportunity or the means to resolve significant emotional, social, or spiritual issues.

Ideally, significant issues would be identified and addressed early in the course of illness, but for some, this is not possible. At times, sedation may be the only means to provide significant comfort and relief of distress. A candid discussion regarding the role of sedation should occur between the physician, the family, and if possible, the patient.

18. What respiratory changes occur as death approaches?

Alterations in breathing occur as a result of the underlying disease process and other comorbid states. Pleural effusions or obstructing lung lesions may create great respiratory distress. The positioning of the patient can be very helpful; support them leaning forward over a bedside table or chair to optimize the workload of the respiratory muscles and utilize gravitational fluid shifts. Studies have shown that the regular administration of small amounts of morphine can decrease the perceived work of breathing without negatively impacting the respiratory pattern.

Respiratory changes commonly occur as the level of consciousness declines. Cheyne-Stokes respiration is characterized by patterns of increasingly rapid breathing alternating with intervals of apnea. Some patients will manifest regular shallow labored breaths called agonal respiration; these patients are deeply comatose, and breathe with an open mouth with much respiratory effort. As patients weaken and become increasingly obtunded, they are no longer able to clear secretions effectively; these may pool in the posterior pharynx, creating a rattling or gurgling sound. Suctioning creates noxious stimulation. It is better to provide repositioning coupled with the use of an anticholinergic such as scopolamine to decrease secretion production. Families and caregivers can continue with mouth care through this time. This may facilitate an active expression of caring and nurturing for those participating in the death process.

19. Is it always necessary to use parenteral medications for symptom management in the last hours of life?

As patients become increasingly weak and changes in mental status occur, most lose their ability to swallow effectively. Physicians must be skilled in adjusting dosages and delivering medications via non-oral routes.

Although symptoms may progress rapidly as death becomes more intermittent, intravenous treatments are rarely indicated and often are not advantageous. Placing an intravenous catheter may be painful and made difficult by the cachexia and dehydration resulting from advanced disease. The fluids infused may create new symptoms such as edema, or may increase existing ascites or effusions. Intravenous fluid support prolongs the dying process. The gadgetry of an intravenous infusion system may further stress a home environment already under duress. The use of concentrated solutions administered via the buccal or sublingual route is preferred when patients can no longer take oral medications. Many analgesics and sedatives can be given rectally. When high dosages necessitate infusion, the subcutaneous delivery route can be accessed via a 25-gauge butterfly needle attached to a syringe driver or small computerized pump. Many medications can be mixed in the infusion pump cassette and infused concomitantly.

20. What role do fluids play at the end of life?

Early in the course of an illness, supportive nutritional therapies are often appropriate when coupled with disease altering treatments. As disease progresses, these therapies may constitute more of a burden than a benefit. Discussions regarding parenteral fluids and nutritional support are particularly likely to arise when patients can no longer swallow. Families often struggle with issues regarding food and fluids, particularly those concerning weight loss and fears of starvation. Thoughtful explanation from the physician regarding the dying process and the potential adverse metabolic effects and fluid overload that may result from feeding can assuage family and caregiver fears of depriving their loved one of sustenance.

The gradual dehydration that occurs prior to death does not always connote diminished mental status or pain. Interestingly, in some circumstances there may actually be a temporary *increase* in the alertness of the patient, despite a steady decrease in oral intake and fluid volume. Patients with end-stage liver disease may experience a reduction in ammonia levels and subsequent encephalopathy with decreased consumption of protein-containing foods. Patients with primary and metastatic brain tumors may exhibit a transient improvement in mental status as the edema associated with the central lesions diminishes with global dehydration. These "improvements" in mental status may be confusing to families and caregivers and require explanation. The easing of peripheral edema may improve comfort by decreasing tissue distention. The reabsorption of ascites or pleural effusions may lessen respiratory difficulty resulting from pulmonary restriction. When a patient is in coma, continuous intravenous infusions will prolong the dying process.

21. Should pain medications be discontinued when patients become unresponsive or comatose?

Pain medications should not be stopped when the patient becomes comatose, but continued around the clock with adjustments made for perceived distress. Most palliative medical physicians feel that is better to err on the side of relief than risk patient discomfort when communication is limited. If urine output becomes significantly limited, the clearing of opioids such as morphine will be diminished. Some physicians would then recommend using alternate opioids, such as hydromorphone, and other renal-cleared medications on an as-needed basis to avoid toxicity.

Nonverbal signs of distress such as grimacing and groaning may be indicative of pain; these must be assessed regularly to facilitate symptom relief. Pretreatment for potential pain with turning, bathing, and changing of clothing and/or linens can be advantageous. Medications for the treatment of chronic diseases such as diabetes and hypertension can be eliminated when patients are clearly dying or when the burden of taking the medication outweighs the potential benefit. The primary focus of care should be on comfort.

22. What role do non-pharmaceutical interventions have when death approaches?

Cognitive work such as imagery and self-hypnosis will not be effective when mental status changes supercede. However, interventions such as massage, music, room fans, or quiet talking may help to alleviate some anxiety and restlessness for the dying patient. Key to ascertaining non-pharmaceutical means of comfort is to obtain insight into past pleasures and comforts of the individual patient. Though jarring to the physician or caregiving team, rock-and-roll booming at the bedside might constitute solace for a dying patient. Research in music for the dying by Therese Schroeder-Sheker, Ph.D. has identified that music without a beat or pulse often facilitates the dying process. Again, key to providing comfort at the end of life is to prioritize the needs of the patient above all others.

23. Does the physician have further responsibilities after the death of the patient?

The physician is responsible for the timely and accurate completion of the death certificate. This document must be completed prior to cremation or burial. It also provides the survivors with the necessary proof of death to complete legal and business affairs. The physician should be well versed in his or her state's requirements regarding death certification.

The involvement of the physician in the period of bereavement will vary. If the physician enjoyed a long-term relationship with the patient and their family, he or she may choose to be included in the personal and community expressions of grief and loss. Certainly, providing opportunities for the family or caregivers to ask questions even months after the death may be very helpful to further facilitate closure in the mourning process. Ideally, the physician will have spurred the early involvement of hospice care for the patient and family. This ensures supportive care throughout the dying process and ongoing bereavement support for more than a year following the death.

24. How do you provide for a "death with dignity?"

"Dying with dignity" is a common phrase used by laypersons and physicians to signify a desired outcome for the dying patient. The meaning of this phrase is not always clear and may not capture for families and patients the essence of their needs and desires in this critical phase of life. Dying with dignity truly implies a judgment—What is dignity? Is it consistent with how the person lived their life? Does the desire for this impose expectations on a dying person and on their family? A more appropriate phrase might be "death with integrity," that is, to die as we have lived, with interpersonal relationships, spirituality, and a sense of self intact. Certainly illness robs us of control, weakens or sacrifices our independence, and threatens us with physical pain and suffering. It is imperative that, as physicians, we provide the optimum of whole-person care at the end of life. Not only must we be diligent in our management of the symptoms of disease and dying, we must also prioritize means of care that respect the completeness of the individual. This would include such issues as the patient's choice regarding the place of death, whether or not sedation is used, and how pain and symptom management is provided. Also key is respect for religious and cultural customs, family traditions, and the patient's value system and their chosen family unit. With optimal symptom management and supportive care, patients can live fully until they die, and can make that transition with integrity.

BIBLIOGRAPHY

1. AAHPM Curriculum on Palliative Medicine and Hospice Care. Module 4, 1998 [in press].
2. Breibart W, et al: Neuropsychiatric syndromes and psychological symptoms in patients with advanced cancer. J Pain Symptom Manage 10:131–141, 1995.
3. Bruera E, et al: Effects of morphine on the dyspnea of terminal cancer patients. J Pain Symptom Manage 5:341, 1990.
4. Byock I: Dying Well. New York, Riverhead Books, 1997.
5. Caralis PV, et al: The influence of ethnicity and race on attitudes toward advance directives, life prolonging treatments, and euthanasia. J Clin Ethics 4:155–165, 1993.
6. Cherny NI, Portenoy RK: Sedation in the management of refractory symptoms: Guidelines for evaluation and treatment. J Palliat Care 10:31–39, 1994.
7. Coyle N, et al: Character of terminal illness in the advanced cancer patient: Pain and other symptoms during the last four weeks of life. J Pain Symptom Manage 5:83–93, 1990.
8. Kubler-Ross E: On Death and Dying. New York, MacMillan, 1969.
9. McCann RM, et al: Comfort care for terminally ill patients, the appropriate use of nutrition and hydration. JAMA 272:1263–1266, 1994.
10. Schroeder-Scheker T: The Chalice of Repose Project. Missoula, MT, Personal communication.
11. Story P, et al: Subcutaneous infusions for control of cancer symptoms. J Pain Symptom Manage 5:33–41, 1990.
12. Twaddle ML: Hospice Care. Dignity and Dying. Grand Rapids, MI, Eerdmans Publishing, 1996.
13. von Gunten CF, Twaddle ML: Terminal care for noncancer patients. Clin Geriatr Med 12:349, 1996.

29. COMMUNICATION IN PALLIATIVE CARE

Geoffrey A. T. Hawson, M.B.B.S., and Kym A. Irving, Ph.D.

1. What information do palliative care patients require?

Diagnosis and prognosis: It is not uncommon for patients to commence the palliative care phase of their treatment with an inadequate understanding of their diagnosis. Lack of understanding may be a result of inadequate communication between physician and patient or may be related to the patient's psychological state or desire not to know. Patients also may lack awareness of the implications of palliative care. Never assume that a patient admitted to a hospice or palliative care unit fully understands the reasons for admission. Carefully assess the level of knowledge and understanding that patients and their families possess and require, in relation to the diagnosis and prognosis of the illness.

Treatment: Information concerning palliative care treatment should include morbidity and likely outcomes so that patients can make informed decisions. Patients may assume that treatments are curative, especially if they involve chemotherapy or radiotherapy.

Death and dying: In most countries, it is acknowledged that patients have the right to know that they are dying. Patients often ask specific questions about their mode of dying and may seek this information at various stages during their illness. As with all communication, physicians should take their lead from patients as to patient requirements in this regard. Once the patient is aware that death is inevitable, observe the patient's verbal and nonverbal cues to determine how extensively the topic of death should be discussed. Consider that for some patients a disservice is done by continuing conversations about death after a desire not to mention or discuss the topic has been clearly expressed.

2. What are the unmet information needs of patients?

Studies have shown that patients with cancer have a high proportion of unmet needs, many of which are related to communication. Generally, patients want more information about their disease, treatment, test results, and symptom control, as well as about self-help and coping strategies. They also report difficulties in obtaining answers to their questions. Ask patients what information and support they require, and seek the assistance of other professionals when a subject is outside your domain.

3. How is information best communicated?

Difficult or complex communications should be planned in advance so that family members or supportive friends can be present. It is best to **arrange a time** when the patient is more likely to be receptive and has fewer problems with pain or sedation.

Respect the **patient's privacy**. The giving of bad news or information of a personal nature should not take place in an open ward. Rooms set aside for counseling and consultation provide a better environment for such interactions. If patients are confined to their bed, arrange an environment to allow as much privacy as possible. Use appropriate nonverbal behaviors, such as aligning yourself with the patient's eye level to convey empathy and concern. Courtesy dictates that mobile phones and pagers (beepers) be inaudible to prevent interruptions during the conversation. Research suggests that interruptions can cause a lack of continuity in the dissemination of information and lead to patient anxiety and suffering.

Medical terminology and jargon confound patient understanding and perpetuate hierarchical divisions between specialists and patients. Therefore, avoid using terms that have no meaning to the patient. At the same time, convey information in an accurate and reliable fashion.

Communication aids, such as diagrams, notes, and video and audiotapes, have been shown to facilitate communication. The recording of information aids patient and family understanding and enhances patient recall. A letter to the patient summarizing important information also can aid memory and strengthen understanding. Moreover, tapes and letters benefit relatives and friends who cannot attend consultations.

4. Why is it important to check the patient's understanding of what has been communicated?
When information is complex and conveyed during times of anxiety and distress, it is not surprising that retention rates are low. Patients themselves are more likely than specialists (71% of patients versus 31% of oncologists) to consider it essential that a review of information occur 24 hours after the initial presentation of bad news. Information often is better retained and understood when provided in stages across sessions.

5. Are there any guidelines for breaking bad news?
There is an increasing number of publications now available, including:
   Girgis A, Sanson-Fischer R: Breaking bad news: Consensus guidelines for medical practitioners. J Clin Oncol 13:2449–2456, 1995.
   Buckman R: How to Break Bad News: A Guideline for Health Professionals. Baltimore, The Johns Hopkins Press, 1992.
The first is a brief but excellent review article with 69 references. The second is a very readable and informative book suitable for novices as well as those with more advanced communication skills.

6. Even when attempts have been made to communicate information clearly, accurately, and empathically, why is it that some patients have difficulty comprehending?
Even when a range of efforts are made to aid the patient's understanding of their illness and treatment, **psychological barriers** such as denial, shock, anxiety, fear of death, and depression may impede comprehension. Psychiatric assessment and pharmacotherapy may be of benefit to these patients.

Problems in communication can be compounded by **biochemical abnormalities** (e.g., hepatic dysfunction, hypercalcemia, or **medication** [e.g., sedation, analgesia]). In these situations, it may be better to delay communication until the underlying biochemical abnormality has been corrected or an adjustment has been made to the sedation/analgesia.

7. What are the information and communication needs of family members?
The information needs of family members are similar to those of patients concerning diagnosis, prognosis, and treatment. Research indicates that family members may infrequently discuss the patient's illness despite spending many hours visiting the patient in hospital. Do not assume that family members gain information from patients. Children and siblings report being the least informed, and professionals skilled in working with these populations may need to be consulted.

Family members, like patients, are a heterogeneous group—some prefer detailed, ongoing accounts of the patient's progress while others are less inquisitive. Such individual differences should be respected. Specialists need to develop skills for dealing with group situations, because consultations involving family members and friends are complex.

Negotiating and understanding health care systems often is a difficult task. Families require information about the palliative care services structure, nature, and staff so that they know whom to contact and when. Brochures, leaflets, and orientation sessions are useful methods for disseminating such information.

8. Why is it important to be aware of family characteristics?
Family characteristics can influence the communication and information needs of patients and family members. For example cultural differences in **attitudes toward illness and death** can affect the exchange of information between patients, family members, and palliative care physicians. One study reports that in Italy cancer is seen as an illness embodying hopelessness and condemnation. In contrast, the prevailing metaphor in the United States concentrates on

"survivors" and "exceptional" patients. These differing metaphors have implications for the interpretation and assimilation of information concerning illness, treatment, and death. In countries that emphasize survivorship, it is not surprising when patients and families have more difficulty with acceptance of information related to death.

Cultural differences also influence disclosure of terminal illnesses to patients, with some preferring that the patient be prevented from knowing. Ask family members specific questions about their cultural practices and beliefs to aid your understanding of their attitudes and concerns.

Communication difficulties in the palliative care setting may be related to communication and relationship problems in the **family environment**. In one study, 15% of families were found to display high levels of psychosocial morbidity and poor social functioning, expressed as conflict ("hostile" families) and low cohesion and expressiveness ("sullen" families). Family-centered intervention programs have identified families at risk using measures such as the Family Environment Scale. When relationship problems are apparent, referrals to family therapists may be indicated.

9. How can a family conference help?

Family conferences are an excellent method of conveying important information to both patient and family and assessing their information needs. Calling a conference draws attention to the problem at hand and allows input and advice from a range of professionals, including doctors, nurses, social workers, psychologists, and spiritual advisors. All attendees should be encouraged to bring with them a list of questions or concerns for discussion. A multidisciplinary approach provides an opportunity for a range of issues to be aired at one time.

10. When should a family conference be held?

• After the diagnosis is ascertained, to discuss prognosis and treatment.
• Any time an issue causes significant difficulties. The conference may be initiated by medical staff or by patients and their families.
• When an important intervention or change of treatment is considered.
• When the patient experiences a significant deterioration that may herald an important change in focus or direction of the medical management.

11. Can discussion about the process of grieving be of benefit before death?

As family members and friends are counseled about the possibility or certainty of the patient's death, it is important to prepare them for the grieving process. Individuals generally accept that grief is normal, but often do not anticipate how profound it can be, or how long it can continue. Providing information about what to expect helps family and friends prepare for bereavement. This counseling can be achieved by analogy or story telling, or by discussion of how other families have reacted to and coped with the death of a loved one. When such communications are awkward, or outside the training of palliative care professionals, referral to or involvement of professionals trained in grief and bereavement counseling should be considered.

12. What mechanisms can be put in place to help families with grief and bereavement?

The increasing importance of addressing bereavement in palliative care services is illustrated by recent developments in Australia, where a **bereavement support service** is now required for accreditation by the Australian Council of Health Standards. Central to the accreditation standards is the recognition that palliative care incorporates not only the patient's needs and wishes, but also the family's. The standards require bereavement risk assessment of primary carers and a funded bereavement services coordinator.

A range of less formal mechanisms can be adopted to communicate support for bereaved carers. **Memorial services** are conducted in many palliative care settings. At the palliative care unit of the first author, a memorial service is held every 6 months at which the families of all patients who have died since the last service are invited to participate. These gatherings provide families with an opportunity to celebrate the life of the loved one and know that they are not alone in their bereavement. They also provide opportunities for staff to share with families the ways in which patients touched their lives.

Remembrance of the patient's death via phone calls and cards acknowledging the anniversary can be helpful to family members.

13. Is it possible to predict who will have difficulties with grief and bereavement?

Bereavement outcome has been linked to demographic variables (e.g., age), personal and psychological variables (e.g., past experience with death and coping skills), relationship with the deceased (e.g., intimacy and quality) and mode of death (e.g., expected versus unexpected). As Sanders points out, although bereavement research generally is problematic with regard to methodology and generalization, risk factors include: poor health before bereavement, concurrent crises, lack of social supports, economic difficulties, and ambivalence and dependency in the relationship. (See also Question 21.)

14. How is bereavement risk assessed?

The most widely cited procedure for risk assessment comes from work undertaken by Parkes and Weiss in the 1970s and implemented at St. Christopher's Hospice in London, where it is now standard practice to interview family members the day after the patient's death. At this meeting, family members' risk of abnormal bereavement is scored according to the eight-item Parkes and Weiss Bereavement Risk Index. The index comprises three demographic variables (e.g., length of preparation for the death) and five items relating to psychological factors (e.g., self-reproach, anger). The items are scored on a 1 to 4 scale or a 1 to 5 scale. Total scores higher than 18 place the person at high risk. The final question on the Index is "How will the key person cope?" Answers indicating a high level of difficulty (4 or 5) place the key person in the high-risk bracket irrespective of the total scores on other items. However, the authors acknowledge that about 33% of those expected to do well have a poor outcome, and 42% of those expected to do poorly have a good outcome, suggesting that a large proportion of individuals requiring ongoing support are not identified by this procedure. A valid and reliable measure of bereavement risk has yet to be developed, although a number of grief inventories are available. Alternative approaches to identifying families at risk after bereavement include assessing the nature of family relationships and employing family-centered interventions.

15. Is the level of communication between health professionals and family and friends related to grief reactions?

The relationships between patients, their loved ones, and palliative care and hospital staff during the dying process are complex, and it is reasonable to expect that the level of satisfaction with care would be reflected in adjustment to bereavement. One study indicates that family and friends who perceive their post bereavement health as excellent or good are more likely to be satisfied with the level of care that their loved one received. There is some evidence that when communication is lacking, grief reactions may be exacerbated. For example, researchers attribute some of the anger experienced by the children of patients dying of cancer to a lack of information concerning treatment. Anecdotal evidence also suggests that when family members have inaccurate understandings of medical interventions, feelings of blame and anger may be heightened. Additionally, grief reactions can be more severe when expectations of a "good" death (peaceful and natural, without unnecessary prolongation of the dying process and with family present) are not met.

A number of variables may influence grief reactions (see Question 21). While an individual's background, personality, and history of relating are beyond the influence of palliative care providers, minimizing stress and trauma and aiding understanding of death through thoughtful and informative interactions with patients, family, and friends are important considerations.

16. Why is it important to maintain good communication among palliative care team members?

- To maintain accuracy and consistency of information
  Regular staff and case conferences enable sharing of patient information and ensure that

information provided to patients is accurate and consistent. Misunderstandings about treatment can occur not only among patients and their families but also among staff. Determine which staff members are responsible for communicating what information, institute reliable procedures for the dissemination of information.

• To manage staff stress and grief

Anecdotal evidence suggests that "bad" deaths (e.g., during which patients experience uncontrollable pain, have no family present, and are unaccepting of their impeding death) require extensive debriefing and may contribute to high turnover rates in the palliative care staff. It may be worthwhile to invite skilled facilitators to manage the debriefing meeting. Debriefing meetings should be held on a regular basis, with special meetings arranged to discuss difficult deaths.

17. What can be done when communication breaks down?

When communication difficulties arise, involve a third party facilitator or mediator. Social workers, psychologists, counselors, and spiritual advisors may fill this role.

18. Why should physicians develop their communication skills?

Communication skills are frequently identified by palliative care providers as an area for improvement. When physicians have well-developed communication skills, the primary benefit is to patients and their families. However, burnout is more prevalent among consultants who feel inadequately trained in communication than among those who feel adequately trained; therefore, there may be personal gains in developing such skills.

19. How can physicians develop their communication skills?

While books and articles are a good starting place, communication skills are best learned through demonstration and controlled practice. In Australia, the National Breast Cancer Centre has commenced workshops on "breaking bad news," aimed at surgeons and others involved in the management of breast cancer. Similar workshops are available in other countries through professional health organizations. In the UK, many workshops for medical specialists are run by Fallowfield.

20. What are the essentials for arranging a communication session with patients and family?

Example Protocol for Communication Session

1. Arrange when, where and who should attend.
2. Assess how much the patient knows (e.g., Can you tell me what you know about your condition?).
3. Assess emotional context. Look for verbal and nonverbal cues.
4. Assess how much the patient wants to know.
   • Are you the kind of person who likes to know exactly what is happening?
   • Would you like me to give you full details of your condition or is there someone else you would like me to talk to?
   • Are you the kind of person who likes full details of what's going on or would you prefer just to hear about the treatment process?
5. Share information.
   • Categorize or consolidate information.
   • Stress important information.
   • Avoid jargon.
   • Check whether the information was received and understood.
   • Reinforce, repeat, clarify.
   • Use communication aids (e.g., audio and videotapes, diagrams, letters).
6. Elicit patient concerns.
7. Respond to patient feelings (e.g., How does what I have just told you make you feel?).
8. Discuss future plan and support.
9. Arrange a review session.

21. What are the major factors influencing the outcome of grief?

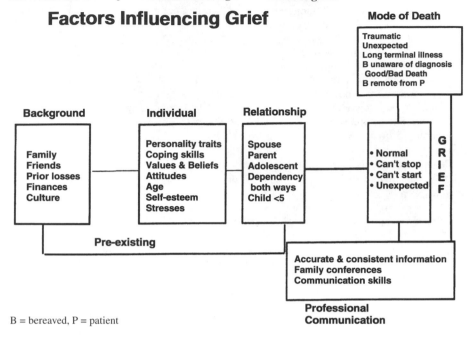

Factors Influencing Grief

B = bereaved, P = patient

BIBLIOGRAPHY

1. Beisecker A, Moore W: Oncologists' perceptions of the effects of cancer patients' companions on physician-patient interactions. J Psychosoc Oncol 12:23–29, 1994.
2. Buckman R: How to Break Bad News—A Guide for Health Care Professionals. Baltimore, Johns Hopkins University Press, 1992.
3. Faulkner A, Maguire P: Talking to Cancer Patients and Their Relatives. New York, Oxford University Press, 1994.
4. Gordon D: Embodying illness, embodying cancer. Culture Med Psychiatr 14:275–297, 1990.
5. Graham J, Ramirez A, Cull A, Finlay I: Job stress and satisfaction among palliative care physicians. Palliat Med 10:185–194, 1996.
6. Hawson GAT, Irving KA: The role of professional-family communication in models of grief. Australian and New Zealand Society of Paliative Medicine Scientific Meeting, Christchurch, United Kingdom, 1996.
7. Kissane DW, Block S, Burns I, et al: Psychological morbidity in the families of patients with cancer. J Psychosoc Oncol 3:47–56, 1994.
8. Mystakidou K, Liossi C, Vlachos L, Papadimitriou J: Disclosure of diagnostic information to cancer patients in Greece. Palliat Med 10:195–200, 1996.
9. Parkes CM, Weiss RS: Recovery from Bereavement. New York, Basic Books, 1983.
10. Sanders C: Risk factors in bereavement outcome. In Stroebe M, Stroebe W, Hansson R (eds): Handbook of Bereavement. New York, Cambridge, 1993.
12. Tattersall MH, Butow PN, Griffin AM, Dunn SM: The take-home message: Patients prefer consultation audiotapes to summary letters. J Clin Oncol 12:1305–1311, 1994.
13. Wiggers JH, Donovan KO, Redman S, Sanson-Fisher RW: Cancer patient satisfaction with care. Cancer 66:610–616, 1990.
13. Wright K, Dyck S: Expressed concerns of adult cancer patient's family members. Cancer Nurs 7:371–374, 1984.

WEBSITE RESOURCES

- UK Communication Workshops
  Professor Lesley Fallowfield
  l.fallowfield@ucl.ac.uk

- NBCC contact for workshops
  National Breast Cancer Centre
  PO Box 572
  Kings Cross Sydney 2011
  Fax 612 9326 9329
  directorate@nbcc.org.au
  http://www.nbcc.org.au

- Contact for Australian Palliative Care Standards
  Australia Palliative Care
  http://www/pallcare.org.au

30. ETHICAL ISSUES

Tadaaki Sakai, M.D.

1. Is it always necessary for health care professionals to communicate the truth of a fatal illness and its prognosis to patients and families?

The basic rule is to tell the truth if patients want to know. The relationship between patients and health care professionals is built on trust. Any deception will undermine the foundation of the relationship, thus hampering treatment and care.

Patients must have true and accurate knowledge to make their own treatment and lifestyle decisions. True communication is critically important to improve quality of life, which palliative medicine and palliative care try to achieve.

Another principle is to communicate as much truth as patients want. For example, a lung cancer patient with spine metastasis knows the diagnosis but does not want to know anything more. If irradiation of the spine is a good treatment to relieve pain, we may tell the patient about the spine metastasis and the treatment we propose. In telling the truth, the clinician must weigh the shock the patient may experience learning unwanted information against the benefit enjoyed from the treatment. It is the responsibility of the medical professional to tell the truth if truth-telling is judged to give greater benefit.

It may not be possible to communicate truth, however, to patients with lowered level of consciousness or confusion. When truth-telling will probably not benefit the patient and simply make him or her fearful, it is better to tell the family only. However, most patients want to know the truth about their disease.

2. How is the truth told?

Directly and *not* incidentally. The physical environment should be constructed to preserve the patient's privacy. Other suggestions include:

- Confirm what the patient knows and how much he or she wants to know.
- Follow the patient's agenda, not yours, and communicate properly several times, if necessary.
- Expect that the patient may express denial or anger when bad news is given.
- Avoid giving false hope.
- Avoid hasty and abrupt truth-telling; it could push the patient into depression.
- Be gentle, select the words, accept the patient's reaction, assure and support the patient.
- The patient must feel real partnership with health care professionals during truth-telling. Providing information on prognosis and treatment options should be followed by effective recommendations for symptom control.

3. How can the caregiver help when the family is opposed to telling the truth to the patient on the grounds that he or she cannot tolerate the bad news?

In Western nations, patients are legally and ethically entitled to receive accurate information from physicians. However, there are many societies in which this practice does not exist. For many reasons, families often ask health care professionals not to tell the bad news to the patients. They think that the patient cannot withstand the news and will become depressed and demoralized, resulting in earlier death. Some families do not know how to cope with the patients' suffering and project their fears on the patient.

Families may ignore the fact that patients need to have accurate information to plan their lives. Except when patients refuse to be informed of the consequences of their diseases, medical professionals should gently explain to families that patients will be isolated if they are not told the truth and relieved when they can share information with their families, and that the news will not hasten death. Occasionally a patient does not want to be informed about a fatal illness, but the spouse wants health care professionals to tell the patient the truth. An extreme example is HIV-positive patients. They have the right to refuse information, but this right cannot be translated as an exemption from responsibility to protect the safety and welfare of the family and society. It is wrong not to tell the patients the truth.

4. When is it acceptable to withhold the truth?

We should honor a patient's request that "I don't want to receive any more bad news." However, if the patient is considered at greater risk by not knowing the facts (as when the patient drives a car without knowing about a brain metastasis that creates risk of a traffic accident), we have to communicate truthfully but carefully. It is also ethically right to tell the truth indirectly when the patient is too optimistic about the illness.

5. Is it acceptable to administer medication to an unconscious, dying patient with death rattle at the request of the family?

Yes, but first explain the mechanism of death rattle to the family. Administration of an anti-cholinergic agent or hyoscine is effective. Death rattle is a noise generated at every breath by semiclosed central airways of a patient in a semi- or deep coma who has lost the cough reflex. It enables him to discharge airway secretions. The presumably unconscious patient is unaware of the rattle and unaffected by it. However, the rattle can torment family members.

6. What is the role of intravenous fluid infusion in a patient for whom oral intake has become impossible in the palliative care setting?

Oral intake frequently becomes impossible for terminal cancer patients, except in transient intestinal obstruction. When patients cannot take food or water by mouth, intravenous fluid infusion may overload the compromised cardiopulmonary system, leading to dyspnea, pleural effusion, ascites, edema, and possibly increased pain. Fluid infusion also limits mobility of the patients, resulting in psychological stress, which acts as a barrier between the patient and the family. The patient should be told both the risks and benefits, if any, to make an informed decision. However, meticulous oral care and keeping the mouth wet at all times is critical if intravenous fluids are withheld.

7. What are the indications for blood transfusion to the chronic or acutely bleeding patient in the palliative care setting?

1. The patient has effort dyspnea, severe fatigue, or lethargy, which are likely to be corrected by blood transfusion.

2. It is expected that the blood transfusion will produce a durable effect, e.g., for 2 weeks.

3. The patient agrees to receive blood transfusions and other tests as needed.

It is not ethical to continue blood transfusions for short-term gains, when it may simply prolong death, or because a family member insists.

8. When the prognosis is too grim, is it necessary to administer antibiotics for infection control in the palliative care setting?

Antibiotics may be withheld when the medical professionals judge that the treatment is medically futile or that the burden and risk to the patient are far greater than any benefit. However, antibiotics may be given to control symptoms that are distressful to the patient, such as high fever and sometimes confusion caused by underlying infections in elderly patients.

9. How should medical professionals deal with the patient and family who wish to pursue alternative therapy to try to cure the disease or slow its progression?

Alternative therapy is not considered an evidence-based medicine. There are tremendous varieties of alternative therapies, and it is difficult to give proper advice on any kind. It is, however, true that placebo effects of any drugs are observed in about 30% of cases. Staunch belief in the alternative therapy sometimes makes the patient feel better without changing the disease process.

The health care professional should (1) ask the patient and or the family to describe the alternative therapy they wish to use and then (2) render an opinion gently and rationally. It is allowable for the patient to use alternative medicine if it is not too expensive for the family.

There is no reason to deny the alternative medicine if it contains less purified or synthesized substances or if it contains vegetable products that are recognized as good in modern nutrition.

It is necessary to monitor the patient closely and objectively and to have occasional discussions to prevent the family from feeling guilty if the alternative therapy fails.

10. What are essential considerations regarding advance directives?

An advance directive is an oral statement or a document to state a person's requests for end-of-life treatment or possible treatment when he or she may have lost the ability to make decisions. Examples are, "I do not want cardiopulmonary resuscitation, intravenous alimentation, a respirator and/or renal dialysis simply to prolong life," or "I want pain and suffering to be removed even if it may hasten death." Advance directives should not be required against a patient's will.

In some cultures, a patient's autonomy is not well established and there is prevalent hesitation, reluctance, or "depending on the situation" among patients. In such cultures, some advance directives are not voluntary. The legal validity of advance directives varies in different countries and jurisdictions within countries.

The most important consideration is that the wishes expressed in the directives are not transient but continuous and consistent. It is difficult for the patient to make statements before knowing how it feels to have advanced disease or to be dying. For health care professionals, it is difficult to know whether the situation described by the patient agrees with the current situation. In the course of the disease, we have to confirm if the wishes stated in the advance directives are still valid or need some modification. When conflicts arise, a multidisciplinary meeting with all family members or the assistance of an ethics committee may be sought.

In advance directives, everything cannot be directed. It is unreasonable to refuse beneficial treatments. Though the primary goal of the advance directives is to select end-of-life issues, death is personal only in the context of family and society. Health care professionals should respect empathy and compassion of the family, which should be taken into consideration in preparing directives.

11. Describe durable power of attorney.

It is difficult to predict end of life because disease states and processes are diverse and complicated. It is natural that the patients feel uneasy making advance directives. Sometimes a person can be designated as a "durable power of attorney" who has good rapport with the patient and who can sympathize with him or her. Usually the patient makes his own health care decisions so far as he is competent. The person with power of attorney makes decisions for health care when the patient becomes incompetent. A limited number of countries have introduced a system of durable power of attorney. Usually a family member or close friend makes the decisions. However, a friend may face conflicts due to having different opinions from family members. The best solution is to prepare a document that serves as both the advance directive and the durable power of attorney.

12. What is the difference between "spokesperson" and durable power of attorney?

A spokesperson represents the family without any legal authority. The durable power of attorney, on the other hand, is designated by the patient under state statutes in the United States and has legal authority.

13. What are the benefits to the patient and family of having a living will?

It assures the treatment or the refusal of a treatment as a patient chooses even when his condition worsens and he becomes unable to make sound judgments. The living will is a means to secure a patient's self-determination. It also helps families and physicians in making critical decisions.

14. How do you tell patients that a "do not resuscitate" (DNR) order may be beneficial in their situation?

The American Heart Association and American Academy of Sciences at the National Conference on Cardiopulmonary Resuscitation and Emergency Cardiac Care stated that "the purpose of CPR [cardiopulmonary resuscitation] is the prevention of sudden unexpected death. CPR is not indicated in such situations as terminal irreversible illness where death is not unexpected." In many palliative care settings, therefore, DNR is considered a proper option and CPR is contraindicated.

There remains a discussion concerning whether the prognosis is hopeless. The decision should be medical. Patients and families requesting apparently futile CPR are denying their presentment of death, expecting more than is possible from medicine, or incorrectly understanding CPR.

15. When the living will and the patient's durable power of attorney are not readily available, how would you decide DNR or life-sustaining treatment for a terminal patient?

It is considered ethical to withhold treatment when sustaining life is physiologically futile, when the cost and the risk of the treatment are far greater than its benefits, or when treatment is expected to produce painful and uncontrollable symptoms. However, we have to save lives of patients when the risks are minimal even if the benefits are not very great.

16. Why do some physicians resist DNR orders?

One of the biggest reasons is as follows. CPR is sometimes indicated for a terminal patient. For example, transient CO_2 narcosis recovers with short-term assisted mechanical ventilation. Physicians are sometimes hesitant to perform this treatment due to the existing DNR. They are afraid of legal prosecution. There should be no concern about the validity of their medical judgment that CPR can maintain a patient's life for awhile.

17. Is it true that the patient who is declared DNR will receive less care?

No. However, there is a widespread misunderstanding among the public and sometimes among physicians that patients who are declared DNR will receive less care or be easily given up.

18. What is chemical CPR?

CPR is sometimes judicially considered to be an invasive and rough action. Chemical CPR is treatment using only drugs, such as antiarrhythmics, without any intubation or chest compression.

19. How can health care professionals treat dying patients whose suffering is so severe that they want euthanasia?

In a good palliative care setting, it is rare to see such patients. First, we have to determine if symptoms and pain are well controlled. Some patients feel it is better to die than to expose their misery to others.

Physician-assisted suicide is illegal except in the Netherlands. In other jurisdictions, a number of issues remain unsolved. First, it is difficult to confirm the voluntary nature of a patient's judgment in severe pain, confusion, or depression at the terminal stage. Second, uncertainty remains concerning diagnosis, dying, or timing of death in any given patient. Thirdly, economic reasons may supersede the clinical indicators.

Health care professionals must decline requests for euthanasia and do so gently but clearly. We have to do our best to relieve pain and suffering first and try to find the intent behind the patient's request. Euthanasia should not be substituted for good palliative care.

20. What are the indications for applying principles of "double effects"?

The principles of double effects are the rules of ethics that actions resulting in unfavorable results are forgiven if the consequences are foreseen but unintended. It is applied in giving higher doses of sedatives to relieve severe suffering, which may cause earlier death. It is difficult to determine if the action hastens death or prevents futile prolongation of life. It is better to make a risk/benefit comparison than simply to apply the principles.

BIBLIOGRAPHY

1. American Heart Association: Guidelines for cardiopulmonary resuscitation and emergency cardiac care. VIII, Ethical Considerations in Resuscitation. JAMA 268:2282–2288, 1992.
2. British Medical Association: Advance Statements about Medical Treatment. London, BMJ Publishing Group, 1995.
3. Buckman R: How to Break Bad News. Baltimore, Johns Hopkins University Press, 1992.
4. Doyle D: Domiciliary palliative care. In Doyle D, Hanks GWC, Macdonald N (eds): The Textbook of Palliative Medicine. New York, Oxford University Press, 1993, pp 629–647.
5. Faden RR, Beauchamp TL: A History and Theory of Informed Consent. New York, Oxford University Press, 1986.
6. King NMP: Making Sense of Advance Directives. Washington, DC, Georgetown University Press, 1996.
7. Randall F, Downie RS: Palliative Care Ethics. New York, Oxford University Press, 1996.
8. Twycross R: Introducing Palliative Care. Oxford, Radcliffe Medical Press, 1997.
9. Wilkinson J: Ethical issues in palliative care. In Doyle D, Hanks GWC, Macdonald N (eds): The Textbook of Palliative Medicine. New York, Oxford University Press, 1993, pp 495–504.

31. FATIGUE IN PALLIATIVE CARE: THE UNIVERSAL SYMPTOM?

Suresh K. Joishy, M.D., F.A.C.P.

1. Why is the symptom of fatigue important in palliative care?

Fatigue, one of the most common complaints heard by physicians, is a nonspecific but serious symptom. It indicates a physical or psychological disease and may be one of the main symptoms leading to diagnosis of cancer, multiple sclerosis, myocardial infarction, chronic renal disease, chronic obstructive pulmonary disease, and depression.

The etiology and pathogenesis of fatigue remain unknown. In cancer patients in palliative care, fatigue can disturb mood, perceptions, concentration, and compliance with medical treatments. As with pain, fatigue appears to have no useful purpose.

The occurrence of fatigue in early diagnostic and treatment phases of cancer and its continuation in the palliative care setting underscore the need for intervention. In this chapter, *fatigue* indicates a symptom that is causing distress to a patient. Modern medicine has no specific pharmacotherapeutic measures to control fatigue.

2. How do patients describe fatigue?

Common terminologies used interchangeably by patients include:

1. Tiredness—patients generally describe tiredness as occurring after some physical activity or due to lack of sleep.

2. Weakness—patients use this term when they are unable to carry out day-to-day activities.

3. Lack of energy—even at rest, patients are feeling tiredness, weakness, or fatigue.

3. How do physicians describe fatigue?

The following medical terminologies are used interchangeably by physicians:

1. Fatigue—usually physiologic, felt by normal individuals after vigorous physical exertion or prolonged intellectual work and accompanying normal sleep/wake cycles. This phenomenon disappears after restful sleep. It is not a symptom.

2. Malaise—the French word for "not feeling well."

3. Asthenia—indicates pathologic fatigue. While some clinicians feel that this word can be substituted for *fatigue, fatigue* is better understood by patients and physicians.

4. Is fatigue a genuine symptom, or is it a subsymptom of other symptoms?

Most diseases and chronic symptoms are associated with fatigue. Hence, fatigue is so nonspecific, one wonders if it is a genuine symptom. Fatigue perhaps could be described as a "medium" in which other symptoms are sustained. Studies have shown that fatigue may persist even after cure of cancers such as Hodgkin's disease. Ultimately, the fatigue can be considered a linking symptom to other symptoms.

5. What symptoms in palliative care patients are known to be associated with fatigue?

Fatigue assessment studies have shown quantitative correlation between fatigue and other symptoms in cancer patients. Fatigue correlates with pain, depression, anxiety, lack of appetite, and higher heart rate. However, correlation does not prove a cause/effect relationship. When patients do not have words to describe fatigue, they may be able to describe the consequence of fatigue, such as lack of appetite, muscle weakness, and exhaustion.

6. What is the prevalence of fatigue in cancer patients?

Although there are no systematic studies of fatigue in the palliative care setting, several studies have addressed the issue in relation to cancer treatments. Chemotherapy results in fatigue in

75–100% of cases. Many patients remain fatigued months to years after treatment has ended. Similar instances of fatigue have been quoted in patients receiving radiotherapy, particularly abdominal radiation. Patients in palliative care generally do not receive chemotherapy, but palliative radiotherapy to control pain and other symptoms is not uncommon.

7. What causes fatigue in noncancer patients?

Several epidemiologic studies have shown that symptoms of fatigue such as tiredness, weakness, and poor concentration are widespread in patients attending general medical clinics. Fatigue is common in all types of common infections. Prolonged fatigue may occur in patients with diabetes mellitus, anemia, surgery, and some viral illnesses. There are some gender differences in the feeling of fatigue. It is three times more common in women of childbearing age. In young women, fatigue may be a presenting symptom of anemia or pregnancy. In older people, fatigue is more commonly associated with circulatory disorders or polypharmacy. Lack of sleep is also attributed to chronic fatigue.

Psychological causes are paramount in 40–51% of patients and physical causes in 31–39% of the patients. Old age, family reasons, natural stress, and home or marital stress are common psychological reasons for fatigue.

8. What is the mechanism of fatigue in palliative care patients with advanced cancers?

We do not know. Several theories, which propose somatic and psychological or combined causes, are listed below.

Proposed Mechanisms Causing Fatigue

CONDITION	MECHANISM
Malnutrition	
Anorexia/nausea/vomiting	Not having enough calories
Dysphagia	Impaired energy metabolism
	Loss of muscle mass and muscle weakness
	Hyper/hypometabolic state
Hormonal conditions	
Accumulation of products of cell destruction due to tumor necrosis or cancer treatments, including chemotherapy/radiotherapy	Release of substances called "asthenins" Tumor necrosis factor and other cytokines
Anemia	Hypoxia
Drugs: antiemetics, hypnotics	Side effects disturbing sleep/wake cycle, akathisia, hiccups
Pain	Altered sleep/wake cycle, disruption of nutrition, immobility
Paraneoplastic syndromes	Myopathy, hypercalcemia, hyponatremia
Psychological factors	
Depression, anxiety, confusion, anger	Loss of function, loss of energy, worry, stress Impaired cognitive functions Attention deficiency

9. What consequence of fatigue do palliative care patients experience?

It is difficult to disassociate the symptoms of fatigue from its consequences. However, fatigue can profoundly affect the quality of life and self-worth.

Decreased activity due to fatigue may cause rapid decline and potentially irreversible loss in energy metabolism. The functioning of every organ system may be affected. The consequences include decreased strength, increase in shortness of breath, and tachycardia with slight exertion. The patient feels the frequent need to slow down, stop, and rest, which again propitiates fatigue. Structural and functional changes in the muscles have been noted in persisting fatigue states.

Impairment of cognitive function is another major consequence of fatigue. Impaired perception and thinking, reduced attention span, and inability to focus and concentrate occur. Hence, activities of daily living become difficult, leading to poor quality of life. Fatigue alters the sleep/wake cycle and causes daytime sleeping, which leads to insomnia.

10. How do you assess fatigue in palliative care?

Characterizing fatigue in the patient's own words is important. Necessary information is obtained on temporal patterns of fatigue, debilitating and relieving factors, and the impact of fatigue on day-to-day activities. The meaning of fatigue to the individual patient and the cultural influences on expression of feelings of fatigue should be noted.

Several instruments to assess fatigue have been reported in the literature, but none of them are considered accurate or patient-friendly in a palliative care setting. The policy should be to adopt a scale to assess the severity of fatigue using a visual analog scale or numeric scale. History taking with simple questions remains the best way to assess fatigue. The following questions may be used:

- Do you get tired easily?
- Do you need to rest frequently?
- Do you feel drowsy?
- Do you find it difficult to start doing things?
- Do you find it difficult to continue doing things?
- Do you get tired when you need to concentrate?
- Do you feel you have enough energy?
- Do you feel weak in the muscles?

Palliative care patients who are still ambulatory are advised to maintain a "fatigue diary" to identify what activities lead to fatigue and periods of rest and sleep.

11. Can fatigue be relieved in palliative care patients?

Although managing fatigue is difficult, there are several reversible causes of fatigue:

Anemia. Red blood cell transfusions are indicated to control fatigue if it is a distressing symptom or is having an adverse effect on activities of daily living.

Chronic obstructive pulmonary disease. Bronchodilators and oxygen therapy can be used to improve patients' quality of life and range of ambulation.

Polypharmacy. Palliative care patients are polysymptomatic and they are on polypharmacy, causing fatigue as a side effect. Hence, the drugs should be thinned.

Insomnia. Correction of the sleep/wake cycle with hypnotics may alleviate fatigue in sleepless patients.

Malnutrition. Practical history taking and explaining to patients the differences in better eating choices for increased caloric intake are appropriate. Appetite stimulants such as megestrol acetate may help. Empiric therapies with methylphenidate, dexamethasone, or prednisone also may be very effective.

Pain and other symptoms. It is important to treat all of the patient's other symptoms as vigorously as fatigue. Good control of pain may relieve fatigue instantly.

Psychological problems. Anxiety and depression can be controlled effectively by psychotropic drugs, which may control fatigue. One should not forget psychosocial support and spiritual counseling in palliative care patients.

12. What measures can be used to conserve energy in palliative care patients who have fatigue?

1. Plan or schedule activities; maintain a fatigue diary to assess how far the patient can ambulate and carry out other activities.

2. Try to reduce or eliminate activities that cause fatigue. Recommend sitting and reading or other activities without physical exertion. Afternoon naps may help conserve energy and prepare patients for the next half of the day.

3. Conserve energy by eliminating nonessential activities. Substitute other activities requiring less energy. Consultation with a physical or occupational therapist is valuable.

4. Increase dependence on caregivers. Emotionally, this approach is not acceptable to patients: feelings of loss of independence further add to the depression. However, patients need to be taught how to "relegate or delegate" activities to their caregivers at home.

13. What further research is needed to understand fatigue in palliative care?

Make fatigue a high-profile symptom in palliative care instead of the last item in a long list of research items. More research is needed to understand fatigue from the patient's point of view. Common ground between patients and physicians for understanding fatigue is also needed and will help us to understand fatigue in different populations, age groups, and cultures. There is need to determine if fatigue is a unique symptom or a cluster of symptoms. Research needs to be conducted to develop pharmacotherapy for fatigue. Fatigue needs to be recognized as a universal symptom in palliative care.

BIBLIOGRAPHY

1. David A, Pelosi A, McDonald E, et al: Tired, weak, or in need of rest: Fatigue among general practice attenders. BMJ 301:1199–1202, 1990.
2. Hünry C, Bernhard J, Joss R, et al: "Fatigue and malaise" as a quality of life indicator in small cell lung cancer patients. Support Care Cancer 1:316–320, 1993.
3. Irvine DM, Vincent L, Bubel N, et al: A critical appraisal of research literature investigating fatigue in the individual with cancer. Cancer Nurs 14:188–189, 1991.
4. Koboshi-Shoot JAM, Hanewald GJFP, Van Dam FSAM, Bruning PF: Assessment of malaise in cancer patients treated with radiotherapy. Cancer Nurs 8:306–313, 1985.
5. Morant R: Asthenia in cancer patients: A double edged inflammatory response against tumor? J Palliat Care 7:22–24, 1991.
6. Morant R, Stiefel F, Berchtold W, et al: Preliminary results of a study assessing asthenia and related psychological and biological phenomena in patients with advanced cancer. Support Cancer Care 1:101–107, 1993.
7. Rhodes VA, Watson PM, Hanson BM: Patient's descriptions of the influence of tiredness and weakness on self-care abilities. Cancer Nurs 11:186–194, 1988.
8. Smets EMA, Garssen B, Schuster-Vitterhoeve ALJ, deHaes JCJM: Fatigue in cancer patients. Br J Cancer 68:220–224,, 1993.
9. Winningham M, Nail LM, Burke MB, et al: Fatigue and the cancer experience: The state of the knowledge. Oncol Nurs Forum 21:23–36, 1994.

32. SLEEPLESS PATIENTS

Suresh K. Joishy, M.D., F.A.C.P.

1. Why is insomnia a neglected subject in palliative care?

Sleep is still a poorly understood phenomenon in physiology. No standards exist for how much sleep an individual needs for normal, day-to-day activities. Research on insomnia, while extensive, has been conducted mainly in otherwise healthy subjects. There is a simple assumption that, if symptoms are controlled, palliative care patients will automatically fall asleep at night. That has not been this author's experience. One of the most common complaints of palliative care patients in our outpatient ambulatory clinic is insomnia. As with pain and vomiting, patients generally do not volunteer information about insomnia. Perhaps they have been suffering from insomnia for so long that they do not feel it worth complaining about. They will, however, complain about fatigue, which may be the result of sleeplessness.

Many palliative care patients are taking hypnotics when they present to palliative care, which usually stops further dialog on insomnia.

There are no physical signs to indicate insomnia. Thus, there are numerous barriers to assessment of sleep quality. The magnitude of sleeplessness and its influence on other symptoms often surfaces when the patient is hospitalized. However, because the patient is usually resting in bed when we observe them, we often forget to ask our patients about sleep. It is also difficult to obtain information about patient sleeplessness from the caregivers who are trying to get their own well-deserved sleep at night.

2. Why is a good night's sleep essential for palliative care patients?

Sleep for a patient in palliative care is precious. Sleep is the only activity that offers them an invaluable respite from the worries associated with physical symptoms. Nighttime sleep also prepares the patient to better tolerate symptoms the next day. For patients who are dependent, it is essential that they sleep at night so that their caregivers can sleep too. There is a patient and caregiver perception that symptoms worsen at night. This makes a good night's sleep even more essential. Insomnia is common in cancer patients and may significantly impair their quality of life. Satisfaction with sleep is the combined result of intact neurobiologic functions and cultural and personal beliefs about the role of sleep in the individual's life. The patient's attitudes toward life, life events, personality, and mood may also determine the patterns necessary for a good night's sleep.

3. What determines the cycle of alertness/sleepiness?

A number of physiological variables affect how alert or sleepy we are at any given point in time. Most important are homeostatic and chronobiologic factors. The homeostatic factor is directly related to the duration of wakefulness. The longer the duration of wakefulness, the greater the pressure to sleep. The chronobiologic factor is determined by the biologic clock, located in the suprachiasmatic nucleus of the hypothalamus. The biologic clock has an inherent rhythm that is maintained by the environmental light/dark cycle.

The sleep pattern may also be genetically determined. The total amount of sleep required may range from 4–10 hours, and the timing of the sleep period, resulting in a tendency to be "early to bed early to rise larks" or "late to bed late to rise owls." The age of the patient is also an important factor. With advancing age, the sleep phase tends to advance in the 24-hour period, and the intensity of the sleep phase decreases.

4. What is insomnia?

Insomnia is not a disorder in itself. It is often a symptom of an underlying medical, psychiatric, or psychosocial condition. It is a syndrome defined as a relative lack of sleep, inadequate quality of sleep, or both. For practical purposes, insomnia may be categorized as transient (a few nights), short term (less than a month), or chronic (longer than a month). Insomnia can be primary or secondary. Primary insomnia, supposedly caused by dysfunction of the sleep mechanisms in the brain, is uncommon. Secondary insomnia can have physical, psychological, psychosocial, and spiritual causes. Secondary insomnia is common among palliative care patients. Aging is also a cause of secondary insomnia, and many palliative care patients are elderly.

5. What patterns of insomnia are common?

Insomnia may begin as a transient disruption of sleep, and in susceptible patients, it can create feedback loops: the inability to sleep for a few nights generates anticipatory anxiety, which in turn perpetuates the insomnia. This has been called the "sleeplessness phobia" and may trigger a habit referred to as "psychophysiological insomnia."

Patients may suffer from difficulties with initiation of sleep, maintenance of sleep, early awakening, or combinations of these.

6. What questions should be asked when assessing insomnia?

- Is your sleep at night satisfactory? Do you tend to fall asleep when you don't want to or when you shouldn't?
- Does anything unusual happen to you during your sleeping hours?

7. How is information about the patient's sleep patterns obtained?

Take a sleep history. Utilize focused physical exams, including cardiopulmonary, neurologic, and psychiatric evaluations. Take a history of wake-sleep function. Question bed partners, family members, co-workers, and caregivers. Ask the patient to maintain a sleep-wake diary.

8. What are the consequences of sleep deprivation?

- Impaired performance
- Difficulty performing tasks involving sustained attention
- Cognitive impairments
- The vicious cycle of insomnia, which also includes fatigue, a lower pain threshold, irritability, and the perpetuation of negative thoughts.

9. How important is the bed for good sleep?

Many people complain that they do not sleep well away from home. Most of the time it is the bed that is blamed.

Palliative care patients with poor performance status are in bed most of the time. This increases the burden of the caregiver as they must move the patient in and out of bed. Although most patients prefer their own bed, for the sake of caregiver convenience they often agree to use a hospital bed at home. Hospital beds improve nursing care but they may not help the patient to sleep better.

As disease progresses, the patient becomes cachectic, less mobile, more helpless, and virtually bedridden.

10. There are special beds designed for orthopedic patients, for intensive care units, and for neurosurgical patients. What type of bed is ideal for palliative care patients?

- The hospital bed should be more comfortable than the home bed.
- The bed should enhance sleep.
- The bed should eliminate frequent turning of the patient.
- The mattress should not increase pressure on the skin and bones of cachectic patients.
- The bed should facilitate the healing process.
- The design should decrease pain if the patient is suffering from incidental pain on movement.
- The controls should be patient friendly (they rarely are).

11. What are the major causes of insomnia in palliative care patients?

CAUSE	SLEEPLESS SUFFERING OR WORRYING
Depression	Loss: physical, companionship, helplessness
Anxiety	Fears of disease and death; treatments and procedures
Pain	When will it end? When will be the next?
Dyspnea	Positioning in bed not conducive to sleep. Sound of O_2 bubbling. Nasal prongs. Labor of breathing
Sleep-wake cycle	Disruption of normal schedule. Excessive time in bed during the day
Psychophysiologic	End of life issues
Spiritual needs	Feeling of abandonment

12. How are sleep disorders classified?

Insomnias. Subjective patient complaint of poor sleep because of insufficient sleep; difficulty in initiating or maintaining sleep; interrupted sleep; poor quality of sleep (non-restorative); or a disrupted wake/sleep cycle. **Note:** Insomnia is not a disease or diagnosis. It is a symptom.

Dyssomnias. These are primary sleep disorders that result from sleep mechanisms involving brain centers and sleep physiology. Examples of these include disturbance of the quality, quantity, or timing of nocturnal sleep, or excessive daytime sleepiness.

Parasomnias. Events or conditions caused by sleep: nightmares, sleep terrors, waking with panic attacks, and eneuresis.

13. How is sleep disturbance in palliative care evaluated?

Because sleep disturbances occur in a large percentage of palliative care patients, and because insomnia occurs in 50% of those patients, sleep disturbances should be suspected when evaluating each patient. Patients may not volunteer this information; thus, it should be sought by the physician.

- **Identify the primary complaint:** Insomnia, excessive sleep, and distribution of sleep/ wake cycle.
- **Characterize the complaint:** Difficulty in initiating sleep; recurrent awakening, or insufficient total sleep.
- **Gather documentation:** Consult with the patient's bed partners and caregivers, or give the patient/caregiver a sleep diary to log activities, naps, and sleeping hours.
- **Perform a focused history taking:** Medications, substance use.
- **Perform a focused physical examination:** Cardiopulmonary, areas of pain, and neurologic examinations.

14. Why do some patients sleep all day and complain about not sleeping at night?

- **To make up:** The patient feels he should sleep when he feels sleepy during the day because he "didn't sleep a wink" at night.
- **To catch up:** The patient is afraid that he may not get any sleep at night and feels he should catch up while he can.
- **The patient cannot help falling asleep during the day** because of medications such as opioids. Some patients appear to sleep more than usual when receiving radiotherapy. Sometimes leaving the home or the waiting periods before hospital treatments will exhaust the patient.
- **Disrupted sleep/wake cycle:** Patients sleep because they are physically inactive or tired at irregular periods.

15. What are the consequences of daytime sleepiness for the patient?

Some patients may not identify daytime sleepiness as a problem (the patient is "compliant" and quiet). Daytime sleeping can become disabling. Patients sleeping during the day become inactive, poorly motivated, and less capable of participating in treatments. Their ability to retain information about their illness and treatments is compromised. Daytime sleeping deprives the patient of family and social interactions. When patients awaken from daytime sleeping, their depression and irritability may worsen. Whereas nighttime sleep is invigorating, daytime sleep has an opposite effect.

16. What about afternoon naps?
Taking an afternoon nap or "siesta" is common in Latin American and Asian cultures. Unfortunately it is considered a sign of laziness in Western culture. In fact, napping may result in better work performance. A nap is a brief period of sleep lasting no more 30 minutes to 1 hour. The afternoon nap *must* be encouraged in palliative care patients. This nap may prevent them from sleeping all day and may prepare them to better face their symptoms for the rest of the day. Napping also may help the caregivers to nap at the same time as the patient, and thus give better care for the rest of the day. Caregiver sleep is important for good patient care.

17. What is a good sleep hygiene protocol to follow?
- Achieve pain relief at night.
- Avoid stimulants such as coffee and tea after 2 pm.
- Drugs such as steroids should be given before noon. If given in divided doses, specify the hours in the order. Do not merely write "BID."
- Encourage a short afternoon nap but *not* daytime sleeping.
- Keep the patient occupied during the day with an active schedule.
- Do not disturb the patient at night unless absolutely necessary. If the patient is hospitalized, avoid waking the patient for recording vital signs unless it is critical for management of that patient.
- Consult with a physical therapist to obtain cognitive and physical activity for bedridden patients.
- Remove unnecessary sights and sounds that either stimulate daytime sleeping or awaken the patient at night.
- After gaining a thorough understanding of the patient's sleep problem, use sleep medications judiciously.

18. What are the adverse effects of sleep deprivation?
Sleep deprivation should be considered to be a contributing factor whenever symptoms seem to be worsening or becoming refractory without apparent cause. The decrease in the pain threshold because of insomnia is a good example. Progressive fatigue, sleepiness, drowsiness, and impaired concentration are obvious consequences of insomnia, unless the patient is already known to be depressed. The symptoms of sleep deprivation and those of depression may be difficult to differentiate.

19. Why do some elderly patients appear to be sleepy during the day although they report sleeping well at night?
It is possible that these patients suffer a condition called "sleep fragmentation." It refers to the occurrence of multiple, brief arousals from sleep, typically without awareness or recollection on the part of the sleeper. To be restorative, it is important for nighttime sleep to be continuous. Even 2–20 second arousals, if frequent, can cause patients to become physiologically sleepy during the day.

20. What is pseudo insomnia?
Pseudo insomnia refers to a poor quality of sleep rather than to real alteration in the sleep pattern. Patients often blame sleep quality for any recently developed feelings of fatigue, depression, irritability, tension, sleepiness, lack of concentration, drowsiness, or muscle cramps. Depression alone may cause all of these symptoms. It may be difficult to differentiate depression from insomnia.

21. How do you record changes in sleep pattern?

Physicians often record sleep-related complaints in one sentence: "Patient complains of sleeping poorly." But, like any other symptoms in palliative care, sleep disturbances should be recorded meticulously. Changes in the sleep pattern may include variations in the total time spent asleep; variations in the time taken to get to sleep; mental activity such as excessive brooding and anxious or repetitive thoughts; panic attacks while waiting to fall asleep; and the number and duration of awakenings during the night. Also note any sensations felt just before and during sleep, such as sweating, feeling hot, feeling "pins and needles," leg cramps, and jerking. Record all of the medications taken by the patient, including recently added drugs. Sleeping pill consumption should also be recorded. A patient's daytime performance may indicate the effects of disrupted sleep.

It is also important to ask the patient about those circumstances in which they are able to sleep better. These may include changes in the temperature or lighting of the bedroom, certain scents and sounds, and the quality of the mattress and pillows.

22. Focused history taking can help the physician to choose the appropriate treatment for insomnia. What should be looked for?

- **Identify the part of the night in which sleep is disturbed.** If sleep disturbance is at the beginning of the night, prescribe a later retiring time. Conversely, if early morning awakenings are problematic, prescribe an earlier rising time.
- **Predisposing factors:** These conditions can set the stage for insomnia and may determine whether the problem becomes chronic. Patients taking therapeutic doses of steroids have a lowered threshold for nocturnal arousal. Change the timing and dosage so that the last dose of prednisone or dexamethasone can be given by noon.
- **Precipitating factors:** Focus on concurrent conditions that may precipitate the problem. These are triggers for insomnia. A good example is depression precipitating insomnia. The problem may ease after resolution of the depression.
- **Perpetuating factors:** These factors develop after insomnia begins. In many cases, the original cause of the sleep problem has long subsided, but the perpetuating factors maintain the sleep disturbance. Common perpetuating factors in palliative care patients include worrying about lost sleep, rising late in the morning, or sleeping during the day to justify sleep lost after a bad night. This irregularity of schedule and oversleeping may make it difficult to fall asleep the following night, and the sleep problem is then sustained. For effective long-term treatment, patient education is key. The patient should understand the sleep problem, particularly that it may have less to do with underlying disease and more to do with worrying about not falling asleep easily at night.
- **Medical factors:** Prednisone, theophylline, and high blood pressure medications may produce insomnia. Changing the time of medications, using drugs with a different side effect profile, or adding a hypnotic drug to the regimen may ameliorate the problem.

23. What are the essential principles in the treatment of insomnia?

- Understanding and modifying the patient's expectations and attitudes via patient education is crucial. Patients expect immediate relief from insomnia after a long suffering. Insomnia may take several weeks to resolve.
- Sleep hygiene
- Hypnotics

BIBLIOGRAPHY

1. Berrios GE, Shapiro CM: I don't get enough sleep, doctor. BMJ 306:846–848, 1993.
2. Mahowald MW: Sleepiness and sleep disorders. Causes and consequences. Minnesota Med 77:27–32, 1994.
3. Pressman MR, Orr WC (eds): Understanding Sleep. The Evaluation and Treatment of Sleep Disorders. Washington, DC, American Psychosocial Association, 1997.
4. Sateia MJ, Silberfarb PM: Sleep disorders in patients with advanced cancer. Progr Palliat Care 4:120–124, 1996.

33. SYMPTOM PROFILE OF ADVANCED CANCER PATIENTS: PROPOSAL FOR NEW STAGING SYSTEMS

Suresh K. Joishy, M.D., F.A.C.P.

1. Who is designated as an advanced cancer patient?

Any cancer patient whose disease has progressed beyond the curable stage. Technically and traditionally, advanced cancer meant stage IV disease. However, in the palliative care setting, the patient presents with continuing progression of earlier-detected stage IV cancer. No additional staging has been considered for patients presenting for palliative care.

2. Should we consider classifying advanced cancer patients in palliative care beyond stage IV?

Cancer continues to progress in patients with stage IV disease who present for palliative care. Earlier-detected metastatic lesions may expand relentlessly. New metastatic lesions may continue to appear. It seems unreasonable to continue to lump these patients in stage IV. This author feels that there is a need for further staging. For example, describing a patient as having stage IV carcinoma of the breast does not indicate if the existing metastatic lesion of the liver is progressing; the patient also might have developed new metastasis in the brain. Another major drawback of the traditional staging system is its lack of description of many symptoms, which actually determine the patient's suffering. Thus, traditional staging is a static process that fails to describe the dynamic nature of the disease when patients come to palliative care.

3. What is meant by "profile of a cancer patient"?

A patient with any disease can be described in clinical terms of diagnosis, extent of disease, and prognosis. The cancer patient is described in terms of histologic diagnosis of the primary and staging for the extent of the disease. For example, stage I ductal carcinoma of the breast indicates that disease is limited to the breast. Stage II generally describes lymph nodal involvement only. Stage III describes extensive locoregional disease. Stage IV describes metastasis to other organs. For most cancers, advanced stage is indicated once the disease has poor prognosis. Disease and description of the cancer patient in terms of diagnosis and staging is considered the profile of a cancer patient. However, there are no terminologies for staging to describe the profile of cancer patients in palliative care.

4. If stage IV cancer means advanced disease, do all palliative care patients belong in stage IV?

No. Cancer patients are entered into palliative care because of symptoms irrespective of extent of disease. However, most cancer patients presenting to palliative care or hospice have metastatic disease and are described traditionally as stage IV. Because most patients in stage I and II can be cured, they rarely enter palliative care. Stage III patients with advanced locore-gional disease refractory to local curative therapies may be managed in palliative care.

5. Why do existing staging systems not go beyond stage IV in describing cancer patients?

The cancer staging system was proposed before the advent of palliative care. Oncologists still try to cure the patients who are in stage IV.

6. Must further staging of cancer be proposed in palliative care?

This author proposes further staging of cancer patients in palliative care, as follows: One need not advance cancer patients beyond stage IV in palliative care unless they show progression. Stage

III patients with refractory, locoregional disease and symptoms may be classified as stage III until they develop progression, at which point traditional stage IV can be indicated. Any time the existing metastatic lesions progress and cause symptoms, the patient would fall into stage V. For example, a patient with breast cancer who presented with liver metastasis in stage IV, and now shows expanding and more numerous liver metastasis and develops hepatic pain or obstructive jaundice, should be considered as in stage V.

Patients with previously known stage IV or V disease who develop new metastatic lesions should be considered as having stage VI. For example, the patient with breast cancer presenting with liver metastasis, stage IV, who develops new metastasis in the lung or brain should be considered as in stage VI.

7. Does it make sense to stage symptoms in palliative care?

Each symptom should be considered a disease entity that has its own etiology, pathogenesis, prognosis, and response to therapies. It has the same descriptors as for any disease. Pain is a symptom that can be staged.

8. Describe an example of staging for pain.

Stage I: Localized or focused
Stage II: Localized in wider area than before
Stage III: Radiation to the corresponding dermatomes
Stage IV: Undifferentiated
The following suffixes could be used to describe the type of pain:
   S: Somatic   N: Neuropathic
   V: Visceral   M: Mixed
For example, cancer pain radiating to the dermatomes with neuropathic pain could be described as stage IIIN.

Numeric suffixes could be used for more than one pain in more than one location. For example, if a multiple myeloma patient has localized pain in stage IIIN, with pain radiating to the left inguinal regions and pain in the right shoulder and right iliac wing, the pain could be staged as stage III, N3.

9. Propose stages for nausea and vomiting, dyspnea, and constipation.

Examples of Staging

STAGE	NAUSEA AND VOMITING	DYSPNEA	CONSTIPATION
I	Nausea only	On exertion only	Dependent on oral laxative
II	Nausea and vomiting	Occurring at rest	Dependent on rectal laxative
III	Nausea and vomiting with bowel obstruction	Oxygen dependent	Impaction
IV	Undifferentiated symptom	Terminal dyspnea or undifferentiated symptom	Refractory to laxatives or due to bowel obstruction

10. What is undifferentiated disease?

Disease that defies definition, as is often the case in patients with advanced cancer in palliative care. If a patient is polysymptomatic, it is often difficult to pinpoint the cause of the symptoms. It also is difficult to disassociate the symptoms from organic or psychosocial causes. When the patient is unable to describe symptoms, the palliative care physician is required to use his or her experience to make a problem list in the order of importance, recognizing symptoms that require immediate treatment and relief. The physician may be cornered into labeling the patient as having undifferentiated disease with undifferentiated symptoms in whatever stage the cancer may be.

11. What is "failure to thrive"?

The term "failure to thrive" is imported from pediatrics and is also applied to some geriatric patients. Pediatricians use the term when the patients fail to achieve weight gain, height, behavioral milestones, and functional status compared to normal children. In geriatrics the term is used to indicate loss of functional status.

12. What are the features of "failure to thrive" in palliative care?

- Loss of appetite and weight
- Decline in initiative, concentration, and drive
- Signs of hopelessness and helplessness
- Tendency to fall, develop decubiti, and become totally immobile (ECOG performance status 4)

13. Do all elderly persons go through a period of failure to thrive prior to natural death?

In the absence of disease, elderly patients may eventually undergo a process of progressive functional decline, apathy, and loss of willingness to eat and drink that culminates in death. Undoubtedly, many cancer patients are proceeding toward "natural death" because of their advanced age and not necessarily because of advanced cancer, particularly when their cancer-related symptoms are being controlled.

14. What other terminologies describe failure to thrive?

Literature reviews show "taken to bed," "the dwindles," "wasting away," "endstage frailty," and "psychobiological failure."

15. What is meant by "pre-death"?

Many deaths in old age may be preceded by a period of "pre-death," during which persons outlive the vigor of their bodies and wisdom of their brains. Clearly, an aggressive diagnostic approach in such situations would not only be futile but could contribute to suffering. In palliative care patients in the pre-death phase, comfort measures are indicated.

16. What interventions are appropriate when palliative care patients show failure to thrive or enter the phase of pre-death?

The basic philosophy of palliative care is symptom control and improving quality of life. This applies to any phase of the patient's life. The following interventions are indicated.

Impaired activities of daily living. Functional status is the most powerful prognostic indicator. Inability to perform a simple act may be due to painful skeletal metastasis, memory loss, or depression. The goal is to control symptoms. Physical and occupational therapy consultation is valuable.

Anorexic cachexia. Undernutrition or hypoalbuminemia is an independent predictor of death in the elderly. If there are easily reversible causes, such as poor-fitting dentures or changes in food preferences, dietary consultation is in order. If dysphagia is a major symptom, surgical intervention with palliative intent may be required.

Depression and social isolation. These are risk factors for poor outcome of any symptom control.

Cognitive impairment. Dementia syndromes are not uncommon in elderly and debilitated patients. Evaluation should include reversible or treatable causes of cognitive impairment. Patients are managed by palliative care team members.

17. Is the term "persistent vegetative state" applicable in describing advanced cancer patients in palliative care?

"Persistent vegetative state" (PVS) is a rare disorder and is a clinical diagnosis. Traditionally PVS has been described in patients with brain injuries due to trauma or infections. The main characteristics are a sleep/wake pattern, response to stimuli only in a reflex way, and evidence that the patient is awake but not aware.

Patients with an advanced central nervous system tumor or a previously resected and heavily treated brain tumor occasionally may be seen in palliative care. Being awake but unaware results from complete loss of cerebral cortical functioning with preservation of at least some hypothalamic and brainstem function. Such patients are often young and taking high-dose steroids and anticonvulsants to prevent seizures. They may appear cushingoid due to steroid therapy and may be receiving artificial nutrition with feeding tubes.

18. How do you evaluate and manage PVS?

With a team approach. The most important item in the assessment of PVS is to determine if the patient is aware of the environment. Assessing awareness in a brain-damaged patient with profound physical disability requires skill, time, and repeated observations. Neurologic evaluation is mandatory. Any motor activity that can be used to communicate with the patient should be identified early. Lack of eye blink to threat or absence of visual tracking are not enough to diagnose PVS. Early identification of awareness is the key to the team's making a difficult decision in the long-term management of PVS patients.

19. Is the cancer patient profile distinct or unique to each different cancer?

Early-stage cancers may show unique clinical features because the disease is limited to a particular organ. For example, a patient with lung cancer may present with cough, shortness of breath, or hemoptysis. Patients with colon cancer may experience altered bowel habits or hematochezia. However, most patients with advanced cancers, irrespective of the primary, in stage III or IV, share several common symptoms or complications related to sites of metastasis.

20. What are the symptom profiles that occur in patients in palliative care?

Symptom Profiles in Common Types of Cancer

TYPE OF CANCER	CONDITIONS	SYMPTOMS
Lung cancer		
Any type	Recurrent pulmonary lesions, residual disease, mediastinal or hilar metastasis, pleural effusion	Dyspnea, cough, hiccups, chest pain, cachexia
Squamous cell carcinoma	Hypercalcemia	Nausea, vomiting, constipation, confusion
Small cell carcinoma	SIADH	Hypotension, lethargy, convulsions
	Procedures: Postthoracotomy syndrome, Pancoast's syndrome	Pain in the chest wall, pain in the shoulder
	Superior vena cava syndrome	Facial congestion, dyspnea, confusion
	Skeletal metastasis, cord compression, pathologic fracture	Pain, weakness, loss of power in corresponding limbs
	Brain metastasis	Blurring of vision, headache, vomiting, seizures
	Liver metastasis	Abdominal pain, anorexia, jaundice, nausea and vomiting, gastroparesis
Breast cancer	Residual, recurrent, locoregional disease	Mass effect, fungation, ulceration, bleeding, lymphedema
	Axillary dissection, axillary radiotherapy, plexopathy	Pain and loss of power in corresponding dermatomes of the brachial plexus
	Lung metastasis, pleural effusion, spread to the lungs, lymphangitis	Chest pain, cough, and dyspnea
	Skeletal metastasis, pathologic fracture	Pain and loss of power in the limbs
	Hypercalcemia with bone metastasis	Confusion, constipation, vomiting
	Hepatic metastasis, peritoneal metastasis, ovarian metastasis, malignant ascites	Abdominal pain, abdominal distention, gastroparesis, anorexia, cachexia

(Table continued on facing page.)

Symptom Profiles in Common Types of Cancer (Continued)

TYPE OF CANCER	CONDITIONS	SYMPTOMS
Head and neck cancer	Local residual disease, radical surgeries in the face or neck, cervical plexopathy	Swelling and deformity of the face or neck, fungating/ulcerative lesions, discharge and bleeding, malodorous tumors, impact on self-esteem due to cosmetic insult
	Tracheostomy and feeding tubes	Nonfunctioning tubes, dyspnea, frequent infections
	Hypercalcemia with or without bone metastasis	Confusion, constipation, vomiting
	Radiation to the head and neck region	Xerostomia, radiation-induced skin changes
Colorectal cancer	Surgery—colostomy	Altered bowel habits, constipation or diarrhea, hematochezia, colostomy-related complications
	Pelvic metastasis, plexopathy, retroperitoneal mass	Pelvic pain, urinary symptoms, retention, or incontinence
	Abdominal metastasis, peritoneal metastasis, malignant ascites	Abdominal pain, abdominal distention, respiratory discomfort
	Hepatic metastasis, hepatomegaly	Obstructive jaundice, anorexia, gastroparesis, vomiting
	Pulmonary metastasis	Asymptomatic or dyspnea

SIADH = syndrome of inappropriate antidiuretic hormone.

21. When should a patient's symptom profile be compiled?

Whenever the patient is admitted to the palliative care service, after establishing the diagnosis and extent of the disease, the next step is to keep an accurate record of symptom profile. To this list one should add a psychological and spiritual profile of the patient. The list should form the basis for daily assessment and periodic assessment of the patient.

BIBLIOGRAPHY

1. Andrews L, Murphy L, Munday R, Littlewood C: Misdiagnosis of the vegetative state: Retrospective study in a rehabilitation unit. BMJ 313:13–16, 1996.
2. Cassell EJ: Clinical incoherence about person: The problem of the persistent vegetative state. Ann Intern Med 125:146–147, 1996.
3. Lewith GT: Undifferentiated illness: Some suggestions for approaching the polysymptomatic patient. J R Soc Med 81:563–565, 1988.
4. Sarkisian CA, Lachs MS: "Failure to thrive" in older adults. Ann Intern Med 124:1072–1078, 1996.

34. A GLOSSARY FOR MORPHINE

Suresh K. Joishy, M.D., F.A.C.P.

What are the theoretical and therapeutic encounters that may occur with day-to-day morphine use? Because the morphine encounters are numerous, the following comprehensive glossary may help as a quick reference guide.

ATC (Around the Clock) Infusion Dose: The continuously infused dose of morphine specified hourly for every 4 hours during titration and q 24 hours during the baseline period.

Agonist: Morphine is an agonist because it acts on *mu* receptors. The drug has an affinity for and stimulates physiologic activity at cell receptors.

Allergy to Morphine: Rare. May manifest with itching. Relieved by antihistamines.

Baseline Pain: The stabilized level of pain experienced for 12 or more hours during the last 24 hours on morphine.

Bolus Dose: That dose of morphine given *in addition* to the ATC and rescue doses on a PRN basis with a specified interval. For incidental pain, for example.

Bradypnea: A reduced respiration rate, seen in some patients, without respiratory failure. If 6/mt or less, naloxone (a morphine antagonist) should be used.

Breakthrough pain: A transitory increase in pain intensity, which is greater than the baseline intensity experienced by the patient on morphine.

Ceiling Effect and Morphine: Increasing the dose of a drug may not be effective after reaching a certain dosage. This is called the "ceiling effect." However, the dose of morphine can be escalated as high as necessary for pain control, with that dose limited only by side effects.

Codeine vs. Morphine: Morphine is far superior to and more potent than codeine. The milligram potency ratio for PO codeine and PO morphine is 13:1. Parenteral codeine is *not* recommended.

Constipation: A common side effect of morphine, constipation responds well to a good bowel regimen.

Cough and Morphine: Morphine's central action makes it a good antitussive in a palliative care setting.

Dysphoria: The restlessness experienced by some patients using morphine.

Dyspnea and Morphine: Morphine is an excellent drug for control of dyspnea.

Epidural: A very effective route for administration of morphine. The potency ratio of IV administration versus epidural administration is 10:1.

Equianalgesic Table: A reference table used to calculate the milligram potency ratio, conversion factors, and different routes for morphine as compared to other opioids.

Escalation Dose: The increased dose of morphine during the titration period.

Family Education: Education is a must for the patient on morphine so that side effects will not be confused with allergy.

Half Life of Morphine: The time required for the plasma level of morphine to fall to half or to a certain measured level. Usually 2–3½ hours.

Hepatic Failure: Should this occur, the morphine dose should be monitored closely or eliminated entirely, and an alternate opioid should be found.

Hydrocodone vs. Morphine: The equianalgesic potency is unclear. Probably 1:1, PO only. Morphine is far superior. Hydrocodone is not available IV.

Hydromorphone vs. Morphine: Hydromorphone is more potent than morphine. The oral milligram potency ratio of IV morphine to IV hydromorphone is 10:1.5. The conversion factor is 6.7. PO morphine to PO hydromorphone is 4:1. The conversion factor is 4. Hydromorphone is a good alternative to morphine, but more expensive.

IV/SQ Rescue Dose: Administration of 50% of the ATC dose for breakthrough pain at variable intervals, 15–30 minutes or hourly during the titration period, and q 2 hours during the stable baseline period.

Incidental Pain: A type of breakthrough pain, precipitated by volitional movement while the patient is on morphine.

Intramuscular Injection of Morphine: Not recommended in palliative care. The PO, IV, or SQ routs of administration are preferred.

Intranasal Morphine: Rarely used for pain control.

Intrathecal Morphine: Very effective in selected cases.

Intravenous: The preferred route of administration for acute severe pain in the hospital setting.

Itching: An uncommon side effect of morphine. This may be the result of the preservatives in morphine rather than the morphine itself.

Kedian: 24-hour, slow release morphine. An American brand name.

Ketorolac vs. Morphine: Ketorolac is the only parenteral NSAID. It is a good adjunct as a parenteral morphine sparing agent.

Levorphanol vs. Morphine: Levorphanol has a much longer half-life than morphine. Morphine is far more superior and versatile. Milligram potency ratio for PO levorphanol to PO morphine is 1:7.5; IV levorphanol to IV morphine is 1:5.

Liquid Morphine: A convenient morphine preparation for PO titration. Liquid morphine is useful when the patient cannot swallow tablets. It may be also absorbed sublingually. Liquid morphine is a good rescue preparation when the patient is on transdermal fentanyl.

Loading Dose: The first dose of morphine for titration.

MS Contin Tablets: Continuous release morphine. An American brand name.

MS-IR: Morphine sulfate immediate release. Tablets or liquid. All injectables are immediate release.

Meperidine vs. Morphine: Morphine is far superior and more potent than meperidine. The milligram potency ratio of PO meperidine to PO morphine is 10:1. The ratio of IV meperidine to IV morphine is 7.5:1.

Metabolites: Different metabolites of morphine cause different side effects. Some are hepatically cleared and some are renally cleared. Each patient handles metabolites differently and toxicity is not predictable.

Methadone vs. Morphine: The milligram potency ratio PO and IV of methadone is the same for morphine. Morphine is far superior and more versatile. Methadone has a longer half-life, which causes delayed toxicity.

Morphine: The principle and most active alkaloid of opium. Morphine sulfate (MS), a pentahydrate sulfate salt of morphine, is preferred in the United States. In Great Britain and Germany, morphine trihydrate hydrochloride is preferred.

Morphine Resistance: Neuropathic pain may show more resistance to morphine than will somatic or visceral pain.

Morphine Sparing Agent: Any drug that will reduce the dose of morphine without compromising pain control.

Myoclonus: A side effect of morphine in debilitated patients on chronic therapy with higher doses.

NSAID vs. Morphine: NSAIDs are good adjuncts with morphine for controlling severe somatic pain.

Naloxone vs. Morphine: Naloxone is a *mu* antagonist. It is used to control respiratory depression by morphine, which is rare in palliative care.

Nausea: A side effect of morphine that occurs only during the initial stages of treatment.

Nebulized Morphine: Very useful to control severe respiratory distress, particularly for lymphangitic spread of malignancy in the lungs.

Opiate: Any derivative of opium. Morphine is the opiate par excellence.

Opioid: Any synthetic drug with opiate-like activity that may bind to opiate receptors.

Opioid Bowel: Dose-related bowel obstruction in patients with risk factors for constipation while on high doses of morphine.

Opioid Naive Patient: A patient who has not received any opioid therapy within the last few days. The starting dose of morphine should be lowest.

Opioid Tolerant Patient: A pharmacologic response in which a patient may require higher doses of morphine for analgesia.

Oral Rescue Dose: Administration of 50% of the ATC dose hourly during titration, and ⅙ of the total 24-hour oral dose. During the baseline period, q 2–4 hours.

Oral Route: The preferred route of administration for morphine.

Orders for Morphine: These must be absolutely accurate for dose route, schedule, ATC dosing, and breakthrough dosing.

Oxycodone vs. Morphine: The milligram potency ratio is 1:1 orally. Morphine is a good choice if oxycodone is ineffective. oxycodone PO:morphine IV is 3:1.

PCA: Patient controlled analgesia. This is a good way to administer morphine parenterally, SQ/IV, in the hospital or at home.

Pain Assessment Scale for Morphine: The simpler the better. A 0–10 numeric analog scale for pain intensity is sufficient in palliative care.

Paradoxical Pain: Higher doses of morphine may paradoxically cause pain. This is a rare event.

Peak Effect: The time taken for maximum analgesic effect. This is 15–30 minutes for IV/SQ morphine and 2 hours for PO morphine.

Pentazocin vs. Morphine: Morphine is far superior as an analgesic.

Renal Failure: Should this occur, monitor the morphine dose closely or eliminate it completely. Find an alternate opioid.

Rescue Dose of Morphine: That dose of morphine given in addition to the ATC dose to control breakthrough pain.

Sedation: A relatively common side effect of morphine. Not a reason to discontinue morphine, however, the dose should be reduced until somnolescence subsides.

Starting Dose: The first dose of morphine for titration.

Step-Down Dose: Decreasing morphine (25% every 24 hours if no rescue doses are needed or if side effects developed during the baseline period).

Subcutaneous Route: Morphine is very active subcutaneously, which is a useful route of administration for PCA in a home hospice setting.

Sublingual: Morphine, in tablet or liquid form, is absorbed well sublingually.

Suppository: Morphine suppositories are as active as oral morphine in selected patients. Slow release morphine tablets may occasional be used as a suppository.

Titration: The method of morphine administration used to determine the optimal dose to control pain with ATC and rescue principles. Titration can be by PO, IV. or SQ routes, with corresponding preparations.

Titration Period: The time taken to determine the optimum ATC and rescue doses to achieve stable baseline pain.

Tolerance: The physiologic effect of morphine may be confused with addiction when higher doses are needed.

Transdermal Fentanyl vs. Morphine: Potency ratios are expressed in different units; for example, morphine at 300 mg/24 hours equals fentanyl at 150 mcg/hour.

WHO Ladder and Morphine: Morphine is recommended for severe pain in the third step of the WHO pain ladder.

INDEX

Page numbers in **boldface type** indicate complete chapters.